ERWIN AMLACHER, Dr.rer.nat.habil., Dip.Biol.,
Laboratorium für Fischkrankheiten,
Berlin — Rahnsdorf

Translated

TEXTBOOK
)F FISH DISEASES

Waterproof Edition
by
D. A. CONROY,

and

R. L. HERMAN

ISBN 0-87666-037-5

Distributed in the U.S.A. by T.F.H. Publications, Inc., 211 West Sylvania Avenue, P.O. Box 27,
Neptune City, N.J. 07753; in England by T.F.H. (Gt. Britain) Ltd., 13 Nutley Lane, Reigate, Surrey;
in Canada to the book store and library trade by Clarke, Irwin & Company, Clarwin House, 791 St.
Clair Avenue West, Toronto 10, Ontario; in Canada to the pet trade by Rolf C. Hagen Ltd., 3225
Sartelon Street, Montreal 382, Quebec; in Southeast Asia by Y.W. Ong, 9 Lorong 36 Geylang,
Singapore 14; in Australia and the south Pacific by Pet Imports Pty. Ltd., P.O. Box 149, Brookvale
2100, N.S.W., Australia. Published by T.F.H. Publications, Inc. Ltd., The British Crown Colony of
Hong Kong.

Translated by

D. A. CONROY, M.I.Biol., F.I.S.T.,
Fish Pathology Group,
Unilever Research Laboratory,
Aberdeen,
Scotland;

and

R. L. HERMAN
Eastern Fish Disease Laboratory,
Bureau of Sport Fisheries and Wildlife,
Leetown, West Virginia

This book is based upon the German language edition of
TASCHENBUCH DER FISCHKRANKHEITEN by Dr. Erwin
Amlacher. It was originally published by Gustav Fischer
Verlag, Jena, DDR.

FOREWORD

This Manual is the result of many years work in the field of fish pathology. Its object is that of presenting in a concise and clear manner the most important facets of the subject. Fish pathology has a vital importance to the fishing industry, as well as to fish farming activities, by virtue of the capital which is invested in these same. Apart from analyzing and presenting the more fundamental information, the themes have been so arranged as to prove of utility both to the veterinarian and to the fish farmer. This latter consideration determined the manner in which the topics were selected.

The present book attempts to be something of usefulness, as well as being easy to handle and to understand, not only to the specialist who is occupied full-time with the study of fish biology, but also for the veterinarian and others who may be interested in the breeding of carp, trout, and ornamental aquarium fishes, and for aquarists and fishermen. The text is presented in an orderly fashion so that it may the better be utilized by the reader. Each important disease is without exception divided as follows: 1. symptoms; 2. diagnosis; 3. etiology; morphology and taxonomy (or biology) of the causative agent; course of the disease; 4. histopathology and histochemistry; 5. therapy, prophylaxis and hygiene. In my opinion such a presentation serves the purpose of facilitating a uniform description, as well as to save time. The Tables for the diagnosis and the treatment of the different diseases have this same object in view. With regard to the figures, I have not made any attempt to be original, and always where it has been possible I have attempted to include data reported by other investigators who have made concrete contributions to the subject. It is for this same reason that the number of figures taken from other works is in the region of a third of the total.

My sincere thanks are due to all those who stimulated my interest and supported me in my efforts during the nine years in which I have been working in the field of fish pathology. I must express my gratitude to my respected Professor, Dr. Schäperclaus, of Berlin, as well as to Dr. Uschmann, of Ernst Haeckel, Jena. I would also like to thank most heartily Mr. H. Weser for my practice in the VEB Binnenfischerei, and Messrs. K. Rehberg (Jnr.), K. Pensel, W. Rudolph, G. Michler, and O. Kronsbein of the VEB Binnenfischerei Königswartha, who encouraged my research throughout these nine years.

In the field of aquarism, I was assisted by Mr. W. Voigt, of Berlin-Steglitz, and by colleagues from the Berlin Zoo. For having furnished me with scientific material, I express my thanks to Prof. Dr. W. Schäperclaus, to Dr. Jara, Mr. Wagner, and to my colleagues in the Institute Messrs. Bandlow and Mattheis. I am grateful to Prof. Dr. H. H. Reichenbach-Klinke, of the Bayerische Biologische Versuchsanstalt, Munich, for a preparation of *Eimeria* and for most useful bibliographical material. My friend Dr. Fey, of the Berlin-Buch Institute for Biology and Medicine, provided me with many new details on the morphology of Teleost blood, and gave his opinion on several preparations of tumors. Dr. Ippen, of the Institute for Comparative Pathology in Berlin, also afforded me considerable assistance in the study of such preparations, and I wish to express my gratitude to him. I should also like to thank Mrs. Ursula Rogowski and Miss Gisela König for having made the drawings.

Gustav Fischer, the publishers, have compiled an attractive and practical book. For this, as well as for their constant collaboration, I render them my gratitude. I do not wish to close without thanking very specially my Technician, Miss Waltraud Rudolph, for the way in which she has helped in the preparation of the illustrations and of the manuscript.

E. AMLACHER

TRANSLATOR'S FOREWORD

At the present time the need for a concise and practical manual on fish pathology has become increasingly apparent to fishery biologists, hatchery-men, aquarists and veterinarians, as well as to others who may have some connection with any one of these activities. The professional fish pathologist is able to keep himself reasonably up to date with recent developments in his field by consultation of the appropriate bibliography, much of which may be highly specialized. However, with the possible exception of the now classical treatise on fish pathology written by Schäperclaus and published in 1954, no one book is available which attempts to include details of laboratory techniques and descriptions of the symptoms, diagnosis, and treatment of the more important fish diseases all in the same volume, and for the benefit of those who may have had no previous experience in this particular field. This unfortunate situation has now been effectively remedied by Dr. Erwin Amlacher, an English translation of whose book is herein presented.

On reading the text, the reader will at once become aware of the variety and depth of Dr. Amlacher's own experience in the field. Here is no mere scholarly rendering of a somewhat specialized topic, but rather an excellent account of the subject based on a first-hand personal experience with it built up over many years. The subject matter is presented in a crisp and orderly fashion, amply supplemented by photographs and diagrams, and the translator has himself used this book as a basic text for courses on fish diseases given in South America to students with no prior knowledge of the speciality.

Every effort has been made in the English translation to present Dr. Amlacher's concepts and ideas in a form as close as possible to that of the original. This latter was intended primarily for use in Central European countries, and I have therefore taken the liberty of incorporating additional material on columnaris, bacterial kidney disease and ulcer disease likely to enhance the value of the book to readers in North America. Where the occasion warrants it, supplementary information has also been given in the form of footnotes, many of which include details of North American publications for the benefit of readers in the United States and Canada. In both instances any responsibility for such inclusions is entirely my own, and every effort has been made to keep such citations in line with Dr. Amlacher's own format.

7

In conclusion I should like to thank those fish pathologists who have given me their comments, and particularly to Dr. Z. Kabata of the Marine Laboratory, Aberdeen, and to my friend and colleague, Dr. Iain Anderson, for their interest and encouragement throughout the preparation of this translation. I should also like to thank Mr. Ainslie Thin, of Messrs. Oliver and Boyd Ltd., for his courtesy and assistance.

D. A. CONROY,
Aberdeen, December 1966

INTRODUCTION

Fish culture is an old branch of animal husbandry but there are few textbooks on diseases of fishes. The first textbook was that of Bruno Hofer published in Germany in 1904. This was followed by several published in Germany, Soviet Union, Poland, and Czechoslovakia.

In the English speaking countries, fishery biology literature is abundant but textbooks on fish diseases are particularly scanty. The best known books are by H. S. Davis dealing with culture and diseases of freshwater game fishes and those by C. van Duijn, Reichenbach-Klinke and Elkan which are general in character but do not give sufficient information on diseases of salmonids.

Dr. Amlacher's book was published in Germany in 1961. Being comprehensive, concise and lucid it became very popular. The German book was translated into Spanish and now an English translation, or more correctly a new edition, is available. Dr. Amlacher brought it up-to-date and expanded it for the English translation which was made by Mr. Conroy from the Spanish translation.

Roger Lee Herman, Eastern Fish Disease Laboratory, U.S. Fish and Wildlife Service added information which will be of particular interest to readers in the United States and Canada.

A textbook on fish diseases is particularly important in North America because fish pathology is not included in the curriculum of most of the schools of veterinary medicine. Let us hope that when a comprehensive text on fish diseases becomes available interest in fish diseases and in fish pathology training will catch up with the rapidly expanding culture of freshwater fishes.

August 7, 1967

S. F. SNIESZKO, Director
Bureau of Sport Fisheries and Wildlife
Eastern Fish Disease Laboratory
Kearneysville, West Virginia
25430

CONTENTS

Sockeye salmon virus disease
Chinook salmon virus disease
BACTERIA
Piscine tuberculosis (tuberculosis piscium)
Bacterial hemorrhagic septicemia; (Infectious abdominal dropsy
or ascites: myo-entero-hepatic syndrome)
"Red Pest" of freshwater eels
"Red Spot" of freshwater fish
"Red Spot" of saltwater eels (red bubonic plague or pestis rubra
anguillarum)
Vibriosis or pike pest
Furunculosis
Bacterial tail rot
Columnaris disease
Coldwater disease (Peduncle disease)
Bacterial gill disease
Bacterial kidney disease
Ulcer disease

Coral fish disease
Velvet disease
Miscellaneous
Ichthyosporidium (Ichthyophonus)
Branchiomycosis (gill rot)
Aphanomycosis (crab or crayfish pest)
Saprolegniasis and achlyasis
FLAGELLATES (MASTIGOPHORA)
Costiasis
Octomitiasis
Octomitus symphysodoni nova species (?)
Trypanoplasma (Cryptobia)
SPOROZOA
Nodular coccidiosis in the intestine of carp
Enterococcidiosis in the carp
Whirling disease
Nodular diseases (Sporozoiasis tuberosa)
Tubero-ulcerous myxoboliasis
Plistophorosis (myolytic sporozoiasis)
Glugea pseudotumefaciens
Glugea anomala Moniez (Figure 125)

NOTE

These plates several times referenced in the text appear on the covers.

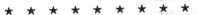

Ichthyosporidium hoferi—Mallory stain (aniline blue-orange G-acid fuchsin); outer capsule layer, blue; inner capsule layer, reddish; nuclei, red-orange; plasma, alveolar structured. ×840   Ziehl-Neelsen methylene blue stain; capsule, unstained; nuclei, red-violet with dark chromatin. ×640   PAS reaction after McManus/Hotchkiss, counterstained with light green; capsule and plasma inclusions, positive, red stained; host tissue and plasmodium nuclei, green. ×560 Glycogen reaction after Bauer; plasma inclusions, positive; capsule layer without reaction. ×840

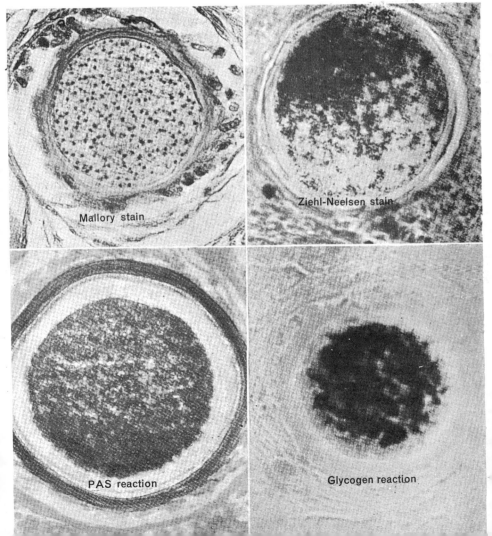

Mallory stain

Ziehl-Neelsen stain

PAS reaction

Glycogen reaction

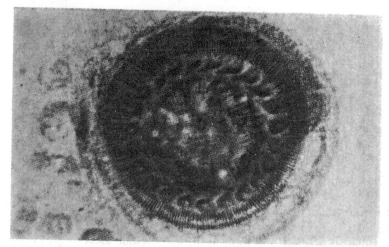

Trichodina domerguei

Plate: (Smears and photographs, Dr. Jara)

Chilodonella cyprini

Myxobolus pfeifferi spore with evaginated polar flagellum

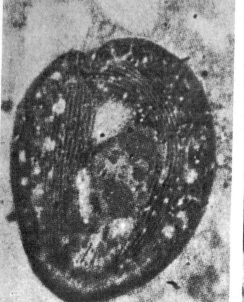

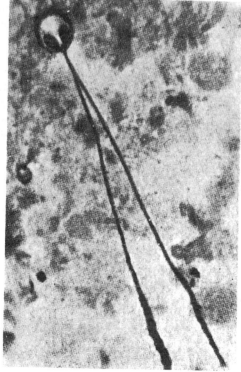

Chapter 1

TECHNIQUE OF INVESTIGATION

To diagnose a disease is to take the first step towards combatting it; but to know what disease it is and to establish a diagnosis requires a method of investigation, which in the great majority of cases starts by making a clinical history of the disease (anamnesis), and following a general study (external exploration) this leads to the investigation *sensu stricto* (autopsy, bacteriological and histological analysis). Without being a professional fish pathologist, the work of whom is precisely that, the interested aquarist or fish breeder may also form an idea of the state of health of his fish by assimilation of the simple techniques for investigation which are described herein, and by the use of an ordinary student's microscope to facilitate minute examination. It follows without saying that in every fish hatchery there should be at least one graduate in biology whose duties lie in the field of fish pathology.

Instruments for autopsy and for the preparation of smears and other material

The following instruments are required (*Figure 1*):
1. Two pairs of straight scissors, the larger pair having rounded ends, and the smaller pair with sharp points;
2. One pair of artery forceps;
3. One spatula;
4. Two pairs of curved forceps;
5. Two bacteriological loops;
6. One or more pipettes;
7. One or more Petri dishes;
8. An adequate number of slides and coverslips;
9. A wooden dissection board;
10. A microscope.

These instruments are kept in a small case or a suitable box.

External examination of the diseased fish

The fishes of particular interest to us are Teleosts, and we shall briefly

17

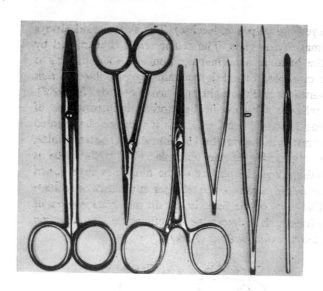

Figure 1. Instruments for post-mortem identification. (Original)

make a study of their anatomy because a knowledge of this is essential in order to undertake a comprehensive investigation. The body of a fish has a torpedo-like shape which enables it to offer the least possible resistance to the water. We may differentiate the following body regions: the head or cephalic region, the trunk, and the tail or caudal region. Between the head and the trunk is found the gill or branchial region. For reasons of convenience we may also distinguish between the neck and the ventral mouth region. *Figure 2* shows the external anatomical details of greatest interest, and no further mention of these in particular will be necessary in the text.

The examination begins with external observation of any fish suspected of having a disease. In the first place we must decide whether the fish is behaving abnormally in the water, paying special attention to the following points:

General symptons: Is the fish listless?, does it show any escape reflex?, is it eating?, is it swimming?, does it swim abnormally?, does it swim around in circles?, does it keep itself to the bottom?, does it tend to scrape against the bottom when it swims?, does it remain at the surface of the water?, does it keep its mouth open and breath air?, are the respiratory movements frequent and rapid? (count the number of gill movements/minute), does it tend to jump out of the water?

External symptoms: After having removed the fish from the water, the color of the body is noted (decoloration, darkening, blackening etc.), as well as the presence of any cloudiness of the skin (grey or white), reddening, ragged or torn fins, raised scales, white spots or parasites visible to the naked eye (e.g. carp lice, leeches). The skin should always be examined with a magnifying glass. The ocular reflex is examined by holding the fish in the hand in a normal position and then turning it towards the right, for example, if the fish maintains its gaze fixed so that the left eye turns downwards and the right one turns upwards (*Figure 3*). The absence of this reflex is a pathological symptom, indicating loss of the labyrinth stabilizing function. Further to this it must be determined whether there are deformities of the vertebral column and of the mandibles, or perforation and/or shortening of the opercula. Finally the anus is examined for any swelling, and the texture of the muscle is determined by making a cut in the dorsal region to see whether any ulcers or inflammation are present. The color of the feces in certain instances is often of great value as a clue with which to determine the etiology of the infection (e.g. *Eimeria cyprini*, see *coccidial enteritis of carp*).

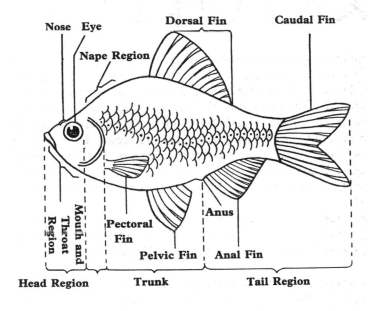

Figure 2. External anatomy of a Teleost fish. (Amlacher)

Sacrifice (or killing)

There are various well proven procedures for the rapid killing of fish. For small individuals the best method is to cut off their heads or cut them in the neck (*Figure 4*), by means of which the brain is cut with scissors at a point just posterior to the eyes, or conversely the incision is made in the region between the brain and the spinal cord. Another procedure is to place them in an anesthetic such as tricaine methanesulfonate (MS–222) or quinaldine. (Bell 1967.) However cutting the neck has the advantage that the fish remains alive and fresh, and any parasites of the skin are not removed as a result of the action of any chemical substances. Larger fish such as carp are killed in the field by a blow on the head, or in the laboratory by an electric current.

Exploration of the skin and gills; smears

The dead fish is placed laterally on a wooden board. We begin with an exploration of the skin. *Figure 5* shows the places from which material may be taken for smears. The best skin smears are obtained from the lateral sides of the body, from the caudal fin, and from the axillae or bases of the fins. Almost on every occasion on which the gills are examined, smears are made.

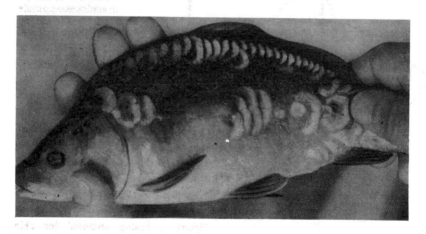

Figure 3. Ocular reflex of a carp infected with ichthyophthiriasis. The fish was turned to the right from the normal position. (Wagner)

The instrument used for this procedure is the spatula, which is scraped along the skin from head to tail (*Figure 6*). In this way mucus mixed with epidermal cells and any parasites present on the skin is obtained.

Cutaneous or gill material obtained by scraping is placed into a drop of water previously put onto a slide, the whole is carefully mixed by means of a pair of mounted needles, and then covered with a coverslip. In this state it is examined under the microscope using a low power objective. At times, especially when there are small protozoans, the addition of a little Indian ink to the water is useful (approximately a tenth part in volume of ink to water). The ink disperses in the water and colors every-

20

Figure 4. Technique of neck incision. (Amlacher)

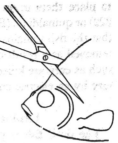

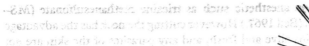

Trunk   Tail

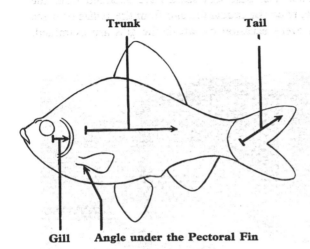

Figure5. The arrows show the direction In which the spatula is moved in taking material for smears.

Gill   Angle under the Pectoral Fin

Figure 6. Taking material for skin smear. (Amlacher)

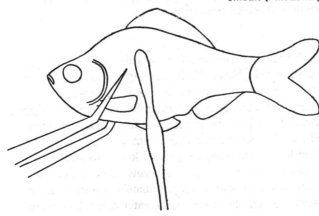

thing black with the exception of any parasites whose form is thus brought out in relief.

Technique of autopsy

Only in very rare instances indeed is it possible to study a diseased fish successfully without the need for killing it beforehand. In clear cut cases of skin disease, such as an *Ichthyophthirius* infection, an ordinary skin smear is sufficient to establish the diagnosis. In the presence of an open ulceration, again a scraping from this may frequently suffice to establish a satisfactory diagnosis. However it is not always quite so easy, especially in the case of internal diseases such as piscine tuberculosis and ichthyosporidiosis, where an autopsy is indispensable. In tuberculosis and bacterial hemorrhagic septicemia where there is any doubt, smears and cultures should be taken from the internal organs so as to demonstrate the presence of acid-fast bacilli (tuberculosis) or the causative agent of dropsy (see the section on bacteriological techniques). Faced with the problem of diseases such as these, an analysis of one or two fish should enable a better idea to be made of the overall state of health of the population, as for example in a fish hatchery.

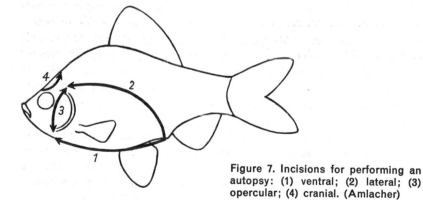

Figure 7. Incisions for performing an autopsy: (1) ventral; (2) lateral; (3) opercular; (4) cranial. (Amlacher)

The form in which the cuts and incisions are made during an autopsy on a fish is shown schematically in *Figure 7*.

Ornamental fish are held fast by means of a pair of large curved forceps as shown in *Figure 8*. Following this, the first ventral or abdominal incision is carried out with a pair of sharp-pointed scissors. To perform this the scissors are introduced into the anus in such a manner that the intra-abdominal point remains steady whilst the cut is made in close contact with the ventral wall so as not to damage any of the internal organs (e.g. intestine). By this means the incision is continued in a straight line in the

22

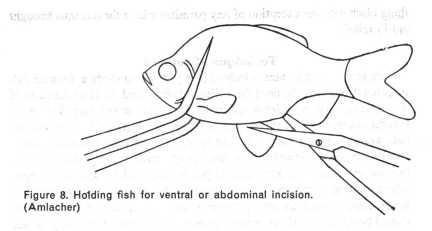

Figure 8. Holding fish for ventral or abdominal incision.
(Amlacher)

direction of the head, between the ventral fins and almost up to the pectoral fins.

Straight away the fish is placed in a lateral position and the second (or lateral) cut is made, in a semi-circle leaving the anus, passing through the lateral surface of the body and above the operculum, to finally penetrate the gill cavity. On doing this the body wall is held firmly and lifted up with a pair of forceps (*Figures 7* and *9*). The tissues adhering to the body wall and peritoneum are carefully cut with a mounted needle or with a flat instrument. Almost always the kidney is found adhering to the body wall on the side which has been removed, and thus may be rapidly removed without any further difficulty. If the second cut is extended to the gill cavity, the strip of body wall may be easily bent forward and downwards. When considered necessary, this strip of body wall may be cut transversely and removed.

The first two cuts serve to enable the internal organs to be removed at will. In larger fish such as two-year-old carp or tench, in place of an ordinary pair of forceps, a pair of artery forceps may be used. One arm is placed into the anal opening of the fish and then the forceps are closed. These forceps hold the lateral body wall as shown in *Figure 9*.

Third we use the opercular cut to free the gills (*Figures 10* and *7*). The direction in which the cut is made is of little real importance. The gill operculum is then raised with forceps.

Finally the fourth or cranial cut is made from front to back with a fine scalpel (*Figures 11* and *7*) so that the brain is exposed. To perform this the fish is held with the fingers or with a pair of strong curved forceps (*Figure 11*).

In this way the dissection as such is completed, and the more important internal organs are thus exposed for study (*Figure 12*).

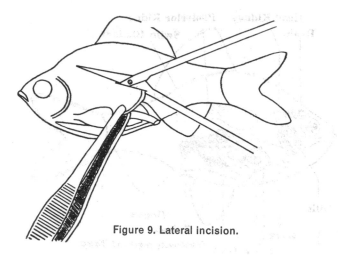

Figure 9. Lateral incision.

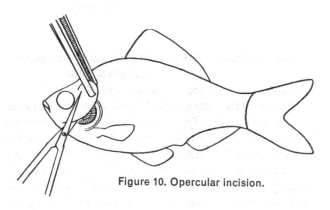

Figure 10. Opercular incision.

Figure 11. Cranial incision. (Amlacher)

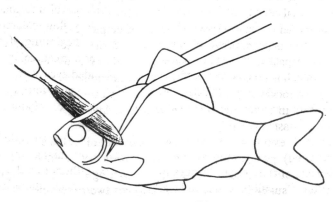

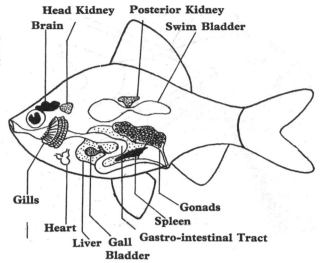

Figure 12. Arrangement of the internal organs of a Teleost fish. (Amlacher)

Head Kidney **Posterior Kidney**
Brain
Swim Bladder

Gills
Gonads
Spleen
Heart
Gastro-intestinal Tract
Liver **Gall**
Bladder

Investigation of the internal organs; maceration and squash preparations

(1) INSPECTION OF THE INTERNAL ORGANS

Before making any slides, the dissected fish is examined with the naked eye or with a magnifying glass, paying special attention to the color and consistency of the organs: pale gills; yellowish coloration of the liver; congestion and reddening of the liver; inflammation of the spleen and splenomegaly; pale coloration of the kidney; transparency and inflammatory reddening of the intestine; hardening of the bile and gall bladder; adipose tissue between the intestine, liver and genitalia; fluid in the peritoneal cavity (in positive cases record whether this is clear yellow or bloody and aqueous); white nodules on the gills, liver, spleen and kidney; odor in the abdominal cavity. All of these lesions furnish useful information for any subsequent examination. Thus for example yellow colored livers indicate a fatty degeneration of that organ and the beginning of a destruction of the hepatic cells. The same may be said of a green coloration of the liver, which is seen occasionally. Finally, extruded eyes or those deeply seated in the socket are indicative of a pathological condition. The swim bladder (absent in some species of fish) may be reddened or inflamed.

(2) MICROSCOPICAL OBSERVATION

For microscopical examinations we can make use of the so-called macerated (or teased) preparations. These are made by taking small pinhead-sized pieces of the organ in question and putting them in a drop of water on a slide. Usually it is possible to carry out two macerations at

25

the same time in one drop of water. The fragments of the organ are teased by means of two mounted needles, the points of which are sharpened previously on a carborundum stone. It is most important that the pieces of organ be well macerated, since only good preparations are of value for microscopical study. On completing the maceration procedure a coverslip is placed on the slide, and should it be necessary this is carefully put into position with the handle of the mounted needle with very light pressure. The same procedure is carried out with all of the internal organs and the body musculature (see plistophorosis). Several gill filaments are removed from the gills and are examined whole, for which it is sufficient to press them very carefully beneath the coverslip, taking care that no cartilaginous parts of the gill arch remain under the coverslip, for in such an instance this will break, since gill arches resist pressure.

In certain cases it is necessary to carry out an examination of the eyes. These are cut out, and the orbits scraped with a spatula. Material obtained by scraping is examined firstly as described above. After this the eyeball is cut open on a slide and the fluid which runs from it is examined. The amount of pigment in the eyes makes any exacting study rather difficult to perform.

Squash preparations are made by squeezing a small piece of the organ between two slides. Both macerated and squash preparations are examined microscopically. With an ordinary Zeiss L microscope, the best results are obtained with a × 10 eyepiece and × 3, × 8, and × 40 objectives. For bacteriological work the oil immersion objective is likewise used. One should always start with low power objectives. The best way is to use a combination of a × 10 eyepiece with a × 8 objective, with which the greater majority of fish parasites may be seen (except for bacterial ones). For the preparation of permanently mounted slides, see the section dealing with histological techniques and rapid methods given below.

Histological and histochemical techniques
(*A special method is indicated for each disease when this is neceesary*)

In the event of it being necessary to carry out a more exhaustive study so as to establish a clear diagnosis on macerated material, pieces of diseased tissue should be fixed. Fixation is a process whereby the vital activities of the tissues are brought to a halt by causing the death of the cells, and with the help of specialized methods the tissue is prepared for microscopical examination.

(1) FIXATIVES

These are almost all liquid. The most common one is commercial 40% formalin, duly diluted. In our laboratory we use a mixture of one part formalin to four parts of distilled water for fixation. A piece of tissue some

26

4 mm. thick is fixed in this for 18–24 hours. In order to treat certain tissues with greater care, a dilution of one part formalin to nine parts of distilled water may be used, this is the routine formalin mixture used in the United States. When it is necessary to carry out a rapid fixation, as for example in a non-routine case, I recommend a hot fixation as used in medical laboratory work. Small blocks of tissue (2 mm. thick) are added to boiling formol saline and then left for one minute; after this they are hardened in 96% alcohol. Stieve's fluid (saturated solution of mercuric chloride 7.6 cc., 40% formalin 2 cc., glacial acetic acid 0.4 cc.) or Bouin's (saturated aqueous picric acid, 75 parts; commercial formalin, 25 parts; glacial acetic acid, 5 parts) are excellent fixatives for fish tissue. Bouin's is said to enhance staining quality.

The fixation of blocks of tissue not exceeding 4 mm. thick is completed in Stieve's fluid within 6 hours or less, since it is of very rapid penetration. An excessively long fixation in Stieve's fluid produces abundant deposits of mercuric chloride in the tissues. The recommended time of fixation with Bouin's fixative is 6–12 hours.

In my own laboratory a mixture of two parts of absolute alcohol and one part of 40% formalin is used for histochemical studies. According to Schäperclaus, protozoa are fixed in smears which are allowed to dry. Where it is wished to stain flagellates (e.g. *Cryptobia*) they must be fixed while still fresh with osmic acid vapor. Wet smears are fixed in alcoholic sublimate (one part of 96% alcohol: two parts of concentrated mercuric chloride solution). Smears from blood and organs are dried in the air and then fixed in absolute methanol.

(2) FURTHER TREATMENT OF FIXED MATERIAL

After fixation in formalin or Bouin's fixative, tissues are passed through the alcohol series to absolute alcohol. Tissues fixed in Stieve's fluid may be placed directly in 90% alcohol and the absolute. From absolute alcohol, tissues are placed in absolute alcohol-xylene (50:50), xylene and then paraffin (58–60° C.). Specific times for each bath vary from laboratory to laboratory. Also, some laboratories prefer solvents other than xylene for clearing, i.e. chloroform, benzene, or dioxane.

Paraffin sections are cut from the blocks at 5–10 microns and floated on warm water (just below the melting point of the paraffin). The sections are lifted from the water bath on microscope slides coated with a minimal amount of Mayer's albumin. These slides are allowed to dry thoroughly and are then ready for staining.

(3) STAINING

For the staining of paraffin wax sections and smears, I recommend the following methods. The best procedure is to run the first and the second simultaneously.

Hematoxylin—eosin

This is the standard, routine histological stain combination.

The sections, duly brought to water by passing through xylol, xylol-alcohol, absolute alcohol, 90%, 70%, 40% alcohol and distilled water, are treated in the following manner:—

(a) stain with Delafield's hematoxylin 2–3 minutes;

(b) wash in distilled water 30 seconds;

(c) stain with 1% aqueous eosin 30 seconds;

(d) wash with distilled water;

(e) take through the alcohols to dehydrate, clear rapidly in xylol, and mount.

Mallory's acid fuchsin—aniline blue—orange G stain

This method is less effective for staining cell nuclei, but it gives a good specific stain for connective tissues. The deparaffinized and hydrated sections are treated as follows:—

(a) stain for 1–5 minutes in a 1% aqueous solution of acid fuchsin diluted 1:10 in water;

(b) wash with distilled water;

(c) leave for one minute in a 1% aqueous solution of phosphomolybdic acid;

(d) wash twice with distilled water;

(e) stain in the following: water-soluble aniline blue 0.5 gm., oxalic acid 2 gm., orange G 2 gm., water 100 cc. The solution is boiled and filtered after cooling. The duration of the stain is from 2–20 minutes;

(f) wash in water;

(g) differentiate in 96% alcohol;

(h) absolute alcohol, xylol, balsam.

Collagen fibers and reticular connective tissues are stained a brilliant and intense blue color, as are mucin and hyaline (cartilaginous) tissues. Smooth muscle fibers are red-violet, and erythrocytes a dirty red. In spite of the general opinion that this staining method does not give good results following fixation of the material in formalin, we have always been quite successful with the technique as outlined above.

Giemsa

For the staining of blood smears and *organ imprint* slides, Giemsa's method is recommended.

(a) leave the smears to dry in the air, and then fix in absolute methanol for 10 minutes;

(b) dry in the air;

(c) stain with dilute Giemsa (one drop of stock stain solution to 1 cc. of boiled distilled water at pH 6.6) for 20 minutes;

(*d*) pour off the stain and wash the smear carefully with boiled distilled water;

(*e*) dry in the air.

Staining of wet smears

For skin and intestinal protozoa (especially flagellates and ciliates) Reichenow's procedure is recommended. The material is smeared with a platinum loop (or with a second slide, whichever is more convenient) onto a coverslip (20 × 20 mm.).

(*a*) fix the smear for three minutes while the coverslip floats face downwards in alcoholic sublimate (one part 96% alcohol: two parts concentrated aqueous solution of mercuric chloride);

(*b*) turn the coverslip round and immerse it in the above liquid for 15 minutes;

(*c*) wash with iodized 70% alcohol for 20 minutes;

(*d*) wash with 70% alcohol for 30 minutes;

(*e*) stain with Giemsa or hematoxylin—eosin;

(*f*) xylol, mount in balsam.

(4) RAPID PROCEDURE

Frequently there remain doubts as to the precise identity of a parasite or tumor after the completion of the autopsy. Since the fish is dead, the autopsy completed, and the macerated preparation ready and covered with a coverslip, one wonders just what may be done. The answer is to put the slide in a Petri dish which contains one part of formalin to four parts of water. After five hours the formalin is thrown away and 40% alcohol added. Following three hours in 40% alcohol, this is changed for 70%. When required the slide may be kept in 70% alcohol for a longer period (e.g. overnight). This is followed with 95% and absolute alcohol respectively. After applying the absolute alcohol, the slide is taken for complete dehydration to methyl benzoate (or xylol) for three hours. In the majority of cases the coverslip becomes detached from the slide at this stage, and the section floats free. On other occasions it remains adhering to the slide. According to what may have happened the following steps are taken. If the tissue has worked free, a drop of balsam is put onto another slide, the tissue is removed from the benzene, mounted in the balsam and carefully covered with a coverslip. If the tissue remains stuck to the coverslip we continue in the same way except that both the tissue and the coverslip are taken out of the benzene together and mounted in balsam. In the event of the tissue being stuck to the slide itself, a drop of balsam is added and a coverslip placed on top of it.

The slides obtained in this way are allowed to dry for three days, after which they may be sent for examination to a fish pathology laboratory.

(5) HISTOCHEMISTRY

Histochemical methods are also applied to fish pathology. We have for some years been successfully making glycogen determinations in liver sections for the diagnosis of infectious abdominal dropsy. For this we use Bauer's and Langhan's methods. The Perls Berlin blue reaction is also used for sections, as well as the peroxidase reaction for blood smears. Important work in the field of analytical pathology is reserved for histochemistry. Thus for example, the McManus and Hotchkiss polysaccharide reaction is useful for the identification of fungal cellulose, and the Feulgen stain is of value for nuclei.

Bacteriological techniques

Bacteriological studies should be carried out before the fish is opened or cut. The research worker must ensure that any infectious material collected has not at any time come into contact with the skin or the intestine of the fish.

(1) OBTAINING MATERIAL AND ITS CULTURE

The techniques for obtaining or extracting infectious material from the diseased parts vary considerably in accordance with the nature of the case under study.

Internal organs

The fish is placed on its right side with the head to the left. With a large needle the caudal peduncle is fixed to a board. The surface of the fish is swabbed with alcohol or other disinfectant. This having been done, a ventral and a lateral incision respectively are made with a sterile pair of scissors. Great care must be taken to ensure that the inside surface of the lateral flap does not come into contact with any sterile instruments or culture media. With a flamed loop the surface of the liver, spleen, heart and kidney is punctured, and a little of the infectious material is plated onto the appropriate culture medium or media. Any instruments used are sterilized by dipping them in alcohol and immediately flaming prior to use.

Blood

Once the fish has been anesthetized, it is hung head upwards, the dorsal and anal fins are cut, and the body is dried with a rag (paying particular attention to the head and gills, to avoid any dripping of water). With a sterile pair of Spencer-Wells forceps the caudal fin is carefully held and the peduncle is completely cauterized with a red hot metal blade. The caudal peduncle is then cut in the sterilized region with a pair of scissors and the tail cut completely away. The blood flows readily from the cut and may be collected in a sterile tube. A sterile needle and syringe may be used to take blood from the heart or caudal muscle after topical disinfection of the skin.

(2) SMEARS

For routine diagnosis the preparation of stained smears of the organs is extremely useful (in tuberculosis for example). The smear is made by pressing the surface of an organ onto a slide, or by taking a piece of it with a sterile pair of forceps and macerating it in sterile distilled water with a flamed mounted needle or loop. The thinner the smear the better it will stain. The slide is air dried and the appropriate data are written at one end with a diamond. In certain cases the material is fixed by passing the slide gently through the flame of a burner.

(3) CULTURE MEDIA

The ordinary culture media used in the study of bacterial fish diseases are as follows:

(a) *peptone water* (1 gm. peptone; 0.5 gm. sodium chloride; 100 cc. water; in the case of marine fish the concentration of sodium chloride is increased to 2 gm.). The ingredients are dissolved by heating in the autoclave for about an hour, then they are filtered, and distributed into test tubes. The tubes are tyndallized for three consecutive days in the autoclave.

(b) *nutrient broth:* 500 gm. of minced, boneless and fat-free meat are placed in one liter of ordinary tap water and held at room temperature overnight, or at 37° C. for one hour. The whole is then boiled for thirty minutes in the autoclave. After this it is passed to a muslin cloth, in which it is pressed, and the liquid filtered. The volume is then made up to one liter. Beef is the best meat to use. To the resulting beef broth are added 10 gm. peptone (added whilst still cold), 3 gm. of sodium chloride (or 10 gm. for marine fish), and 2 gm. of sodium phosphate. This mixture is heated to dissolve for thirty minutes in an autoclave, filtered through a double layer of filter paper (the best method is to leave it until any larger particles have sedimented out, and then to decant the clear fluid). The pH is adjusted to 7.5 with sodium hydroxide solution, the medium is then reheated and the pH adjusted again. The liquid is distributed into test tubes provided with cotton wool plugs (or into large bottles) and then tyndallized for twenty minutes on each of three consecutive days at 120° C. for 15–20 minutes.

(c) *nutrient agar:* The broth described above is boiled in an autoclave together with 2.5% powdered agar until this latter is dissolved (about an hour is required for this). The agar should previously have been left to soak for several hours. The pH is adjusted to 7.6 and the medium is left to sediment in the autoclave and the clear portion decanted. The agar is best stored in special bottles (milk bottles are satisfactory). From these are taken the quantities required to pour Petri dishes or to make agar slants (6 cc. of agar per tube).

Should the agar be turbid, it may be cleared by adjusting the pH, filtering, and adding an egg white well mixed with 50 cc. of water.

(d) *fuchsin—sucrose—agar*: 100 cc. of neutral nutrient agar are melted in a water bath, mixed with 1 cc. of 10% sodium hydroxide solution, and cooled to 60° C. 1 gm. of sucrose is dissolved in 2–3 cc. of sterile distilled water in a sterile cylinder and the whole briefly boiled and added to the agar. Following this 0.5 cc. of an alcoholic fuchsin solution is added with a sterile pipette. 1 gm. of sodium sulfate (Na_2SO_3 $7H_2O$) is dissolved in 10 cc. of sterile water, heated without boiling, and from this 2.5 cc. are added to the medium in such a way as to make the red color disappear. Shake the medium and pour it in 10 cc. quantities into sterile Petri dishes.

(e) *Jensen's egg medium*: 600 cc. of Loewenstein's stock solution (4.0 gm. monopotassium phosphate, 1.0 gm. magnesium citrate, 0.4 gm. magnesium sulfate, 6.0 gm. asparagine, 20.0 gm. double distilled glycerine, and distilled water to 1.000 cc.) are boiled for two hours in a 1 liter flask. Allow to cool. Add 30 gm. of potato starch. Boil in a water bath with continual shaking until a pasty consistency is obtained. Leave for one hour at 56° C. Add a liter of egg emulsion, shake well and add 20 cc. of 2% malachite green solution. Distribute in tubes and allow to solidify. Sterilize for the first day 30 minutes at 85° C., the second day 30 minutes at 75° C. The glycerine concentration should be 0.74%.

(f) *Amlacher's egg medium*: 160 cc. of egg emulsion, 95 cc. of 0.64% NaCl solution, 5 cc. of glycerine (double distilled), 5 gm. flour of potatoes or 1 gm. peptone, 2 gm. asparagine, 10 cc. of a 10% solution of malachite green.

For obtaining pure cultures and for studying the fermentative activities of bacterial fish pathogens a number of special media such as litmus—casein—carbohydrate are required (consult "Fischkrankheiten" by W. Schäperclaus).

(4) BACTERIAL CULTURES

In the majority of cases, cultures are incubated at 22–26° C. Before a precise bacteriological study may be carried out it is necessary to ensure, that one has obtained pure cultures with which to work. To obtain these a loopful of a fresh liquid culture is streaked onto agar in such a way as to produce individual colonies. These latter may be subsequently maintained on agar slopes.

If we have impure cultures (for example, in the case of *Aeromonas liquefaciens*), a small quantity of the initial culture is added to a drop of water and suspended therein. A loopful is taken from this and added to another drop of water, from which a further loopful is taken and added to a tube of melted gelatine and the whole mixed. Following this the gelatine is poured into a Petri dish. Any typical colonies which develop are picked off with a sterile wire and streaked onto agar slopes. For the obtention of truly unicellular cultures the book by Schäperclaus should be consulted.

(5) STAINING OF BACTERIA IN SMEARS

The principal staining methods used in fish pathology are Gram's, methylene blue and Ziehl-Neelsen (for acid-fast bacteria). Histological sections are also stained. This latter method, when performed by an expert, can also yield a great deal of useful histopathological data.

Gram's stain

This stain allows bacteria to be divided into Gram positive (stained by aniline derivatives and treated in such a manner that they do not decolorize with alcohol), and Gram negative (which lose the stain and must be demonstrated with a counterstain). The following modification of Gram's method, by Habs, is the most frequently employed: the smears are fixed by heat and stained for three minutes with a phenicated gentian violet (10 cc. saturated gentian violet solution are mixed with 90 cc. of freshly prepared 2.5% phenol solution) and mordanted for one minute with a potassium iodide-iodine solution (1 gm. iodine and 2 gm. of potassium iodide are mixed together in a mortar and dissolved in 5 cc. of water; the volume is then made up to 300 cc. with water). Following this the smear is decolorized with 96% alcohol until no more stain runs freely away. Then it is stained for a few seconds with carbol fuchsin solution (10 cc. of a saturated alcoholic solution of fuchsin are mixed with 90 cc. of a 5% phenol solution, and the resulting mixture is diluted 1:10 with water). The smear is finally washed well with water and dried. Gram positive bacteria stain bluish-violet and Gram negative ones stain red. The phenicated gentian violet solution is allowed to fall drop by drop onto the smear through a filter paper. In the case of the iodine solution and the carbol fuchsin, it is better to first moisten the filter paper with the stain before filtering.

Methylene blue

For this stain an alkaline solution of methylene blue (Löffler's) is used. To 30 cc. of a saturated alcoholic solution of methylene blue are added 100 cc. of a 0.01% potassium hydroxide solution (prepared by diluting 1 cc. of 1% potassium hydroxide solution in 99 cc. of distilled water). In order to use it as a counterstain in the demonstrain of acid-fast bacilli, one part of Löffler's methylene blue is mixed with 4–9 parts of water. This solution stains intensely and rapidly (1–2 minutes) and stores very well.

Polychrome methylene blue is used chiefly to stain bacteria in sections. This consists of 1 gm. of methylene blue in 100 cc. of distilled water, together with 20 cc. of 96% alcohol and 1 gm. of potassium carbonate. Allow this to evaporate slowly in a water bath until its volume has been reduced to about 100 cc.

Carbol fuchsin

Carbol fuchsin is used in conjunction with methylene blue in a special method used to stain acid-fast bacilli (tubercle bacilli, organisms causing tuberculosis in cold-blooded animals). These bacteria, which possess a waxy sheath, do not take up the usual stains, but Ziehl-Neelsen's method places them in a state wherein they retain the dye even when treated with acid and alcohol (acid-alcohol resistance), while other types of bacteria and tissue cells are decolorized and are only visible after staining with a counterstain (methylene blue). The following modification is commonly used: the smear is heat fixed for 2–3 minutes with strong carbol fuchsin (10 cc. of a concentrated alcoholic solution of fuchsin are mixed with 90 cc. of a 5% phenol solution), heating the slide with a flame until steam rises (do *NOT* boil!!). Decolorize with acid-alcohol (3 cc. of 25% hydrochloric acid mixed with 100 cc. of 69% alcohol) for 5 seconds. Wash twice in 70% alcohol until the smear is decolorized. Wash with distilled water. Stain with a very dilute solution of methylene blue for 30 seconds. Wash with distilled water and dry. Acid-fast bacilli appear red on a blue background. The counterstain should be the palest blue possible.

(6) STAINING OF FLAGELLA

In order to be able to identify certain species of bacteria and protozoans it is necessary to demonstrate the presence of flagella. Flagella do not stain with the ordinary methods and even special techniques do not always give the results anticipated. Slides and coverslips must be scrupulously clean and completely free from grease. The bacteria are taken from surface cultures. Three spots of water are placed at different points of the slide. In the first of these the material on the point of a mounted needle is diluted after having been taken from the culture, and the smallest amount of this is transferred to the second and third drops respectively. The drops are spread so as to allow them to dry quickly.

The best method for demonstrating flagella is that of Zettnow, which Habs describes as follows: a drop of water is put onto a slide and to this is added the culture adhering to the point of a needle. A larger drop of water is placed onto a second slide and a loopful of 2% osmic acid is added to this. A small portion of the first drop is taken and mixed with the second one. From this a loopful is taken and spread over the surface of a coverslip, allowed to dry, and passed twice through a flame. The coverslip is put into a dish, face downwards, supported by glass or wooden rods. 3 cc. of well shaken tannin-antimony mordant are heated in a test-tube until clear. This is then poured onto the coverslip until it becomes opaque (the mordant is prepared by heating 10 gm. of tannin in 150 cc. of boiling distilled water, filtering and cooling to 50° C. 36 cc. of a 5% antimony tartrate solution are added until a permanent precipitate is formed. A part of this mordant should be cleared on boiling in a test-tube and cloud up on cooling again. If it remains clear when cool, more antimony tartrate is added;

but if on the other hand it acquires an intense milky white turbidity, then more tannin solution must be added. The mixture may be preserved by adding a crystal of thymol. Finally the coverslip is washed with water, drop by drop, and a solution of silver is added slowly and heated with a weak flame until steam rises (the edges of the smear become black in color at this point). After this the smear is washed and dried. The silver solution has the following composition: 5 gm. of silver nitrate and 6 gm. of sodium sulphate are shaken with 30 cc. of distilled water. The precipitate which forms is washed three times with water. 500 cc. of distilled water are then added and the whole is shaken. When it has sedimented, 25 cc. of the supernatant solution are mixed with the same volume of water and a few drops of 33% ethylamine are added carefully until the precipitate has become dissolved. This solution keeps fairly well.

General methods are available and can be found in microbiology texts. Experience will tell the individual which works best for him.

(7) STAINING OF BACTERIA IN SECTIONS

For bacteriological studies sections are stained in the same way and with the same stains as are used for smears. The staining time is usually longer. There is no uniform criterion with regard to the most suitable fixative to be used. All that is required is that the bacteria should be quickly killed. The best fixatives with which to accomplish this are mercuric chloride, formalin or alcohol. Too long a time in alcohol is unfavorable to the staining of bacteria, and usually makes it more difficult to section the organ. Paraffin wax is the best material for embedding.

Staining of sections by Gram's method

Weigert's modification is used: there is a preliminary nuclear stain in Kernechrot solution for 5–10 minutes (dissolve 5 gm. of aluminum sulfate in 100 cc. of distilled water and to this then add 0.1 gm. of a good red nuclear stain, boil, cool and filter); wash in 0.6% sodium chloride; stain with gentian violet in aniline solution for 5–20 minutes (vigorously shake 5 cc. of aniline with 100 cc. distilled water for several minutes; filter the milky liquid through a filter paper moistened with water, mix 100 cc. of the fat-free filtrate with 11 cc. of a saturated alcoholic solution of gentian violet. The stain should be used only if clear (as it rapidly becomes useless); wash in 0.6% sodium chloride; dry with filter paper; immerse 1–2 minutes in potassium iodide-iodine solution (see Gram's method above); dry completely with filter paper; decolorize with aniline oil until the sections appear red; clear in xylol and mount in balsam.

Staining of tubercle bacilli in sections

The Ziehl-Neelsen method is used as the Habs modification: stain with carbol fuchsin for 24 hours at room temperature, or from 30 minutes to 2 hours at 37° C. Decolorize with 1% acid alcohol for 30 seconds to 2 minutes. Wash with 70% alcohol for 2–3 minutes until the section appears colorless. Counterstain with a dilute alcoholic solution of methylene blue for 2–5 minutes. Wash briefly with 0.5% acetic acid. Take through the alcohols, clear in xylol and mount in balsam.

Virological techniques, Cell culture

VIROLOGICAL TECHNIQUES

For the demonstration and transmission of a virus infection, the infected tissue is generally homogenized (homogenizers such as Waring Blender, Potter-Elvehjem). In an emergency, the tissue can also be pulverized with sterile quartz sand in a mortar. All operations should be carried out in the cold (0–4° C.).

As a suspension medium, physiological saline serves in its simplest form, sterile 0.85% NaCl solution at pH 7.2 for poikilotherms. Fresh pathological material stored at −20°C or material held in 50% glycerol at 4°C can be used for examination. The material is suspended in the proportion of 1:10 (one part by weight of infectious material to 10 volumes of suspension medium) and the homogenate centrifuged 2 or 3 times for 10 to 20 minutes at 2000 g. The supernatant is filtered through a cell retaining filter (Schott G5, G4; Seitz asbestos, Coors P3—porcelain). The cell free filtrate can then be injected or put in cultures. For the concentration of the virus, the cell free filtrate must be centrifuged at 4° C. for 10 to 15 minutes at 12,000 or 26,000 g. The "virus pellet" found in the sediment is resuspended in 100 cc. of 0.005M Na citrate solution (pH 7.2) and applied in quantities of 0.1–1.0 cc.

The cytopathogenic effect (CPE) in cell cultures is only characteristic for cytocidal viruses. Therefore, with every attempt to demonstrate virus, the cell free filtrate must be injected into healthy fish. The CPE is also necessary as complementary for the determination of the nature of the virus. Also, the electron microscope is required for confirmation of the virus.

CELL CULTURE FOR VIROLOGICAL INVESTIGATIONS

Fish gonads (especially ovaries, e.g. from carp) are trypsinized at pH 7.2 for several hours. The trypsinization is carried out according to Wolf et al (1960) in a modified PBS (phosphate buffered saline). The buffer is after Dulbeco and Vogt (1954) whose composition is as follows:

(a) NaCl 8.0 gm., KCl 0.2 gm., Na_2HPO_4 1.065 gm., KH_2PO_4 0.249 gm., water 800 cc.;

(b) $CaCl_2$ 0.1 gm., water 100 cc.;

(c) $MgCl_2 \cdot 6H_2O$ 0.1 gm., water 100 cc.

These are autoclaved separately. After they have cooled, they are mixed. This solution mixture makes up 87.5% of the digestion liquid. It is made up to 100% with 2.5% trypsin solution. In addition, calcium penicillin G and streptomycin sulfate are added in an amount of 200 units/ml.

The trypsinized cell material can be removed at hourly intervals. The trypsinized cells are centrifuged for 20 minutes at 200 g and cultivated in Demeter flasks in Parker medium 199 plus 10% calf serum at 27° C. after the addition of 1 unit of penicillin and 1 milligram dihydrostreptomycin per cc. (Wolf and Dunbar 1958). From carp ovary, a thick cell sheet forms after 1–2 days (Pfitzner 1966). These can be retrypsinized or better (Pfitzner 1966) pipetted off or scraped off (rubber scraper) and changed to subcultures which live up to 4 weeks without medium change. She succeeded in establishing only up to three subcultures from carp ovaries.

In the U.S.A., a permanent line from the gonads of the rainbow trout (RTG–2) has been established. It consists of a pure line of fibroblasts.

Hematological and serological techniques

At the present time hematological investigations have been ever increasing in importance not only in basic ichthyology but also in practical fish pathology. Usually any hematological study is based upon the examination of smears, although hemoglobin and total protein estimations, serum electrophoresis and other biochemical determinations are also carried out.

(1) EXTRACTION OF BLOOD

The fish is killed by a blow on the head or by an electric shock, and is then hung with the head uppermost (see techniques for the extraction of infectious material). After cutting the dorsal and anal fins, the body, head and gill covers are cursorily wiped with a cloth. The tail is cut off along the caudal peduncle with a pair of bone forceps.

The first five drops of blood are allowed to go to waste and the remainder is collected into long and narrow test-tubes. For making smears a small drop is taken directly onto a slide. It is also useful to take up a 0.02 ml. quantity in a pipette for the hemoglobin estimation. The whole procedure of taking blood lasts for about three or four minutes. Another way of taking blood, according to Jara (1958–9), is by cardiac puncture. The fish are killed by an electric shock; the thoracic cavity is opened, the branches of the vagus are cut, and the heart is exposed. The blood is taken by means of a syringe cooled on ice, the point being introduced into the bulbus arteriosus. Aspiration should last from a minute or two up to a quarter of an hour. Any blood obtained is voided from the syringe into refrigerated and paraffinized or siliconized tubes. Blood may also be taken from fish by cardiac puncture without any need to dissect out the heart region. A further technique is to puncture the gill arches with fine-pointed glass canulae. These latter should have a large diameter at the open end. They are heparinized internally to prevent coagulation. As and when required, the blood for analysis is removed from the canula (for example, in order to perform a hemoglobin estimation).

(2) BLOOD CLOTTING

In the majority of cases fish blood clots with great rapidity at the surface of the wound. It takes some 3 minutes to clot in watch glasses at room temperature (Jara, 1958–9). According to this same author coagulation depends to a great extent on contact between the blood and the glass, for which reason clotting is delayed when the blood is collected into paraffinized glass tubes.

(3) PREVENTION OF CLOTTING

Blood clotting may be prevented by the addition of calcium fluoride, sodium acetate, sodium oxalate, EDTA, or heparin. 2% sodium oxalate solution is used in many laboratories. A 0.5 cc. quantity of this is allowed to evaporate in a test-tube in an oven at 150° C. The oxalate prevents clotting on the sides of the tubes, and infallibly prevents clotting when no more than 3–4 cc. of blood are taken. For larger amounts of blood a proportionately larger amount of sodium oxalate is used. 0.5 cc. of evaporated 2% sodium oxalate solution is sufficient to prevent the clotting of each 3–4 cc. of blood. Oxalated blood may be used for smears, hemoglobin determinations or blood sugar estimations without the production of any intereference. It has the added advantage of enabling the blood to be stored for up to 48 hours in the refrigerator, and in addition to being precise, allows comparative analyses to be made on any one fish without the necessity for urgent haste on the part of the fish pathologist.

(4) OBTAINING SERUM

Recently collected blood is left untouched for 6 hours in large narrow tubes, in a vertical position and at refrigerator temperature. During this time retraction of the blood clot (erythrocytes and fibrin) takes place, and gives clear yellow serum. Where the specimen is not going to be used immediately, it may be kept in the refrigerator. The serum is tipped into a small centrifuge tube. On doing this a little hemoglobin is inevitably carried with it, but this may be separated by centrifuging at 3000–4000 r.p.m. Serum held in the refrigerator may be used for up to 5 days and more for blood sugar and electrophoretic determinations.

(5) BLOOD SMEARS

Blood smears may be prepared from fresh material or from that to which an anticoagulant (oxalates may cause artifacts) has been previously added. To make the smear, slides should be taken with forceps from a 1:1 mixture of ether and alcohol, and then dried with a clean cloth. The same procedure should be carried out with any coverslips used for making smears.

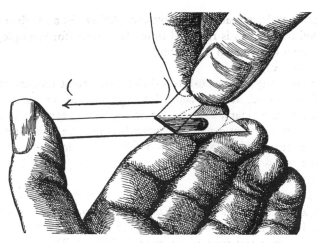

Figure 13. Preparation of a blood smear. (Schilling)

To make a smear from uncoagulated blood, the tube is shaken and a small drop taken out with a glass rod which is then touched onto the slide. The amount of blood thus obtained is usually of a type which gives a good smear. The slide bearing the drop of blood is held in one hand with the drop uppermost, at elbow length, while with the other hand the edge of the coverslip is placed on it at an angle of 45° (*Figure 13*). This is then moved backwards until it just touches the drop of blood which is thus smeared along the slide by capillary attraction in a uniform layer. All of the blood must be used in making the smear, otherwise the smear itself will be thick and irregular. If there be too much blood on the slide, it may be repeatedly touched with the edge of the coverslip, and then the smear made. In the event that small bubbles appear in the smear this means that the slide was too greasy prior to use. On no account should the smear reach the end of the slide. When working with fresh blood the smear should be made rapidly to avoid clotting, a disadvantage not possessed by blood to which a suitable anticoagulant has been added previously. To make a smear without a slide and a coverslip, two scrupulously clean coverslips alone may be used. A drop of blood is placed onto one of them (the drops should be about the size of a pinhead), and the other coverslip is placed on top. The blood spreads by capillary attraction, and then both coverslips are drawn apart and separated by pulling them in opposite directions (*Figure 14*). Once made, the smear is dried in the air and stained. Dried preparations are very sensitive to humidity and should be maintained in a dry, dust-proof place free from flies. They may be mounted in balsam.

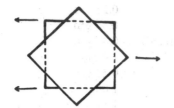

Figure 14. Use of two coverslips in preparation of a blood smear. (Hallman)

(6) STAINING SMEARS

A simple and rapid staining method which fixes the smear at the same time is that of May–Grünwald. The stain is made up of one part of acetic methylene blue, 100 parts of methyl alcohol, and 50 parts of glycerine (for Giemsa's stain see histological techniques).

STAINING TECHNIQUE

(a) the smear, well dried in the air, is put onto a staining rack, flooded with May–Grünwald, and left for 5 minutes;

(b) an equal quantity of distilled water is added, and left for a further 5 minutes;

(c) the whole is well washed with distilled water;

(d) dry well with filter paper;

(e) mount in Canada balsam.

May–Grünwald solution should be kept in a tightly closed bottle to prevent evaporation, as well as to preserve its staining powers.

Leishman's or any other Romanowsky stain may also be used for work with fish blood. In the case of Leishman's stain, the stain is added to the air dried smear and left for one minute, after which the same volume of buffered (pH 7.0) distilled water is mixed with it. The stain is allowed to act for 15 minutes, when it is washed off with distilled water and the slide dried with filter paper prior to examination.

(7) RED AND WHITE CELL COUNTS

These counts may be carried out either with fresh or with heparinized (or oxalated) blood. Special diluting pipettes are used. For the red cell count, blood is drawn up to the 0.5 mark (up to the 1.0 mark in cases of anemia). The point of the pipette is carefully wiped with a clean cloth, and Hayem's fluid drawn up to the 101 mark. Hayem's fluid has the following composition:

sodium chloride	1.0–2.0 gm.
sodium sulfate	5.0 gm.
mercuric chloride	0.5 gm.
distilled water	200 cc.

Wolf (1963) recommends the use of the Cortland salt solution, the composition of which is as follows:

sodium chloride	7.25 gm.

calcium chloride (hydrated)	0.23 gm.
potassium chloride	0.38 gm.
sodium dihydrogen phosphate (hydrated)	0.41 gm.
sodium bicarbonate	1.0 gm.
magnesium sulfate (hydrated)	0.23 gm.
glucose	1.0 gm.
distilled water	1 liter

Other workers have used similar diluting solutions such as that of Hendricks, but the Cortland formula gives reproducible results.

In cases of emergency a 1.5% sodium chloride solution may be used. The blood is diluted 1:200 in the red cell pipette.

For marine fish Conroy and Rodriguez (1965) have recommended Young's marine teleost saline, the composition of which is:

sodium chloride	13.5 gm.
potassium chloride	0.6 gm.
calcium chloride	0.25 gm.
magnesium chloride	0.35 gm.
distilled water	1 liter

A small quantity of mercuric chloride may be added to this where required so as to inhibit the growth of molds.

The white cell pipette is somewhat smaller than that used for red cell counts. Blood is drawn up to the 1.0 mark (or in cases of leucocytosis up to the 0.5 mark). The tip of the pipette is dried and then filled up to the 11 mark with Turk's fluid:

glacial acetic acid	1.0 cc.
distilled water	100 cc.

or Yokoyama's white cell fluid. The composition of this is as follows:

Solution A :	sodium chloride	4.0 gm.
	potassium chloride	200 mgm.
	dextrose	1.25 mgm.
	sodium bicarbonate	250 mgm.
	40% neutral formalin	50 cc.
	water	200 cc.
Solution B :	methyl violet	75 mgm.
	pyronin B	75 mgm.
	water	250 cc.

The water used for freshwater fish will be distilled, and that for marine fish should preferably be either sterile sea water or a saline solution isotonic with sea water (35‰). Equal quantities are added together immediately before use, and the dilution made with the blood in the pipette.

The blood undergoes a 1:9 dilution. After reaching the upper mark (101 or 11 as the case may be) the pipette is removed from the rubber sucking tube and the contents mixed for 30 seconds between the thumb and forefinger. The formation of air bubbles should be stringently avoided. Immediately after this the count proper is performed by means of a Bürker or Schilling counting chamber.

(8) Hemoglobin determination

Larsen and Snieszko (1961) and Larsen (1964) recommend the cyanmethemoglobin method for the determination of hemoglobin in trout and catfish. This actually is not the most accurate method but it has the advantages of commercially available standards for calibration, the reagent is extremely stable, and reproducibility is high. The cyanmethemoglobin method is a colorimeteric procedure. With a "Spectronic 20" instrument, 0.02 cc. whole blood is mixed with 5 cc. of the reagent (Drabkins' solution) and the transmittancy read at 540 mu. The reagent contains cyanide so caution must be used in handling this compound. Larsen and Snieszko (1961) and Larsen (1964) found the oxyhemoglobin method to be the most accurate, requiring no correction, and the acid hematin method the least accurate.

(9) Microhematocrit method determination

The microhematocrit is the volume of packed red cells as a percentage of the total sample measured in a capillary tube. The tubes are filled to 80–90% of their length, one end sealed with plasticine, and centrifuged until a constant reading is obtained. Commercial scales allow direct reading. Millimeter scales may be used and the hematocrit computed from the millimeter measurements. The capillary tubing used is usually 1 mm. inside diameter. A special centrifuge head is required.

Histology of the most important internal organs

The chapter on diagnostic methods must ideally be closed with some fundamental and basic indications as to the normal histology of fish internal organs. In this context it should be borne in mind that there is a great difference between the appearance of an ordinary preparation and that of a section of an organ which has subsequently been stained. Stained microscopical sections allow much more of the finer structure of the organ to be observed. In an ordinary preparation, or in teased material, very little can be recognized of the microscopical structure, as for example is the case with the gills and the kidney.

(1) Skin

The skin is composed of an external layer or epidermis, colorless and completely transparent when healthy, and which does not measure more than a few fractions of a millimeter in thickness (*Figure 15a*). On necrotization (for example as a result of the action of ectoparasites) it becomes opaque and falls away in pieces. Underneath the hard epidermis is found a compact dermis in which the scales are formed (*Figure 15b*), and these come to the body surface after being covered by an epidermal sheath. In the epidermis are to be found numerous mucilage cells, the mucosity of which covers the surface of the fish, increases its powers of movement, and at the same time performs a protective function. Together with the scales are to be seen pigment cells or chromatophores, which contain very small pigment granules and determine the color and the spots on the fish. For this reason we find scales and pigment cells mixed together in smears from the skin. Nerves and blood vessels traverse the dermis. Underneath the dermis is the hypodermis (*Figure 15c*). *Figure 15* shows a transverse section of an area free from scales taken from the skin of a carp. In the epidermis the clear mucilage cells are apparent, and both the dermis and the hypodermis may also be seen. A smear of the skin (*Figure 16*) has quite a different microscopical appearance: together with free scales one does not observe anything more than epidermal cells with part of their contents in the form of droplets, and in some places with occasional dispersed pigment cells.

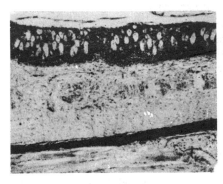

Figure 15. Transverse section through the skin of a carp, in an area free of scales. (Original)

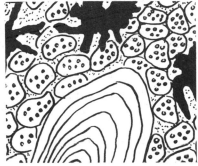

Figure 16. Diagrammatic skin smear— black pigment cells, numerous cutaneous cells, and a loose scale are seen in the figure. (Amlacher)

(2) GILLS

The gills (*Figure 17*) are characterized by the presence of gill filaments, which themselves show numerous tiny folds which serve to further increase the efficiency of the respiratory surface. The gill filaments are connected to the branchial arches. The blood arrives at the gills by an afferent vessel (afferent branchial artery or arteria branchialis) and passes to the general circulatory system by means of an efferent vessel (arteria branchialis efferens). The afferent and efferent branchial vessels break into small capillaries which are distributed throughout the respiratory folds of the gills.

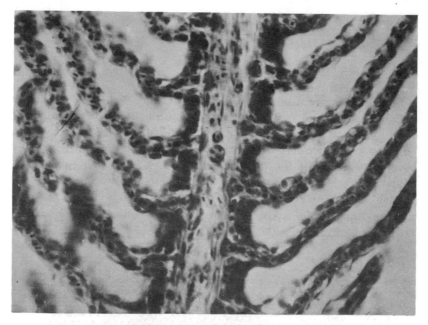

Figure 17. Section through a gill filament of a Teleost. (Amlacher)

(3) HEART

Among the internal organs, the heart is rarely studied. In teleost fishes it is situated inside the pericardium, whose parietal sheet constitutes the pericardial sac which holds the heart, while the visceral sheet or epicardium covers the external face of the same organ. The epicardium is a reticular tissue which contains collagen fibers and elastic fibers in small numbers, and is covered on the outside by a single layer of smooth cells (epicardial epithelium). Towards the interior the most important layer is continued as the myocardium, which forms the heart muscle. The myocardium, in bony fish, is formed of two layers which are clearly differentiated. The external or cortical layer is compact, and the internal one is spongy. The cortical layer is built up of a series of muscular fibers arranged longitudinally, and by a further layer on the inside made up of circular muscle fibers. The spongy layer originates from the circular fibers in the cortical zone. The interior of the heart is covered by the endocardium, which is a simple layer of plane or smooth cells on fine elastic fibers (*Figure 18*).

44

(4) BLOOD

The blood of teleost fishes has the following composition:

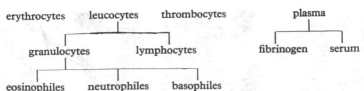

Blood smears are stained by Giemsa's or May-Grünwald's methods (see histological and hematological techniques). The blood undergoes serious changes, especially in the case of bacterial infections (see bacterial hemorrhagic septicemia), but feeding and starvation also affect its composition (changes in the total protein level, hemoglobin, number of erythrocytes). When the presence of trypanosomes is suspected, fresh heart blood smears should be obtained and mixed with 0.64% sodium chloride, using this for analysis and microscopical examination. *Figures 19* and *20* are typical blood smears.

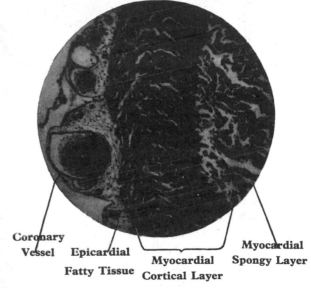

Figure 18. Transverse section through the heart wall of a carp. (Amlacher)

Coronary Vessel — Epicardial Fatty Tissue — Myocardial Cortical Layer — Myocardial Spongy Layer

(5) SPLEEN

The spleen is surrounded by a fine capsule of connective tissue, in the interior of which is found the splenic parenchyma, made up of the following elements:

(*a*) splenic pulp: this is composed of a reticular tissue proceeding from the capsule; red and white pulp is not always easily seen.

(*b*) splenic sinuses: these are cavities prolonged longitudinally and anastomosed, and full of blood (principally erythrocytes). They are smaller at the periphery, since the pulp forms a clearer network here.

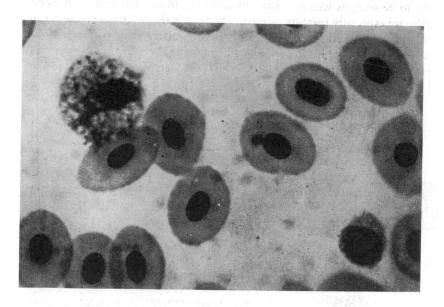

Figure 19. Blood smear from a bream (*Abramis brama* L.) To the left and above is a basophilic granulocyte, with the partially dissolved granules. To the right and below is a lymphocyte; the remaining cells are erythrocytes. (Flemming)

The spleen of teleosts is a deep red color, in practice it is almost black, and its organization is much simpler than is the case with mammals; however there are no joint anatomical and histological details available at present on its normal structure and physiology.

It is an organ which frequently becomes diseased. This is explained by its richness in blood, since numerous pathogenic organisms are spread throughout the body via the blood stream. Histological sections of the spleen do not differ greatly from those made by squash preparations or by maceration (*Figure 21*). The latter are of a clear red color and contain pale granules of a uniform size. Pathological changes have an immediate repercussion on the spleen. It is the most important organ for diagnostic purposes in the case of tropical aquarium fish, since according to previous experience it is the organ which most frequently becomes diseased.

(6) LIVER

The color of the liver is reddish to light brown. In histological sections (*Figure 22*) numerous darkish-brown colored nuclei of the hepatic cells are to be seen, as well as a few blood vessels, inside which the red blood cells are especially brightly stained. The liver is the most important organ of metabolism and for this reason it is particularly subject to metabolic diseases (for example, faulty diet). Furthermore, because the liver is well vascularized (portal circulation), many pathogenic organisms become localized there.

Figure 20. Blood smear from a bream (*Abramis brama* L.). In the top left-hand corner is an esinophilic granulocyte. In the lower right-hand corner are two thrombocytes; the remaining cells are erythrocytes. (Flemming)

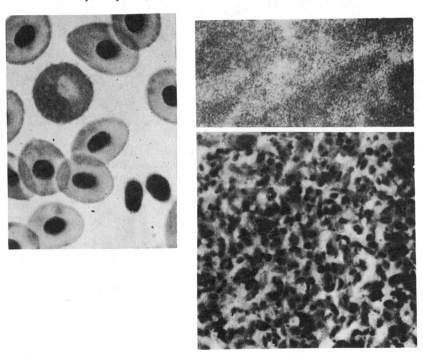

Figure 21. (a) Squash preparation of a piece of spleen from *Mollienesia velifera*; (b) Histological section of the spleen of *Cyprinus carpio*. (Amlacher)

The liver and the pancreas constitute, in carp and other cyprinids, a topographical unit in the sense that the pancreas penetrates into the liver

47

(intrahepatic pancreas, *Figure 23*) and curving and following the branches of the portal it extends throughout the whole organ. The hepatic cells, in a normal state, show well defined limits and form the hepatic strings which are surrounded by blood capillaries. In the interior of these strings of hepatic cells are found the bile caniculi. The normal intact hepatic cells always give a positive glycogen reaction (*Figure 24*). Toxic lesions, for example those of bacterial hemorrhagic septicemia, produce a rupture of the cellular membrane and disappearance of the glycogen.

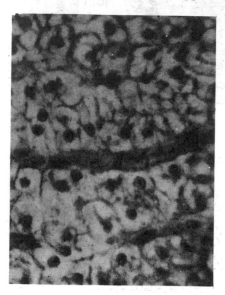

Figure 22. Section of liver of a carp; the center is crossed by a large blood vessel, and the nucleoli of the liver cell nuclei may be seen. (Amlacher)

Liver   Pancreas

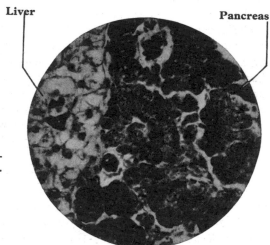

Figure 23. Intra-hepatic pancreatic tissue of the carp. (Amlacher)

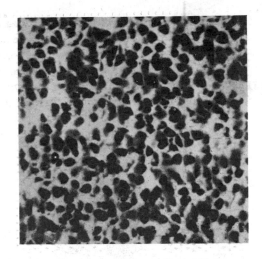

Figure 24. Liver of a carp; the glycogen appears in the form of granules and corpuscles in Bauer's glycogen reaction. (Amlacher)

The exocrine cells of the pancreas (trypsin-diastase) are cylindrical and conical. Their nuclei are situated in the basal zone, in an area of dense cytoplasm, and all of the cell is filled with large secretory granules (zymogen granules). In normal histological preparations, the abundance of secretory granules reduces transparency, the acini of the pancreatic tissue are seen to be dark and their cellular limits are not to be seen in any but the thinnest sections. In squash preparations, the liver of normally fed animals appears as a homogenous mass, of a yellowish color, and which may be crossed by ramified blood vessels. In the event of fatty degeneration, we see fat droplets with a bluish sheen with the naked eye, juxtaposed and with dark borders.

(7) KIDNEY

The kidney is composed of renal tubules and interstitial lymphoid tissue. It also has abundant blood, and its cephalic or anterior portion is the organ of hematopoiesis in bony fishes. Within it numerous pathogenic organisms become localized. The renal tubules commence in a glomerulus (Malpighi's corpuscle), inside which is a small network of blood vessels where urinary secretion takes place. The urine is conveyed to the ureter by means of the uriniferous tubules. *Figure 25* shows a histological preparation, and in this may be observed the cut renal tubules in the very midst of interstitial tissue.

According to Krause (1923) it is difficult to obtain a clear idea on the structure of the kidney based on transverse and longitudinal sections, because the interstitial lymphoid tissue which separates the renal and the uriniferous tubules respectively is extremely rich in cells (which gives rise to many nuclei in the section). The same interstitial tissue is, according to

Krause, a highly ramified stroma of anastomosed cells which cover the numerous blood capillaries. The threads of this reticulum are profusely dotted with small lymphoid cells.

In squash preparations (*Figure 26*) coiled renal tubules are seen, and some glomeruli in the midst of the interstitial tissue. This latter shows granules of a color which varies from chestnut brown to yellow, and with a hyaline sheen.

We shall examine as best we think fit the dorsal portion of the kidney, which as will have been seen above, is extracted on opening the abdominal walls of the fish body. The kidney also is very likely to become diseased.

(8) INTESTINE

The intestine is composed of a double muscular layer, of smooth fibers, and an intestinal mucosa (*Figure 27*) with folds or small crypts to increase the total surface area. Under the mucosa follows a submucosa of elastic connective tissue which is highly vascularized. In the muscular layer a ringed internal layer and an external longitudinal one are seen. The serosa, highly vascularized, is a fibro-elastic layer which serves to isolate the intestine from the peritoneal cavity (*Figure 28*). In squash preparations a mark formed by the crypts (intestinal relief) is to be seen, and this differs in every species.

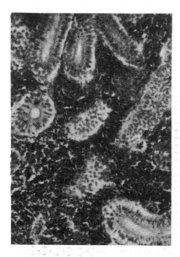

Figure 25. Section through the kidney of a carp. (Amlacher)

When faced with a possible *Octomitus* infection (for example in Angel fish and rainbow trout) it is very important to analyze the rectal contents, since many of these particular flagellates live there.

The brain, genitals and the swim bladder are less frequently subjected to disease, in accordance with the experience which has been gained up to now, and for this reason we shall not consider them further here, in spite

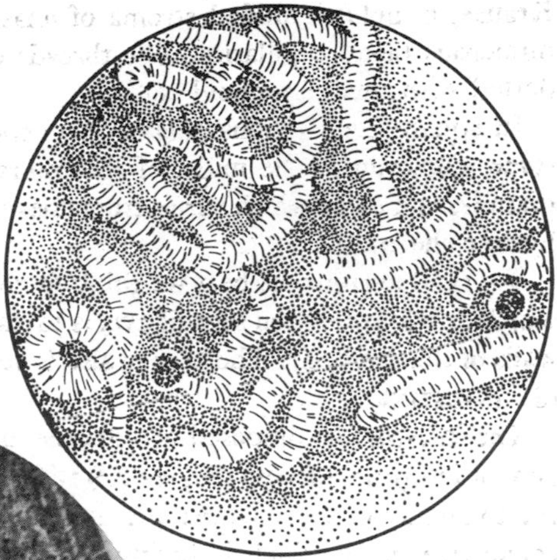

Figure 26. Teased preparation (diagrammatic) of a Teleost kidney. (Original)

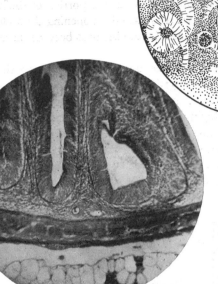

Figure 27. Transverse section of a teleost intestine. (Amlacher)

Figure 28. Transverse section through the intestine of a two-year-old carp, showing the entry into the serosa of two veins of the intestinal musculature, and the peritoneal cavity. The veins are enveloped by pancreatic tissue almost immediately on leaving the intestine. (Amlacher)

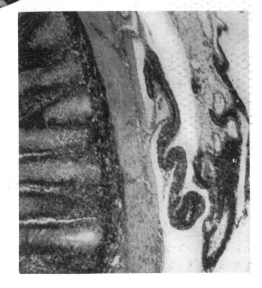

51

of the fact that from the point of view of breeding degeneration of the ovaries, retention of the sperm etc. are of great importance. This will all receive consideration in a special section.

The brain, the color of which is white, is easily macerated and the result of this, on microscopical examination, gives the appearance of an homogenous mass in which fine branches, the cerebral blood capillaries, are from time to time visible.

When the presence of *Octomitus* is suspected, the bile freed on removal of the gall bladder is also analyzed, because this nearly always contains numerous flagellates of the aforementioned genus.

Step by step guide to a post-mortem examination of a fish

(1) External examination: study of the reflex responses;

(2) preparation of smears from the skin and the gills;

(3) for bacteriological examination make a ventral and a lateral incision with sterile scissors (fix the fish firmly onto a wooden board). Whenever the presence of an infectious disease is suspected, make cultures onto agar of all of the internal organs. If it is thought that any fastidious bacteria may be present, culture also into peptone water. To investigate a case of bacterial hemorrhagic septicemia, culture onto sucrose-fuchsin-agar, especially when the presence of many species of bacteria associated with *Aeromonas liquefaciens* is feared (for example, in the case of the intestine);

(4) after having made a bacteriological study, the autopsy proper is begun following an opercular and a cranial incision respectively. If no further cultures are made the final post-mortem examination is started. Teased and squash preparations are made and studied with the microscope. Suspected pathological material is fixed in formalin Bouin's or Stieve's fluid. For histochemical studies the material should be fixed in alcohol-formalin (2 parts of alcohol to 1 part of formalin);

(5) for hematological analysis, follow the direction given in the appropriate section above.

Chapter 2

DIAGNOSIS

General considerations

In the foregoing chapter consideration has been given to the techniques used in fish pathology and research; however once again we must emphasize that any detailed investigation involving the preparation of slides, smears and sections, must first of all be preceded by a close external examination which includes a study of the internal organs of the fish as well as the external appearance on autopsy. To perform this, attention is paid to the natural openings and to the skin, in order to detect the presence of areas of trauma, ulcers, abcesses, loss of color and parasites. The mouth, head and opercula may show deformities or moldy places, and the nasal orifices may also be affected by fungi. A mycosis, a turbidity of the eyes, exophthalmos or a sunken appearance of the eyeballs (see techniques of exploration) are important criteria for certain types of diagnosis. It is important to observe whether the gills are pale in color or whether they are swollen and necrotized. The musculature may be softened in certain places, and the anus may be red, inflamed and prolapsed.

Fraying, inflammation and breaking up of the fins also provides important data for diagnosis, as does the presence of a yellowish colored inflammation of the liver; the occurrence of white nodules in the gills, skin, internal organs, a yellowish colored intestinal fluid etc. In order to complete these data, any information on the previous behavior of the fish prior to death should be included. The anamnesis is always of great importance in the establishment of a correct diagnosis. The pathologist should always be fully acquainted with details as to the source or origin of the animals (fish hatchery, sea, fresh water, marine or freshwater aquarium etc.). He must also be told of the prevailing water conditions, the number of fish lost, and the general development of the infection. *Table 1* gives a useful orientation which aids diagnosis. In the left hand column is indicated the appearance and general behavior of the fish; in the center the possible diseases from which the animal may be suffering; and at the right the appropriate treatment to be applied. I have already said that this Table cannot be treated as a "philosophers' stone", but only as an auxiliary tool to supplement a detailed microscopical study of the skin, gills, and internal organs.

Table 1. DIAGNOSIS OF FISH DISEASES

SYMPTOMS AND BEHAVIOR OF THE FISH	DIAGNOSIS		PROPHYLAXIS AND TREATMENT (see also TABLE 2)
1. Skeleton and body form			
deformities in the longitudinal axis of the body	(a)	deformities of the vertebral column (may be hereditary)	no suitable treatment known
	(b)	whirling disease	no suitable treatment known; the tanks must be disinfected
	(c)	piscine tuberculosis	no suitable treatment known
	(d)	bacterial hemorrhagic septicemia	no suitable treatment known
	(e)	vitamin deficiencies (rickets)	no suitable treatment known
softness and extreme flexibility of the vertebral column	(a)	pox disease	3 intra-peritoneal injections of 1 cc. of a 1% aqueous solution of Arycil and, afterwards of a 5% solution
deformities of the upper and lower jaws	(a)	whirling disease	no suitable treatment known; the tanks must be disinfected
blockage of mouth	(a)	hypertrophy of the thyroid glands	bath in potassium iodide
	(b)	whirling disease	no suitable treatment known; the tanks must be disinfected
fraying of the fins	(a)	bacterial fin rot	Aquarol, sulfadiazine, chloramphenicol acriflavine, Aquarol, malachite green
	(b)	costiasis	
	(c)	alkalosis	lower the pH
red coloration of food fish due to cutaneous hemorrhages; in aquarium fish sudden raising of the scales and fins; swimming around in circles; shimmers; death in a normal position, between plants	(a)	acidosis	raise the pH

54

Signs	Diagnosis	Treatment
marked reduction of the fins until they are reduced to a stump	(a) bacterial fin rot	Aquarol, sulfadiazine, chloramphenicol
destruction of the fins	(a) trauma (b) ectoparasites (c) bacterial fin rot (especially the caudal fin) in aquarium fish	mercurochrome, iodated alcohol Acriflavine, Aquarol, sodium chloride, malachite green Aquarol, sulfadiazine, chloramphenicol
retracted fins; restricted swimming movements	(a) costiasis (b) *Ichthyophthirius*	Acriflavine, Aquarol, malachite green (prolonged bath), sodium chloride solution (1% as a short bath) Aquarol. In fish farms place in spacious tanks. In trout hatcheries, use malachite green (except in those fish destined as human food), formalin
swollen belly	(a) bacterial hemorrhagic septicemia (b) tumefaction of the internal organs of aquarium fish following feeding with bloodworms	chloramphenicol, oxytetracycline, streptomycin change the feeding schedule
emaciation	(a) piscine tuberculosis (b) *Octomitus* (c) ascarids	no suitable treatment known carbarsone parachlorometaxilenol
raised scales	(a) bacterial hemorrhagic septicemia (b) tumefaction of the internal organs following feeding with bloodworms	chloramphenicol, oxytetracycline, streptomycin change the feeding schedule

SYMPTOMS AND BEHAVIOR OF THE FISH	DIAGNOSIS	PROPHYLAXIS AND TREATMENT (see also Table 2)
red tumefaction, punctiform, in the floor of the mouth; occasionally the operculum may be spotted	(a) thyroid tumor (b) cancer of the thyroids	bath in potassium iodide; iodine in diet not curable
exophthalmos	(a) piscine tuberculosis	no suitable treatment known
sunken eyes	(a) bacterial hemorrhagic septicemia (b) *Trypanoplasma* (*Cryptobia*) (c) hunger	chloromycetin, oxytetracycline, streptomycin destroy the leeches
reddened anus, escape of a yellow mucoid intestinal content	(a) enteritis (b) *Eimeria* in the intestinal mucosa	according to etiology no suitable therapy known

2. Skin

SYMPTOMS AND BEHAVIOR OF THE FISH	DIAGNOSIS	PROPHYLAXIS AND TREATMENT
bluish-white turbidity of the epidermis	(a) infection by *Costia, Chilodonella, Trichodina* or *Gyrodactylus* (b) alkalosis	Acriflavine, Aquarol; malachite green against *Gyrodactylus*; methylene blue or short baths in a solution of formalin or sodium chloride reduce the pH
cotton wool-like formations	(a) mycosis (*Saprolegnia*); also in *a frigore* lesions (particularly in the nares)	Aquarol, potassium permanganate, collargol, sodium chloride
rounded and reddened areas on the skin	(a) bites of carp lice (b) bites of leeches	see the corresponding chapter see the corresponding chapter
gelatinous infiltrations in the skin, milky turbidity and pox-like	(a) carp pox	3 intra-peritoneal injections of 1 cc. of a 1% solution of Acyil, following these by a 5% solution

white spots, the size of a sand grain and up to 1 mm. in diameter	(a) *Ichthyophthirius*	Acriflavine, Aquarol, malachite green, formalin
	(b) invasion by green algae (favored by a rise in the pH)	no suitable treatment known
whitish-grey to dirty yellow colored nodules on the skin and fins; the skin falls away in strips; visible with a magnifying glass	(a) *Oodinium*. In freshwater fish, *O. pillularis*. Coral fish disease (*O. ocellatum*)	bath in chlortetracycline or in copper sulphate
pearl or strawberry-like skin proliferations	(a) lymphocystis	in aquarium fish, isolate the diseased ones at once and keep them under observation for at least 2–4 months. In sea-fish, never throw diseased ones back into the sea
desquamation	(a) piscine tuberculosis	see this
red, pink or black growths	(a) tumors	no suitable treatment known; goiter may be treated by a bath in potassium iodide
cauliflower-like papillomas, especially in the mouth region	(a) cauliflower disease	no suitable treatment known
sand-paper effect on the skin	(a) *Ichthyosporidium* (particularly in the herring	see the corresponding chapter
ulcers, spots or ulcerous areas on the skin, scales raised	(a) *Ichthyosporidium*	no suitable treatment known
	(b) bacterial hemorrhagic septicemia	chloramphenicol, oxytetracycline, streptomycin
	(c) furunculosis	chloramphenicol, oxyletracycline, sulfas
	(d) eel pest	see the corresponding chapter
	(e) ulcer disease	chloramphenicol, oxytetracycline
	(f) exanthemic plague	see the corresponding chapter
	(g) kidney disease	erthromycin, sulfas

SYMPTOMS AND BEHAVIOR OF THE FISH	DIAGNOSIS	PROPHYLAXIS AND TREATMENT (see also Table 2)
hemorrhagic points and marks	(a) cercarial infestation (furcocercariae of the Trematodes); aquatic snails are the vectors	destroy the snails
	(b) too acid water	raise the pH
punctiform black spots in the dermis	(a) metacercarial infestation	no suitable treatment known
loss of color of the pigment band in neon tetras (not a certain symptom)	(a) Plistophora	no suitable treatment known
bubbles of air underneath the skin	(a) gas bubble disease	no suitable treatment known
reddening	(a) bacterial hemorrhagic septicemia	chloramphenicol, oxytetracycline, streptomycin
	(b) red pest	see the corresponding chapter
	(c) eel pest	see the corresponding chapter
	(d) acidosis	raise the pH
black coloration	(a) intestinal disturbances	according to the etiology
	(b) whirling disease (if the caudal region is black)	see the corresponding chapter
	(c) melanosis	no suitable treatment known
external welts, tiny unbroken pimples	(a) kidney disease	erythromycin, sulfa drugs
3. Gills		
bluish-white turbidity	(a) infestation by Costia, Chilodonella, Trichodina, Dactylogyrus	acriflavine, Aquarol, malachite green (prolonged bath), short bath in sodium chloride
necrosis and discoloration, especially at the extremes of the gill lamella; discoloration of the gills	(a) alkalosis	reduce the pH
	(b) acidosis	raise the pH
	(c) injuries produced by free chlorine	sodium thiosulfate
	(d) columnaris	sulfas, oxytetracycline

58

gasping at the water surface	(a) lack of oxygen	in tanks, increase the entry of water; in aquaria, increase the aeration and renew the water
spotted discoloration	(a) *Ichthyophthirius*	in aquaria, acriflavine, Aquarol; in fish farms, place the fish in large tanks; in trout hatcheries, malachite green formalin
pale coloration, anemia	(a) the result of many diseases, or as a symptom of disease	according to the diagnosis
white pearl-like nodules (spherical or elongated)	(a) sporozoans	no suitable treatment known
small oval white spots on the gill filaments, which in summer have two small ovaries	(a) parasitic copepods (usually *Ergasilus sieboldii*)	no suitable treatment known
in smears: small worms of up to 1 mm. long	(a) *Dactylogyrus*	in aquaria, long bath with acriflavine; in fish farms, short bath with formalin or sodium chloride
open opercula in young fish and in aquarium fish	(a) suspect the presence of *Dactylogyrus*	in aquaria, long bath with acriflavine; in fish farms, short bath with formalin or sodium chloride
anemia, clear patches. In smears are found eggs with a black mark	(a) eggs of *Sanguinicola*	destroy all aquatic snails
dark and clear coloration, necrosis and destruction of the gill filaments	(a) suspect gill disease	see the corresponding chapter

4. Muscles

ulcerations	(a) *Ichthyosporidium*	no suitable treatment known
	(b) piscine tuberculosis	no suitable treatment known

SYMPTOMS AND BEHAVIOR OF THE FISH	DIAGNOSIS	PROPHYLAXIS AND TREATMENT (see also Table 2)
	(c) bacterial hemorrhagic septicemia	chloramphenicol, oxytetracycline, strepto-mycin
	(d) furunculosis	sulfas, chloramphenicol, oxytetracycline
	(e) vibrio disease of eels	no suitable treatment known
	(f) ulcer disease	chloramphenicol, oxytetracycline
	(g) coldwater disease	sulfa drugs
spotted discoloration	(a) *Plistophora*	no suitable treatment known
swellings with microscopical spores	(a) bubonic plague of fishes	no suitable treatment known
coiled worms detected microscopically	(a) Nematodes	no suitable treatment known
5. Internal organs and visceral cavity variable nodules in liver	(a) hepatoma	no suitable treatment known
whitish nodules in the liver, ovary, spleen, heart and brain. Sand-paper effect on the surface of the heart	(a) *Ichthyosporidium*	no suitable treatment known
white nodules in the liver and heart; nodules in the internal organs	(a) sporozoans	no suitable treatment known
	(b) piscine tuberculosis	no suitable treatment known
liver green colored	(a) biliary stasis	no suitable treatment known
brownish or yellowish coloration of the liver	(a) bacterial hemorrhagic septicemia	see the corresponding chapter
cysts in the liver	(a) cysticerci of *Triaenophorus*	no suitable treatment known
microscopically many small motile parasites are seen in the bile and the rectal contents; the fish frequently show abnormal swimming movements	(a) *Octomitus*; see if *Pterophyllum scalare, Cichlasoma severum* and *Symphysodon discus* are present in the aquarium	carbarsone

60

encysted helminth eggs in the kidney	(a) *Sanguinicola*	destroy all the snails
necrotized tubules detected microscopically in the kidney	(a) VHS; piscine tuberculosis; pike pest	see the corresponding chapters
loss of pigment in the kidney in salmonids	(a) VHS	see the corresponding chapter
extremely motile parasites, about the size of the red blood cells, detected microscopically in the kidney	(a) *Trypanoplasma, Cryptobia*	see the corresponding chapter
inflammation of the swim bladder	(a) bacterial hemorrhagic septicermia	chloramphenicol, oxtyetracycline, streptomycin
	(b) VHS	see the corresponding chapter
concentric layers of growths in the ovary, liver and kidney	(a) *Glugea anomala*	no suitable treatment known
small microscopic worms in the bulbus of the heart	(a) *Sanguinicola*	destroy all snails
white nodules in the heart	(a) encysted worms	see the corresponding chapter
	(b) *Ichthyosporidium*	see the corresponding chapter
appearance of yellowish feces	(a) intestinal coccidiosis (*Eimeria*)	see the corresponding chapter
nodules in the intestine	(a) nodular coccidiosis	see the corresponding chapter
reddening of the rectum, flaccid and transparent intestine	(a) enteritis	according to the etiology
liquid intestinal contents	(a) bacterial hemorrhagic septicemia	chloramphenicol, oxytetracycline, streptomycin
	(b) *Octomitus*	carbarsone

SYMPTOMS AND BEHAVIOR OF THE FISH	DIAGNOSIS	PROPHYLAXIS AND TREATMENT (see also TABLE 2)
visceral cavity filled with fluid	(a) bacterial hemorrhagic septicemia	chloramphenicol, oxytetracycline, streptomycin
	(b) tuberculosis	no suitable treatment known
	(c) kidney disease	see the corresponding chapter
	(d) VHS	see the corresponding chapter
white worms in the visceral cavity	(a) ligulosis or schistocephalosis	see the corresponding chapter
kidney swollen, liver appears pale, internal organs and peritoneal cavity are hemorrhagic. Intact lesions filled with pus	(a) kidney disease	see there
	(b) bacterial hemorrhagic septicemia	see there
6. Blood anemia	(a) blood parasites	see the corresponding chapter
	(b) gill parasites	see the corresponding chapter
	(c) intestinal coccidiosis	see the corresponding chapter
	(d) bacterial hemorrhagic septicemia	see the corresponding chapter
in blood smears, parasites the size of red blood cells, very motile	(a) *Trypanoplasma, Cryptobia*	destroy all leeches
7. Nervous system nodules in the brain and spinal cord, abnormal position of the body, zigzag movements in swimming	(a) *Ichthyosporidium*	no suitable treatment known
extremely motile flagellates in the cerebro-spinal fluid	(a) *Trypanoplasma, Cryptobia*	destroy all leeches
parasites in the blood capillaries of the brain	(a) *Myxosoma*	no suitable treatment known
	(b) *Myxobolus neurobius*	no suitable treatment known

Symptom	Diagnosis	Treatment
the fish are in a head-downwards position	(a) brain infections	according to the etiology
spasms and convulsions	(a) intoxications	according to the toxin
	(b) *Octomitus*	carbarsone
	(c) whirling disease	no suitable treatment known

8. Eyes

Symptom	Diagnosis	Treatment
exophthalmos	(a) kidney disease	erythromycin
	(b) piscine tuberculosis	see the corresponding chapter
	(c) *Ichthyosporidium*	see the corresponding chapter
	(d) infestation by *Diplostomum volvens*	see the corresponding chapter
opacity of the cornea and lens	(a) tuberculosis	see the corresponding chapter
	(b) infestation by *Diplostomum volvens*	see the corresponding chapter

9. Alevins and young fish

Symptom	Diagnosis	Treatment
vitelline sac swollen like a bladder	(a) ascites of the vitelline sac	see the corresponding chapter
open opercula; red tumor in the throat	(b) goiter or cancer of the thyroid	treat the goiter with potassium iodide solution

10. Eggs

Symptom	Diagnosis	Treatment
turbidity of the egg	(a) unfertilized egg	remove
	(b) egg damaged by factors in the environment	remove
radial threads in the egg surface	(a) mycosis produced by *Saprolegnia*	remove the eggs and treat the water

It is not always easy to decide whether a fish is ill or not. There are fish which appear to be perfectly healthy yet are nevertheless candidates for diseases such as tuberculosis and ichthyosporidiosis. Others are carriers of disease germs which themselves do not show any symptoms of disease (i.e., carriers of bacteria and parasites). Sudden mass mortalities may also occur due to a worsening of the quality of the water, for example in cases of intoxication or a complete disappearance of dissolved oxygen.

The foregoing serves to indicate that disease and death in fish may be due to one or another of the following chief causes: parasites, bacteria, chemical and physical factors, metabolic disorders, genetic factors etc.

In cases of a sudden worsening of the condition of the water, the greater part of the fish die all at once, and within a very short period. If, on the other hand, such a condition is of slow development, or parasites and bacteria are involved, the mortalities are more isolated. Certain diseases such as bacterial hemorrhagic septicemia may give rise to mass mortalities. The avoidance of all temperature changes is the basis of large scale fish culture and aquarism. If this last factor is not taken into account, then the fish will die as a result of thermal shock. Such shock may be brought about by sudden chilling, and the fish die as it were with a snap of the fingers.

Annotation of the facts

As much as in the case of field studies as in that of laboratory investigations, it is of prime importance to have a methodology. Well written and suitably filed, such details may allow valuable conclusions to be drawn by analogy in the future. The formation of a methodical filing system may vary according to individual requirements and the wishes of the fish pathologist. The following is an example which may serve as a model:

locality: file number:
proprietor: date:
fish species:
anamnesis:

1. EXTERNAL LESIONS

deformities   protrusion of the anus
scars   swollen belly
visible ulcers   boils
exophthalmos   ectoparasites
sunken eyes   sporozoan swellings

2. INTERNAL LESIONS

number	gills	visceral cavity	liver	intestine	spleen	kidney	heart
1							
2							
3							
4							

cultures:	yes/no (organ):	number:
fixation:	yes/no (organ):	number:
blood smears:	yes/no (organ):	number:
hemoglobin determination: 1	gm./100 ml.	
2	gm./100 ml.	
3	gm./100 ml.	
4	gm./100 ml.	

evaluation of the analytical results (using those of any water analysis):
diagnosis:

Chapter 3

PROPHYLAXIS, HYGIENE AND THERAPY

Prophylaxis

(1) FISHERIES PROPHYLAXIS

In fish farming one of the most important preventive measures is to obtain a suitable source of clean water for all the different necessities of the fish. As will have been seen from the diagnostic table given above, apart from those diseases caused by bacteria and parasites, there are others such as acidosis and alkalosis attributable to water deficiencies. In hatcheries supplied with an acid water, every attempt must be made to keep the pH at approximately neutral (pH 6.5–7.0) by means of a continual or at least a periodical calcification. Lack of oxygen may be the cause of catastrophic mortalities among fish. In trout breeding, special attention must be paid to an adequate oxygenation of the water. Food and population density are also other important factors to be taken into consideration. Recent observations have shown for example, that the food given to trout is frequently insufficient and lacking in vitamins; this is one of the factors which paves the way for infectious nephritis or fatty degeneration of the liver in rainbow trout. The salt concentration in trout foods (for example in fish meal) should never exceed 2%. In carp farming, attention must be paid to increasing the resistance of the fish during hibernation. Apart from facilitating spacious tanks during the winter period, it is important to prolong as much as possible the feeding period. In spring the fish must be fed, or at least encouraged to feed, as soon as is possible and should never be allowed to suffer from any lack or deficiency of natural foods in their new tanks. It is indispensable that the ·natural resistance of cultivated carp be raised by biological means, with the object of reducing losses due to bacterial hemorrhagic septicemia to an absolute minimum. With the same prime object in mind, it is necessary to administer medication (initiated by Schäperclaus) with due attention to the law of epidemiobiological equilibrium formulated by Schäperclaus in 1937. This law states basically:

For example, in the case of bacterial hemorrhagic septicemia the fish develops a specific immunity against the pathological agent; the carp becomes accustomed to it, and an epidemio-biological equilibrium is thereby established. In the case of carp from other regions being suddenly introduced, they bring in bacteria to which they have themselves become immune, but they are not immune to the bacteria already present in the water any more than the carp already living in this water are immune to the new types of bacteria introduced with the new carp. Carp A has become accustomed to bacterium "a"; carp B to bacterium "b". If we place them together bacterium "b" infects carp A, and bacterium "a" likewise infects carp B. The epidemio-biological equilibrium is thus broken and an epizootic results (*Figure 29*).

Sufficient attention can never be paid to the maintenance of this equilibrium. The periodical careful ensuring that adequate draining and disinfection of tanks and raceways is carried out are not merely hygienic measures but also indispensable prophylactic ones as well.

Another of the final objects of prophylaxis is that of preventing infection due to parasites and similar biological factors which give rise to disease problems in cultivated waters. Certain intermediate hosts of such parasites must be systematically eradicated, including, for example, leeches (vectors of trypanosomiasis) and snails (intermediate hosts of trematodes such as *Sanguinicola* sp. and *Diplostomum volvens*). With reference to all of this, it is also important to destroy certain forage fish such as sticklebacks, gudgeons, roach, rudd, catfish, perch etc. which frequently carry numerous trematodes and other skin parasites in large numbers, and which may also infect the water with organisms producing gill rot and bacterial hemorrhagic septicemia. Leeches and fish lice have been shown to carry bacteria of the genus *Aeromonas* which are fish pathogens. These types of fish may be removed by draining and disinfecting the ponds, and placing fine mesh at the point where the water enters to prevent their re-entry into the system. In trout hatcheries one of the gravest dangers is that of the entry of fish suffering from whirling disease, furunculosis or viral infections; for this reason the production of one's own stock is always to be preferred as the best preventive measure available.

The bottom of the tank may easily become converted into the focal point for infection by parasites. *Aeromonas liquefaciens* and certain sporozoans such as *Eimeria* and *Myxosoma* are all to be found in the bottom mud of the ponds or tanks. Fish leeches and *Dactylogyrus* deposit their resistant eggs in the mud. Disinfection is carried out by means of quicklime or calcium cyanamide, at a level of 1000–2500 kg./hectare of carp tank (or in trout hatcheries should whirling disease break out), and 1 kgm. of calcium cyanamide/square meter of the bottom of the tank.

(2) PROPHYLAXIS IN THE BREEDING OF AQUARIUM FISH

The suggestions made for fish hatcheries are in most respects also valid

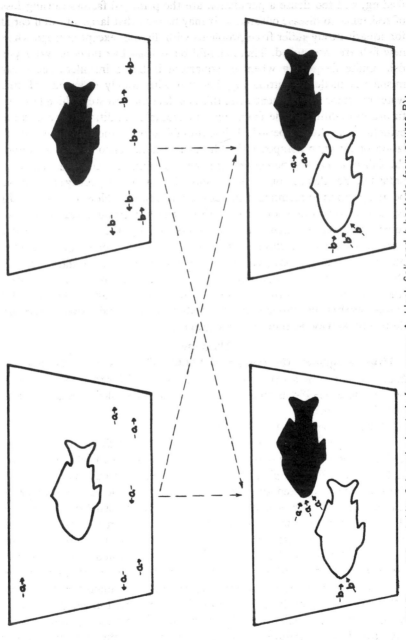

Figure 29. Repopulation (white fish and a bacteria from source A, black fish and b bacteria from source B): Failure to observe the rule of epidemio-biological equilibrium by mixing fish from two sources. (Littrell after Amlacher)

for aquarium tanks. Experience shows that water in bad condition, bad feeding, and too dense a population are the principal factors causing loss of resistance to disease outbreaks. It may be seen that large and well cared for aquaria rarely suffer from problems with disease, except perhaps when new fish are introduced. There should be at least five liters of water per fish. Quite frequently when an aquarium is being installed, the great mistake is made of putting together fish with widely differing pH and water hardness requirements, and this is in fact the first step which leads to future mortalities. Aside from this, unfavorable conditions may become evident after a longer period of time (modification of the pH and accumulation of nitrogen compounds). These slow modifications may debilitate the fish in a scarcely perceptible manner and diminish their resistance to parasites. For this reason the water should be frequently analyzed so as to be in a position to maintain it in optimum conditions. New arrivals should be kept in quarantine for at least three weeks. Certain diseases such as tuberculosis seldom manifest their presence during the quarantine period because they have a chronic and slow course, only becoming apparent under special conditions (see the corresponding section). Sanitary controls should be carried out at frequent intervals, particularly in large aquaria, since controls such as these are of real practical value and utility. By this means diseased individuals can be spotted in time, and either treated or destroyed as may be thought most fitting.

Hygiene

Hygiene signifies the science of health. There is no such thing as fisheries hygiene as a strict scientific discipline, and for this reason it must be considered herein as an absence of epizootics coupled with a complete overall cleanliness.

(1) HYGIENE AND FISH FARMING

In fish farming, it is hygiene of the hatchery which counts above all, and this means that the tanks or ponds must be most carefully maintained and cared for. Aquatic plants and tree trunks must be cut, the water conduits kept clear, cleaned, dried out and disinfected. The fight against snails and leeches and lice is a very important aspect of fisheries hygiene. It should be realized, from the very beginning, that in uncared for fish tanks snails, leeches and fish are, as it were, in their own house. Fisheries hygiene requires that the entry of wild fish be prevented, contributing in this fashion to the maintenance of the natural biological equilibrium. In trout farming, such infections as whirling disease, furunculosis, VHS and IPN must be rigorously and studiously avoided. When infectious diseases do occur (for example bacterial hemorrhagic septicemia), hygiene requires that dead fish be carefully removed and buried, and the tanks disinfected (see prophylaxis).

All hatchery utensils such as nets, buckets, waders etc. must be disinfected, as for example in cases of ichthyophthiriasis, in order to destroy any parasites adhering to them. Immersion in a concentrated solution of sodium chloride (common salt) or potassium permanganate is sufficient to accomplish this.

(2) HYGIENE AND THE REARING OF AQUARIUM FISH

In those establishments dedicated to the rearing and breeding of aquarium fish, hygiene is of even greater importance than is the case with fish farming. There are most disturbing indications at the present time that as a result of a general lack of attention to the basic principles of hygiene some branches of this business are being seriously threatened. This is the case for example in the breeding of neon tetras, which is in grave danger owing to the rapid propagation of plistophorosis, and indeed almost all export orders are being returned for this very same reason. In the official wholesale business, much stricter measures must be taken to ensure that the hygienic conditions are adequate and effective. All aerator tubes, diffusors and filters must be painstakingly disinfected with concentrated potassium permanganate solution or with trypaflavine. The bottom of the aquarium tanks should preferably be flamed with alcohol prior to use. In ornamental aquaria the number of aquatic plants should be reduced to the minimum absolutely necessary. Whenever sanitary inspection reveals the presence of diseased animals, according to the nature of the particular infections, the fish must be immediately placed into quarantine or destroyed. In official fish breeding centers, the authorities must without hesitation put into practice frequent sanitary controls so as to ensure the health of their stock.

Therapy

The cure of certain fish diseases is therapeutically possible; however therapy in general, as much in aquarium fish rearing as in fish farming, is of secondary importance to prophylaxis and hygiene. The same may be said for the breeding of tropical fish, although in this particular case the treatment of protozoan skin diseases is somewhat easier than in large scale hatchery operations. Therapy does not necessarily mean the treatment of isolated cases but rather of a whole population, either in a tank or in an aquarium. The secret of successful therapy is to discover the existence of the disease in time. A limited number of suspect fish are studied, and these specimens selected at random so as to give a good idea of the general state of health of the entire population. No other way exists in fish pathology, contrary to what is the case with human and veterinary medicine.

(1) THERAPY AND FISH FARMING

Of all those diseases which respond to treatment, parasitic infestations of the skin and gills figure first. Among those produced by protozoans are the diseases caused by *Ichthyophthirius*, *Chilodonella*, *Trichodina* and *Costia*; among the worm diseases are those produced by *Dactylogyrus*, *Gyrodactylus* and leeches; and of the crustacean diseases the most important are those brought about by carp lice and the like. Of all the many bacterial fish diseases, bacterial hemorrhagic septicemia is one which may be both avoided and treated successfully, thanks mainly to the researches of Schäperclaus. Certain gill and skin parasites such as *Ichthyophthirius* are combatted by purely biological means. Parasitic crustaceans such as *Ergasilus* and *Lernaea* (with the exception of the carp louse) may generally be combatted by good hygiene and by prophylaxis. The fight against skin and gill parasites consists of short baths or total immersion of the fish in chemical solutions. Infectious bacterial diseases such as dropsy are treated by means of intra-peritoneal injections of antibiotics and by curative baths. The different types of bath, together with details of their preparation and length of duration, are given in *Table 2*.

(2) THERAPY AND THE REARING AND BREEDING OF AQUARIUM FISH

Diseases caused by ecological factors can be eliminated by eliminating the cause (incorrect feeding, bad water etc.). Bacterial and parasitic diseases must be treated with drugs, as in the case of fish farming practice. Unfortunately fully effective drug preparations are not universally available as yet for the treatment of the most dangerous disease of all, fish tuberculosis; for this reason above all great emphasis must be placed on careful hygiene. For goiter and skin parasites, suitable medications are known. In the majority of cases, the treatment of aquarium fish diseases is accomplished by means of a bath, especially in the case of parasitic infestations of the skin and the gills. When long baths are called for, the tank itself is well disinfected with malachite green or trypaflavine. Long term baths are to be preferred to short ones. On the whole, because they are more effective in the removal of parasites the long term baths are to be preferred. Short term baths last only a few minutes, but are stressing to the fish. As soon as these are seen to be acting in an abnormal fashion, they should be removed.

An increase in the temperature of the water, for 5–7 days, has given good results in the case of many types of skin parasites. The temperature may be increased up to 31° C., but always ensuring at the same time that there is a strong and effective aeration of the tank. This treatment kills *Costia*, but other parasites such as *Chilodonella* are only partially destroyed. *Ichthyophthirius* is obliged to detach itself more quickly from the body of the fish. Stolk recommends that the water be heated to 33° C. for 6 hours, and then cooled to 21° C. overnight (repeating this procedure 3–4 times in

71

succession). This technique has given very good results in the treatment of ichthyophthiriasis.

Having detailed the different diseases, the appropriate data regarding their treatment have been subsequently given in *Table 2*. The treatments are given in synopsis and in alphabetical order, giving the composition and dosage of the medication in the left hand column, the duration of treatment in the center one, and the disease (or diseases) against which each is effective in the right hand column.

(3) TECHNIQUES OF CURATIVE BATHS

Wherever possible no therapeutic bath should be given in other than wooden or plastic containers, so as to eliminate any possibility of there being a reaction between the chemical components of the bath and the container itself. In aquarium practice glass containers are used for the same reason. The temperature of the bath should preferably be some 2° C. higher than that of the pond or aquarium (test this with a thermometer). Immersion baths for large numbers of fish are carried out with strong solutions and for an extremely short period of time. Following the bath (with lysol and priasol 5–15 seconds; potassium permanganate 30–45 seconds) the fish are carefully washed several times in a second bath containing clean water. In this way the fish are freed of leeches and lice. Any parasites which remain in the vessels are taken far away from the hatchery and killed with quicklime.

(4) TECHNIQUE OF MASS INJECTION

Preventive mass injections, utilized in the fight against disease, have had very ready acceptance in fish farming practice. Essentially mass injections are those which are carried out in spring to prevent dropsy in carp farming establishments. They are the result of many years of methodical research by Prof. Schäperclaus and members of the Department of Fish Pathology under his capable direction. At the present time they are also carried out in many other countries, a sure proof of their effectiveness. The instructions which follow below are taken from an explanatory pamphlet edited in Prof. Schäperclaus's Department. In the case of mass injections for the prevention of bacterial hemorrhagic septicemia, a solution of chloramphenicol (chloromycetin, Parke-Davis) is used. This solution is prepared in such a way that 3 mgm. of antibiotic which the fish receives are dissolved in 1 cc. of water.

(*a*) Stock solution: 600 mgm. chloramphenicol is dissolved in 10 cc. butylene glycol.

Table 2

DRUG	ADMINISTRATION	DIAGNOSIS
Acriflavine (trypaflavine) 1 gm./100 liters of water	long duration bath	skin parasites
Aquarol: 2 gm. in 25 liters of water	long duration bath; repeat every 3 days. This should be repeated on 3 occasions	*Ichthyophthirius, Costia, Saprolegnia, Chilodonella*, bacterial fin rot
Iodated alcohol: 10% solution	with an artist's paint brush	skin wounds
Arycil (arsenical preparation with a 36.4% arsenic content)	intra-peritoneal injection of 1 cc. of a 1% solution, and then of a 5% solution, three times	carp pox
Atebrine: 1 gm. in 100 liters of water	long duration bath	skin parasites
Aureomycin (chlortetracycline): 13 mgm./liter of water	long duration bath	*Ichthyophthirius*, bacteria, *Oodinium*
Methylene blue-B: 3 cc. of a 1% solution in 10 liters of water	long duration bath	*Chilodonella, Costia, Gyrodactylus*
Quicklime	disinfection: 10–15 Qm./Ha.	against snails and fish leeches. Disinfection of tanks in the case of whirling disease
calcium cyanamide	disinfection: 1 kgm./sq. meter	disinfection of tanks, especially in the case of whirling disease
Carbarsone	0.2% in feed for 4–7 days	*Hexamita (Octomitus)*
Chlorine (bleach)	disinfection: 200 ppm.—1 hr., 10 ppm.—24 hours	disinfection of tanks and equipment

DRUG	ADMINISTRATION	DIAGNOSIS
Chloromycetin (chloramphenicol) 3 mgm. d-chloromycetin/150–400 gm. body weight. Dilute in water by means of butylene glycol. 1 cc. of the solution should contain 3 mgm. of antibiotic	intra-peritoneal injection of 1 cc. of an aqueous solution in 150–400 gm. fish, in bigger fish a little more	bacterial hemorrhagic septicemia
chloromycetin: dissolve 80 mgm. of the antibiotic per liter of water	long duration bath (24 hours minimum)	bacterial hemorrhagic septicemia
in feed—75 mg./kg./day	feed 10 days	furunculosis ulcer disease
chloromycetin: dissolve 50 mgm. of the antibiotic per liter of water for fish of 10 gm. weight	long duration bath; do not use an aquarium, but rather a special container	bacterial hemorrhagic septicemia, bacterial fin rot
sodium chloride: 10–15 gm. per liter of water (for aquarium and small food fish)	short bath of 20 minutes, a special receptacle must be used	*Chilodonella, Trichodina, Gyrodactylus, Dactylogyrus, Saprolegnia*
sodium chloride: 25 gm. per liter of water	short bath (10–15 minutes), never use a zinc recipient	*Chilodonella, Costia, Trichodina, Gyrodactylus, Dactylogyrus, Saprolegnia*
Collargol (silver oxide–78% Ag): 1 mgm./ liter of water	short bath of 20 minutes, a special recipient must be used	*Saprolegnia*
Dipterex (Dylox)	0.25 ppm. (active) once a week for 4 weeks	Copepods, monogenetic trematodes
Ethylmercuric phosphate: 1–2 ppm. (6.25% active)	1 hour bath	bacterial gill disease

Erythromycin: 100 mgm./kg./day	in feed 21 days	kidney disease (*Corynebacterium*)
Formalin: 20–25 cc. commercial formalin for each 100 liters of water 15 ppm. in ponds	short bath of 30–45 minutes (specially recommended for *Costia*) long bath	*Costia, Trichodina, Gyrodactylus, Dactylo-gyrus, Ichthyophthirius*
Furazolidone: 2.5 gm./100 kg./day	in feed for 20 days	furunculosis
Potassium iodide—iodine: dissolve 0.1 gm. iodine and 10 gm. potassium iodide in 100 cc. distilled water. Add 0.5 cc. of this per liter of water	long-duration bath	benign tumors of the thyroid (goiter); ineffective in cancer of the thyroids
Kanamycin: 20 mg./kg.	i.p. injection in feed	*Aeromonas, Pseudomonas, Mycobacterium*
Lysol (cresol derivative) 2 cc. of lysol per liter of water	bath for 5–15 seconds	carp lice, leeches
malachite green: 1 gm./10 sq. meters tank surface, 2–3 times on alternate days, up to a concentration of 0.15 mgm./liter	in trout hatcheries and carp ponds	*Ichthyophthirius, Chilodonella, Costia*
Ammonium nitrate: 0.5 gm./10 liters of water. Repeat after 2 days	long duration bath	to remove hydras
Potassium permanganate: 1 gm./100 liters of water	short bath of 90 minutes, the use of a special receptacle is imperative	*Saprolegnia, Costia, Chilodonella, Tricho-dina*, bacteria
Potassium permanganate: 1 gm./liter of water	immersion bath for 30–45 seconds	*Argulus, Trichodina*
Potassium permanganate: 1 gm./10 liters of water	short bath, 5–10 minutes	*Argulus, Costia, Trichodina*, and *Chilodonella*

DRUG	ADMINISTRATION	DIAGNOSIS
Priasol (cresol derivative): may be used in place of lysol. 4 cc./liter of water	immersion bath, 5–15 seconds	carp lice, leeches
Quaternary ammonium compounds: 2–4 ppm. (active ingredient)	1 hour bath	bacterial gill disease
Rivanol: 1 gm. in 500 liters of water	long duration bath	skin parasites
Streptomycin: 5–10 mgm./150–400 gm. fish body weight	intra-peritoneal injection	bacterial hemorrhagic septicemia
Sulfadiazine: 100–250 mgm./liter of water	long duration bath	bacterial diseases
Sulfamerazine, sulfamethazine, sulfisoxazole: 22 gm./100 kg./day	in feed for 14 days	Furunculosis, cold-water disease, columnaris disease, kidney disease
Sulfanilamide: 100–250 mgm./liter of water	long duration bath	bacterial and fungal diseases
Copper sulfate: 1 gm./10 liters of water	short duration bath of 10–30 minutes. Special recipient must be used	*Costia, Saprolegnia, Gyrodactylus*
Copper sulfate: stock solution of 1 gm./liter of water, use 1.5 cc. of this for each liter of aquarium water	long duration bath (3–10 days). If unsuccessful, repeat. Special recipient must be used	*Oodinium.* Has been used with great success in marine aquaria
Terramycin (oxytetracycline): 3 mgm. per 150–400 gm. fish body weight; 75 mg./kg./day in feed	intra-peritoneal injection, feed 10 days	bacterial hemorrhagic septicemia, furunculosis, ulcer disease
Sodium thiosulfate: 1 gm./10 liters of water		for water containing an excess of chlorine
Tin oxide, di-n-butyl: 25 gm./100 kg. total dose	in feed, dose spread over 3 days	intestinal cestodes, trematodes

76

(*b*) This stock solution is diluted with water so that 1 cc. of the final solution contains 3 mgm. chloramphenicol, *id est* 10 cc. of butylene glycol + 190 cc. of water. With this quantity 200 2-year-old carp of 150–300 gm. may be injected. If we wished to inject 2000 2-year-old carp, then we would dilute 100 cc. of butylene glycol (containing 6000 mgm. of chloramphenicol), in 1900 cc. of water. As a little is always lost when the fluid is being taken up into the syringe, an amount approximately 5% greater than the minimum requirements is prepared (in our example 2100 cc.), for which we would dissolve 150 cc. of butylene glycol in 1950 cc. of water.

(*c*) The necessary amount of water required to prepare the solution is boiled for 5 minutes. The butylene glycol is measured into a small clean glass cylinder, and then poured into a 1 liter measuring cylinder. Any butylene glycol remaining is washed out with boiled water, and the volume made up to 1 liter. This is then placed into a large flask and a further 1100 cc. of boiled water added to it (see our example above). The flask must then be well shaken. The resulting solution should be used up within 3 days, since it does not keep well.

(*d*) For the injection, the chloramphenicol solution is taken from the large flask and put into small beakers from which the syringes are filled.

(*e*) The injections are best given with 10 cc. nylon syringes fitted with Record needles, 3 cm. long. Several of these No. 2 needles are prepared in such a way that they may be frequently changed as and when they become obstructed. The syringes and needles are boiled for 10 minutes prior to use (the plunger and the barrel are separated for sterilization). The little wire must always be removed from the needles before these latter are boiled. Distilled water or rain water should always be used for boiling syringes. Relatively cheap disposable syringes and needles are now available in different sizes.

(*f*) One person performs the injection itself, while another holds the fish. This procedure must be done in a continual fashion, without any interruptions or waste of time. Two people should be able to inject between them, a minimum of 400 2-year-old carp within 1 hour. The fish for injection are put onto a special table, and following this are at once transferred to wooden containers full of water.

(*g*) The carp should be placed in such a position as to have the belly facing towards the person who is actually performing the injection, with the head on the left hand side. The needle is introduced to a depth of approximately 2 cm., at a point shown in *Figure 30*, inserting it very obliquely so that the internal organs are not damaged. According to the present writer, it is not necessary to remove the mucus coating with a cloth, firstly because carp do not have very much mucus and secondly because such an operation cannot be carried out with all the necessary aseptic precautions. The germicidal function of the mucus in fish is to be preferred to cleansing with a cloth. 1 cc. of the antibiotic solution is injected into fish of up to 350 gm., and a little more in bigger fish (for example, 1.5 cc.).

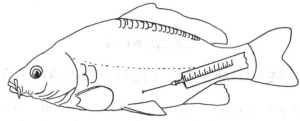

Figure 30. Site of injection. (Original)

(*h*) The syringes are filled on a table situated away from that where the injection is to be performed. The operator should always have several syringes prepared.

(*i*) Immediately following the injection, the fish are returned to the water. The protective effects of this injection last for about 3 weeks, and it should always be performed before releasing the fish into open waters.

To complete the section of therapy, a few words of special interest to aquarists may be added: it is erroneous to administer to fish any drug which promises to be effective when it is suspected that they are ill, since there is no panacea in fish pathology. Only a very precise knowledge of the etiology of any disease authorizes the use of any specific drug or other medicament. To summarize briefly: first know the cause of the disease, and then—only then—commence treatment.

Chapter 4

THE SENDING OF FISH FOR ANALYSIS

Diseased fish and those suspected of being diseased should be sent alive whenever possible. In Germany there are two centers occupied with the study of fish diseases: The Bavarian Institute for Biological Research, Munich, and the Fisheries Department of the German Academy of Sciences. In England game fish such as trout and salmon may be sent to the Freshwater Fisheries Laboratory, London; in Scotland they are forwarded to the Marine Laboratory, Aberdeen. In the United States diseased fish may be forwarded to either the Eastern Fish Disease Laboratory, Leetown (West Virginia) or the Western Fish Disease Laboratory, Seattle (Washington). Aquarium fish may be forwarded in a clean bottle, two-thirds full of water. In this way the oxygen is continually renewed during transit. Neither plants nor dead fish should be included with this water. For large fish, screw-capped bottles or jars may be used. A shock-proof wrapper should always be provided. Nylon or polyethylene bags are of practical utility in the forwarding of living fish for examination.

Recently dead aquarium fish should be sent in hermetically closed screw-capped bottles containing formalin (1 part 40% formalin in 9 parts of water).

Aquarium fish which have been dead for some time tend to decompose rapidly in tropical aquarium tanks, and this makes an accurate and precise investigation impossible (the so-called secondary parasites appear, bacteria and fungi, and this masks the true cause of death). The same thing happens in the case of food fish during the warmer months of the year. The dispatch of fish in such conditions is totally useless in the great majority of cases.

The dispatch of live or recently dead fish is of the utmost importance, since in preserved specimens certain monocellular parasites cannot be detected and this casts doubt on the validity of the final diagnosis. In summertime, the food fish must be sent packed in ice. Recently dead ones are placed in a nylon bag, and this is then surrounded with ice and put into a second larger bag. The whole is sent in a box together with sawdust. If the sender wishes to have the water analyzed simultaneously, this must be sent apart from the fish, in a perfectly clean, preferably sterile bottle. The bottle and cork may be sterilized in an emergency by a vigorous boiling in water prior to adding the sample. No precise analysis of the water can be made if it is sent together with live fish for diagnosis.

Both the water sample bottles and those containing the fish must bear a label indicating the date of taking the sample (in the case of the water sample the hour at which it was taken should also be added). In the event of their being any drainage leaking into the stretch of water, samples of this should be taken as described above, in, and below the point of entry.

Finally, special importance is attached to the necessity of complete details with regard to the history of the case under consideration. Any observations made should be carefully noted, as well as the amount of water in the tank or pond, numbers of fish and their species. The last and most recent change of water of the aquarium must be noted, and details of the pH, hardness and clarity of the water added whenever this is feasible.

Note must also be taken of any color changes which have been observed in the fish (paleness, darkening); if they gasp, if they swim in circles; if the fins are normal or are held tightly to the body; whether they swim actively or inactively. It is of interest to know the composition of the food which they have been given during the preceding 10–20 days, as well as the amount given. In the event of mortalities having occurred, an indication should be given as to whether this occurred suddenly or over the course of a longer period of time. All the data mentioned herein are of inestimable value to the fish pathologist, and may prove of vital importance to him in order to establish the correct diagnosis.

Chapter 5

VIRAL AND BACTERIAL DISEASES

Bacterial diseases are of frequent occurrence in fish. Quite often mixed infections may occur in the aquarium. In such an instance the diagnosis has to be made taking into due account histological, histochemical and bacteriological data with a view to distinguishing between the different types of symptoms present. Work is really only just beginning in this particular field of research.

To this, one has to add certain types of diseases which cannot directly be attributed to parasites and bacteria. Under these conditions one has to accept the possibility of a viral infection, unless of course the disease can clearly be shown to be due to a metabolic or glandular disorder.

Viruses are very small microbes living inside live cells, and which cannot be cultured on ordinary bacteriological media. Their size is less than 0.3 microns, and they are normally only visible by electron microscopy. They may be separated from bacteria by means of filters, from which property comes the name "filterable viruses". The study of fish viruses and virology is only just beginning, quite the opposite to what is occurring with regard to certain bacterial diseases.

The following is a synopsis of viruses and bacteria pathogenic to fish.

(A) VIRUSES: size less than 0.3 microns; visible only by electron microscopy; can only be cultivated in living cells.

(i) lymphocystis virus: induces great enlargement of fibroblasts; size up to 200mu; has been isolated in cell culture; occurs in Pleuronectidae, Percidae, Centrarchidae and many other important families.

(ii) VHS virus: virus of viral hemorrhagic septicemia; size 70–180mu; virus particles formed in connection with cell membranes and membranes of intracellular vacuoles. Cytopathogenic in cell culture.

(iii) IPN virus: agent of infectious pancreatic necrosis; an RNA virus of 18mu; multiplication occurs in cytoplasm; cytopathogenic in cell culture; first fish virus isolated.

81

(iv) Sockeye salmon virus: causes epizootics in young sockeye salmon; over 100mu; supposed to be very specific.

(v) Chinook salmon virus: agent of Sacramento River Chinook disease; less than 50mu; very heat labile; cytoplasmic inclusions in pancrease.

(vi) Pox virus: agent of carp pox; formed in cell nucleus and transferred to cytoplasm; size in nucleus—110mu, in cytoplasm—150mu.

(vii) Papilloma viruses: virus has been associated with several papilloma diseases but have not been fully proven as yet.

There are several other diseases, presumptively viral, which are limited in distribution or are of doubtful cause.

(B) ORDER ACTINOMYCETALES: fungus-like bacteria; may or may not show branching.

(i) *Mycobacterium piscium*: Gram positive bacilli, slender and non-motile; acid-fast; from 1–4 microns in length; optimum growth temperature 25° C.; cultures in meat broth produce a thin and fragile pellicle; orange-yellow colonies on egg medium; causes piscine tuberculosis.

(C) ORDER EUBACTERIALES: straight or curved rods and cocci.

(1) Family: Pseudomonadaceae

(a) *Aeromonas*: straight gram negative rods with polar flagella.

(i) *Aeromonas liquefaciens*: straight rods with one polar flagellum; has many different bio-types; a most important fish pathogen.

— *forma ascitae*: produces infectious abdominal dropsy; measures 0.5 × 0.9 microns.

— *forma sarcowiensis*: causes freshwater eel pest; measures 0.5 × 0.9 microns.

— *forma pellis*: gives rise to Red Pest in pike, perch and carp; measures 0.5 × 0.9 microns.

(ii) *Pseudomonas fluorescens*: more than one flagellum; causes ulcers and lesions in different species of fish; measures from 0.5 × 1.6 microns to 0.5 × 3.0 microns.

(iii) *Pseudomonas putida*: more than one flagellum; may be motile or non-motile; possesses a capsule; causes hemorrhagic septicemia ("Red Pest") in eels and carp.

(iv) *Aeromonas salmonicida*: non-motile and very short rods (cocco-bacilli); produce furunculosis of salmonids; measure 0.5 × 0.8 microns.

(2) Family: Brucellaceae
    (a) *Hemophilus piscium*: Gram negative, non-motile; requires media enriched with fish peptone or cocarboxylase.
    (b) *Vibrio*: curved and spiral-shaped rods.
        (i) *Vibrio anguillarum*: comma-shaped rod with one solitary flagellum; causes Red Pest in saltwater eels, as well as pike pest; measures 0.5×1.5 microns.
(3) Family: Corynebacteriaceae
    (a) *Corynebacterium*: small Gram positive bacilli, occurring in pairs as diplo-bacilli; asporogenous; non-motile; cause bacterial kidney disease and Dee disease in salmonids.
(D) Order: Myxobacteriales
  (1) Family: Cytophagaceae
    (a) *Cytophaga psychrophila*: long, thin, flexible; Gram negative; no microcysts.
  (2) Family: Myxococcaceae
    (a) *Chondrococcus columnaris*: long, thin, flexible; Gram negative form microcysts; arrange in "columns".

VIRUSES AND BACTERIOPHAGES

Viruses are ultra-microscopic bodies which only on rare occasions may come to have the size of the smallest bacteria known, but which are usually very much smaller than this. They are only capable of reproduction in living tissues. They may join together to form filaments and networks, or crystallize in isolated macromolecules. As regards their chemical composition, they are nucleoproteins, which means a combination of proteins and nucleic acid in a relatively constant proportion. The protein component closely resembles albumin, and the nucleic acid can be deoxyribonucleic acid (DNA) or ribonucleic acid (RNA). Certain of the viruses have been found to contain lipids and lipoproteins. Viruses as a group are unstable and tend to decompose readily (with the exception of the tobacco mosaic virus). On introduction into healthy living tissues, they multiply rapidly at the expense of tissue metabolism, forming as a result a new viral protein similar to the original with regards to its physical, chemical and serological properties. Viruses do not possess a capacity to carry out their own metabolism, but utilize that of the host tissues. Spontaneous generation is unknown, although mutations have been observed.

Viral Hemorrhagic Septicemia of Rainbow Trout (VHS); entero-hepato-renal syndrome; infectious trout anemia or Egtved disease

The increasing importance of trout farming, a business proposition concerned principally with obtaining the greatest possible yield by the shortest possible means, with consequent heavy population densities and maximum feeding, greatly favors the increasingly obvious spread of *viral hemorrhagic septicemia* (VHS). It would seem that alimentary deficiencies and the physiological conditions produced by the same are primarily responsible for the entry of the causative agent of this particular infection. CLINICAL PICTURE AND SYMPTOMS: the external clinical picture is very variable. Klingler differentiates three pathological forms:

(i) *chronic or sub-acute form:* this gives a clinical picture of fairly easy recognition and diagnosis. The following symptoms are characteristic of this particular variety: listlessness, little effort made to escape; the fish swim slowly at the surface of the water; they tend to congregate at the edge of the tank; darkish coloration; bilateral exophthalmos; anemia characterized by a gray-brown paleness of the gills which at post-mortem turn white almost immediately; swelling of the belly; yellowish-colored anus; spongy texture of the dorsal muscles.

On autopsy it is frequently possible to detect an ascites in the body cavity, of a clear or slightly yellow coloration, odorless or at the most with a somewhat rancid smell. Punctiform hemorrhages are seen in the peritoneum, meninges and muscles. The color of the liver varies from gray-brown to yellow; its general consistency is broken up and the bile is often gelatinous in appearance. The kidney is swollen and generally has the appearance of one broad red band. In the stomach a yellowish or colorless fluid may be seen, the pH of which is neutral or alkaline. The mucous layer of the rectum may be reddened and inflamed. The fish die off one by one over the course of a few months. The losses are not quite so important if the temperature of the water is around 20° C. and little food is administered to the fish. Growth is generally retarded.

(ii) *Acute or hyper-acute form:* again the typical clinical picture is fairly easy to diagnose.

The symptoms of the acute and hyper-acute form are that it frequently appears in a so-called "whirling form." Tack considers this symptom to be characteristic of VHS. The trout show whirling movements, going head over heels as it were, or rotating on the longitudinal axis of the body. Death may occur within a very short time, and is accompanied by muscular spasms; for example as occurs when the fish are removed. These trout have a wide open mouth and an extremely rapidly occurring *rigor mortis.* Neither exophthalmos nor anemia are particularly pronounced. Autopsy shows a ruptured liver, partially decolorized but usually gray to yellowish-gray. Losses normally reach more than 50%. A sudden decrease in the temperature and fatigue brought on by transportation bring about a rapid death in the greater majority of cases.

(iii) *Latent form:* this is very difficult to diagnose.

It has the following symptoms: in some cases there is a very slight exophthalmos and incipient anemia, which does not become apparent until after death has already occurred. Autopsy shows a pale liver. The kidney may be definitely swollen along its entire length, or partially so (for example in the posterior third, *Figure 31*). The gastric juice has a neutral or weakly alkaline reaction. The latent form may pass to those forms described above as a result of an inadequate feeding, lack of oxygen, a decrease in the temperature, or through fatigue brought on by transportation.

Figure 31. Viral hemorrhagic septicemia in the posterior third of the kidney of a rainbow trout. (Mattheis)

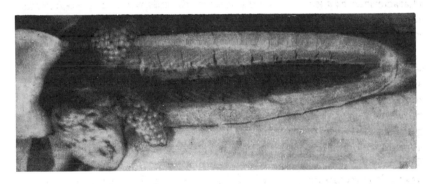

TECHNIQUE OF INVESTIGATION: The diseased fish should be carefully observed and studied in the tank itself. It must be shown whether they have pale gills. On performing the autopsy one should look out for the presence of liquid in the abdominal cavity, the color of the liver, and the size of the kidney. In macerated wet preparations from the liver, observation is made as to whether any pigment is present; the same procedure is carried out with the spleen (*Figures 32* and *33*). The gall bladder and rectum are examined for the presence of *Octomitus truttae*. For histological and histochemical studies, fixation of the liver, kidney and spleen is carried out in formalin and water 1:4, in Stieve's fluid or in alcohol 2:1. Should the nature of the case so require, cultures of the liver and kidney may be taken to determine whether there is any secondary infection present such as furunculosis.

Figure 32. Normally pigmented spleen of a rainbow trout. (Original)

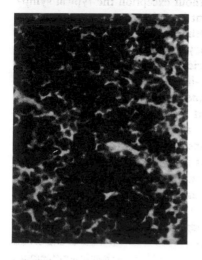

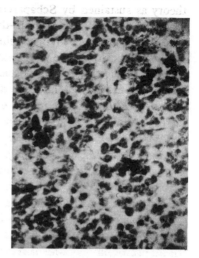

Figure 33. Spleen of a rainbow trout attacked by viral hemorrhagic septicemia and showing marked lack of pigmentation as well as formation of edematous spaces in the splenic tissue. (Original)

For electron microscope studies, fixation is in gluteraldehyde and post fixation in osmium acid. Embedding is in Epon.

ETIOLOGY; MORPHOLOGY AND TAXONOMY OF THE CAUSATIVE AGENT; COURSE OF THE DISEASE: Schäperclaus (1954b) was the first to defend the theory that VHS is a viral disease. In accordance with his observations, the activity of the virus was directed chiefly towards the kidney, but in addition it frequently attacks with some measure of intensity the liver or the intestine (nephrotropism hepatotropism and enterotropism respectively). Deufel (1958b) calculated its size between 100–150mu approximately, by means of ultrafiltration; Zwillenberg and Zwillenberg (1964) and Zwillenberg, Jensen and Zwillenberg (1965) succeeded in determining the size of the virus electronmicroscopically at 60mu × 180mu after it was cultivated in permanent growing fish gonad cells (RTG-2 line). Pfitzner (1966) used, for the demonstration of virus, tissue cultures from ovaries of *Tinca vulgaris* (Tench), and *Cyprinus carpio* (carp). Infection experiments of this author with this trout virus were successful in the goldfish (*Carassius auratus*). On the average, cytopathogenic effects occurred in the tissue cultures 1 to 3 days after infection.

An indirect proof of its viral nature is the injection of organic filtrates free from bacteria, which reproduce without exception the typical symptoms of the disease. All of the most recent investigations confirm the virus theory as sustained by Schäperclaus. Other authors, Besse in particular, maintain that this is a vitamin-deficiency disease. Besse (1955) believed it to be a vitamin B_{12} (cobalamin) deficiency, through a lack of Castle's factor and a disturbance of the extrinsic-intrinsic factor relationship. The disease, characterized by a pernicious anemia, is produced by foodstuffs with a sea-fish base. These are deficient in vitamins and have a slightly alkaline reaction which makes difficult the absorption of the extrinsic factor; in its place anemia-producing substances cross through the gastric mucosa. The same dietary theory, albeit in a slightly modified form, was put forward by Lauridsen (1958). He considers that the cause of the disease is due to a deficiency of vitamin B_1 and vitamin E. Pescheck (1958) arrived at a similar conclusion. Bellet (1958) categorically defends the theory of irrational feeding. In this regard we should remember the importance attached recently by Liebmann (1959) to nutritional factors as provoking certain diseases (for example, bacterial hemorrhagic septicemia). In all probability, irrational feeding plays an important role which favors the appearance of VIIS; for example in Denmark a food based exclusively on fresh herring gives rise to a destruction of thiamin (vitamin B_1) because of the high concentration of the enzyme thiaminase in the herring flesh itself. Be this as it may, we may fully admit that on the basis of our present-day knowledge, this is a viral disease affecting susceptible trout, as is confirmed amply by electronmicroscopy and cell culture. It is classed as an Arbovirus.

The course of the disease depends on many factors. Generally it is characterized by a listless bearing of the diseased fish. The losses reach some 10–15 fish per tank per day. Sick trout do not eat at all. In 50% of all cases a secondary infection with *Octomitus truttae* is to be seen, the distribution of this parasite being chiefly in the rectum.

Viral hemorrhagic septicemia is widespread and is almost always of a slow development. According to Schäperclaus it confers an immunity which may last for several years. It generally coincides with a low water temperature, and as a result breaks out chiefly during the colder months of the year. New trout may bring the disease with them into the hatchery. The loss of fry may be between 9–25%, or (according to Schäperclaus) even as high as 78%.

HISTOPATHOLOGY AND HISTOCHEMISTRY: The parenchymatous organs, and especially the liver and kidney, and also the brain and muscles, show edema. The cells display a clear case of toxic degeneration and there is a barely visible defensive inflammatory reaction in the connective tissue;

only the kidney shows this connective tissue reaction to a marked degree. One's attention is drawn to the clearly defined edema of the lacunae of the lymphoid tissue as well as to its lack of pigmentation (*Figures 34* and *35*). The interstitial tissue is fatty, and is responsible for the renal tumefaction which is apparent macroscopically. At the same time there is an obvious necrosis of the renal tubules. The liver shows fatty degeneration. Its cells are hypertrophied and have the appearance of vesicles, partially affected by a vacuolar degeneration and with partly atrophied nuclei. In seriously affected trout, Bauer's glycogen reaction gives a negative result.

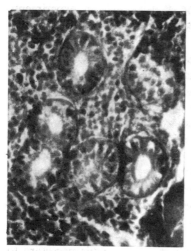

Figure 34. Normal tissue of a rainbow trout kidney, with tubuli and lymphoid interstitial tissue. (Original)

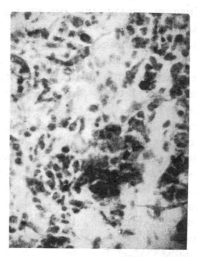

Figure 35. Kidney of rainbow trout infected with viral hemorrhagic septicemia, showing edematous spaces, marked tubular necrosis, and necrotic destruction of the lymphoid tissue. (Original)

Clear edematous spaces and atrophy of the muscular fibers are to be seen in the cardiac muscle. The isolated inflammatory foci are distinguished by a lymphatic infiltration. The skeletal muscles are especially characterized by edematous spaces surrounding the masses of fibers; in sections these appear as clear halos. The nuclei of the muscular fibers remain intact in the great majority of cases. According to Japanese workers, the blood undergoes changes in its morphology. The erythrocytes of diseased trout are smaller and their nuclei are larger than those of normal trout. The red cell count reaches 300,000/cmm. in sick trout as opposed to 1,300,000/cmm. in healthy ones. No variation occurs in the leucocytes. The lymphocytes show an increase of 3–18% of the red cell number in contrast to 1% in normal fish. Should this be the case it may be considered that an increase of more than 2% in the lymphocytes suggests a diseased fish. In sick trout the hemoglobin concentration is considerably decreased, as shown in *Table 3*.

TABLE 3: Hemoglobin concentrations of rainbow trout (normal and diseased with VHS—data from Deufel and Schäperclaus).

STATE	RANGE OF HEMOGLOBIN IN GM./100 ML.	MEAN HEMOGLOBIN CONCENTRATION IN GM./100 ML.
normal	13–16	14
slightly diseased	8–14	11
seriously diseased	2–13	5

THERAPY, PROPHYLAXIS AND HYGIENE: Of all the numerous experiments carried out with a view to avoiding VHS, it will suffice to mention only the more promising.

The work carried out by Deufel (1958c) in aquaria is interesting, since he used Goetsch's vitamin T complex and obtained a marked reduction in the losses when this was administered together with the food. However Deufel indicated at the same time that his measure should be applied principally with a view to the prophylaxis of the disease rather than its treatment. The same may be said of the mixture of vitamins A, B_1 and E prepared by Klingler under the name of "Vitola." On the other hand the results obtained by this worker (Klingler, 1957) were not confirmed by Rasmussen (1959) who doubts the efficiency even of those successes claimed for vitamin B_{12} injections as proposed by Besse (1955). Recently Tack has reported on the successes obtained by the application of terramycin and the F_{100} preparation of vitamin T via the intragastric route. However, apart from the possibilities indicated above, it is necessary to devote much more attention to the physio-pathological factors at the beginning of an outbreak of VHS, and so combat the disease. In practice this means that one must exercise great care to ensure that a defective feeding schedule does not damage the liver, since this is the most important organ for a correct and efficient metabolism. Such care is even more important when there are symptoms of the disease and the presence of a hepatic lesion is suspected. In such an event the feeding ration must be reduced so as to help the liver in its function and avoid, for example, the accumulation of oxidized non-saturated fatty acids. In the colder weather, above all, the retarded metabolism of the trout liver must be borne in mind (fish are poikilotherms), and they should be fed with every possible care. The appearance of the disease during the cold season suggests that there exist a number of predisposing circumstances. For this reason it is fundamental to employ a rational feeding which is not in excess of 5% per day. It goes without saying that on taking these measures the vitamin content of the diet must be carefully watched (supplementing it when necessary with yeast), since we know that vitamin B_1 (or thiamine) positively influences the metabolism of fats. This is of great importance, above all, when the water temperature is low. The cooking of meat is also recommended since this renders it more easy to digest, and the digestive organs are not obliged to work to the same extent as would be the case with raw meat. Any cooked meat should obviously always possess a complement of yeast or bran.

The strictest hygiene must be maintained in the tanks. Any seriously affected trout should be removed, destroyed and either burned or buried. Infected tanks are disinfected with quicklime or with calcium cyanamide (see the list of drugs and their application). In infected fish hatcheries the nets and other utensils should frequently be disinfected. Scrupulous hygiene is a factor of major importance in the case of this disease. Not only newly arrived trout, but also water, nets and similar objects may serve as sources of contagion. We do not at the present know the extent to which the sending of trout eggs from one place to another may be responsible for an outbreak, and thus it is preferable to avoid this as much as is possible. Newly purchased trout should always be placed in quarantine tanks, and in the event of these being intercommunicating, the fish are placed in the lowest one of all. At the slightest suspicion of disease the feeding rations should be immediately reduced or temporarily suspended. Great importance is placed on rational and intelligent feeding, since according to Klingler much fewer losses are sustained by them (less than 10%) in the event of their becoming diseased. Care should always be taken to ensure that the oxygen supply is adequate and the number of fish per cubic meter of the tank should always be within prudent limits.

Papillomatosis ("cauliflower disease")

Cauliflower-like tumors were first studied and described scientifically by Christiansen and Jensen (1950), Schäperclaus (1953a), Amlacher (1957b), and Lühmann and Mann (1957). They occur principally in eels. In the bleak (*Alburnus alburnus*), Amlacher observed a tumor with a cauliflowerlike appearance, the histological structure of which bore a close resemblance to that of the tumors in eels.

The disease has been known to fishermen for a long time, and appeared in 1910 in Jasmund Bay. It was also seen in 1947 occurring on the eastern coast of Sweden, in Polish waters, to the south of Bornholm, and on the east coast of the Danish islands of Seeland and Laaland, as well as in Jutland. At the beginning the number of diseased eels caught was 0.1–2%, but in 1950 the condition appeared with epizootic proportions in the Oder gulf, when five out of every hundred eels were found to be affected. It was also registered in 1953 on the North Sea coast, especially in the lower Elbe at Cuxhaven. From 1954 to 1956 the frequency of diseased eels, both large and small, has increased among the fish landed at Hamburg. According to Lühmann and Mann the eel may be affected when it grows larger than 9 cm. In Hamburg, up to 10% of the eels used in the restocking of waters showed symptoms of the disease, which occurs as much in freshwater as it does in the sea.

CLINICAL PICTURE AND SYMPTOMS: principally the younger fish are attacked. The eels show growth of skin proliferations over the whole body, and particularly on the upper and lower jaws (*Figure 36*). The appearance of these growths resembles that of a cauliflower and for this reason Schäperclaus called it "cauliflower disease." Frequently there are proliferations on the pectoral fins, and as has been mentioned above, the disease also affects the back, the belly and sides, and the caudal region (*Figure 37*). At first the tumors are white, then clear brown, and finally they become darker when the pigmentation is increased (particularly on the back). In advanced cases nothing more than white tumors are to be found.

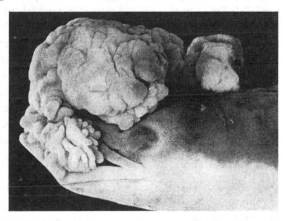

Figure 36. Eel with papillomas in the form of a cauliflower, the result of a marked proliferation in the upper and lower jaws. (Original)

Heavily infected individuals show signs of total exhaustion. Usually the mouth is not attacked, and eels kept in aquaria showed a normal interest in their food. In the same way, the water used in respiration was found to pass freely through the buccal cavity. In spite of all this the sick eels are in no condition to feed themselves properly, and they gradually become more and more emaciated.

TECHNIQUE OF INVESTIGATION: fixation of the papillomas may be carried out in formalin (formalin 40% one part: water four parts) or in Stieve's fluid. Paraffin wax sections are stained with hematoxylin—eosin, Heidenheim's iron hematoxylin, and Mallory's acid fuchsin—aniline blue—orange G, or with Domagk's kernechrot—aniline blue—orange G.

ETIOLOGY; MORPHOLOGY AND TAXONOMY OF THE CAUSATIVE AGENT; COURSE OF THE DISEASE: it is believed that a halophilic virus is the causative agent of cauliflower disease in eels (Schäperclaus), even though no positive results have been so far obtained from attempts to reproduce the condition experimentally. Schäperclaus experimented in sea-water aquaria, inserting small pieces of the papilloma under the skin of eels and goldfish. He further took scrapings from the tumor tissue, placed them into sterile water, and after filtering through cotton wool and bacteriological filters, injected the resulting fluid by the sub-cutaneous, intra-peritoneal and intra-cardiac routes into healthy eels. No papillomas were formed even after 15 months.

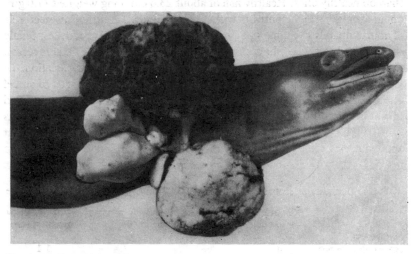

Figure 37. Eel with cauliflower-like growths in the pectoral fin region; those in the dorsal region were hyperemic and darkly pigmented but in the lateral and trunk regions were of white, yellow, and pink coloration. (Amlacher)

In a series of similar experiments, Christiansen and Jensen likewise obtained negative results. My own experiments have also given nothing of any great importance. In spite of all this it would appear that the disease is contagious. The first external symptoms begin on the lower jaw and nasal orifices, and the initial size is approximately 1 mm. From my own unpublished histological investigations, I have formed the impression that the first external manifestations appear as small microscopic folds of skin which multiply and grow. Lühmann and Mann state that these primary foci of proliferation may anastomose and by this means give rise to larger papillomas. The same workers proved that in benign cases the fat content of the eel is not abnormally reduced, although there is never so much as in healthy fish. While healthy eels measuring 19–28.5 cm. in length and 9–29.5 gm. in weight had 1.6–5% fat, in seriously diseased eels of the same size the fat content was less than 1%. Lühmann and Mann gave the following average figures corresponding respectively to eels with lesions of light, medium and heavy intensity respectively.

It is believed that the ingestion of food becomes more difficult some 3–6 months at most after the first appearance of the disease. Since the effects of hunger and starvation do not make themselves felt in the eel until quite some time has elapsed, Lühmann and Mann believe that definitely damaged individuals have had the disease for at least a year, if not longer. Diseased eels, as shown in *Table 4*, weigh considerably less than do healthy ones. Healthy fish of about 23.6 cm. long weighed 17.0 gm. on an average, which contrasts with 11.6 gm. and 10.2 gm. of diseased eels of approximately the same size (see *Table 4*). The internal organs, especially the liver and intestine, show considerable changes. It is clear for this reason that papillomatosis finally leads to death due to complete emaciation. In 1958, I was able to make an interesting observation with regards to an eel affected by this disease. The fish had lived in an aquarium during a period of about 6 months, when suddenly—in the spring—several papillomas broke out all over its body. It died approximately one month after the first appearance of the symptoms. The course of the disease thus appears to resemble that of cancer followed by metastasis.

TABLE 4: Lengths, weights and fat content of eels affected by cauliflower disease.

	NUMBER OF EELS	MEAN LENGTH (CM.)	MEAN WEIGHT (GM.)	MEAN % FAT IN FRESH FLESH
first group (growing number of papillomas)	6	20.7	7.1	1.1
	7	24.7	11.6	1.5
	12	28.5	20.2	2.4
second group (large tumors)	1	21.0	7.7	0.5
	4	24.4	10.2	0.7
	6	27.7	15.9	0.9

HISTOPATHOLOGY AND HISTOCHEMISTRY: the papillomas described by Schäperclaus were clearly different histologically from those in the eel and the bleak, as I have been able to show in a case which I studied personally. We shall not concern ourselves any further with them here, since I do not consider them to be typical "cauliflower disease" tumors. According to Amlacher (1957b), the following histopathological lesions are present in the papillomas of eels and bleak.

In sections the epidermal cells constitute the greater part of the mass of the tumor. As a result of a folding process, the epidermal layer is placed on top of the epidermal layer, and the cylindrical layer on top of the cylindrical layer respectively (*Figure 38*). As a rule the topmost epidermal cells from each fold grow into each other, while between the cylindrical cells grow connective and vascular neoformations at the expense of the remains of the dermis, which in the eel has a reticular appearance (*Figures 39* and *40*). These folds are complicated in the extreme. In simpler cases the folds remain as something more or less resembling a folded carpet, the upper face of which we may consider as the upper epithelial layer of the epidermis, and the under surface as if it were the cylindrical cell layer. Frequently these series of folds are mixed together like the teeth of two cog wheels,

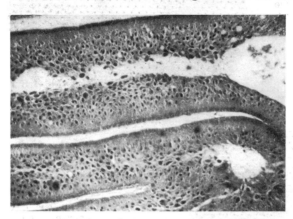

Figure 38. Section through a papilloma in *Alburnus alburnus*, showing the different epidermal elements in an opposite position as a result of fold formation. (Amlacher)

Figure 39. Vascular neoplasms in the remains of skin found between the adjoining layers of the cylindrical layers of the dermis, with simultaneous fusion of the more superficial layers of the epidermis. (Amlacher)

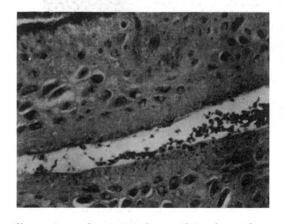

but characteristically the cells are not always stuck together along the whole surface in contact, but rather small spaces are left which may be filled with remains of mucilaginous or epidermal cells (*Figure 41*), without our being able to tell up to what point this conclusion may be valid and generalized. They are particularly well formed, and are extremely numerous in eels suffering from this disease. The origin of this network of connective tissue and blood vessels, described by Schäperclaus

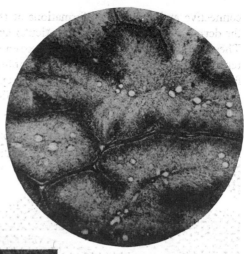

Figure 40. Transverse section through a papilloma in an eel, showing a tumorous mass composed of epidermal cells between which the dermal remains form a connective structure provided with capillaries. (Original)

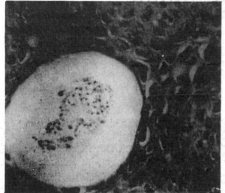

Figure 41. Formation of hollow spaces between the strongly joined upper layers of the epidermis. (Amlacher)

as a great network of collagen fibers acting as a support, is explained in my own work by the fact that the epidermal folds are followed by constrictions which in section give the appearance of epidermal islands (*Figure 42*). This process was found to be rare in *Alburnus alburnus*, although it is regularly observed in eels. One of the aforementioned epidermal islands consists of epithelial cells in the center, and a multistratified peripherous layer of cylindrical cells. The cylindrical cells of neighboring tissues lean against those of the island. Probably this is the manner in which the papilloma is formed. In opposition to the observations published by Schäperclaus, I would like to mention the presence of black pigmented granules in sections through the papillomas. Although none of the material which I examined personally was found to have such granules, I share the opinion of Christiansen and Jensen in that such pigmentation may be observed in the connective tissues of the capillaries, probably in the form of skin remains.

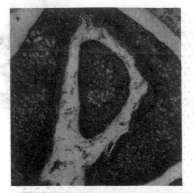

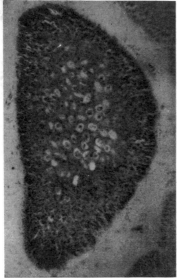

Figure 42. (a) Formation of an epithelial island within a papilloma, caused by constriction; (b) Highly magified epithelial island with a cylindrical layer in the periphery and epidermal cells in the interior. (Amlacher)

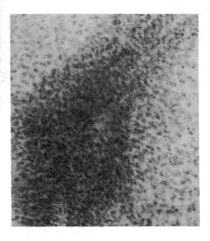

Figure 43. Feulgen's nuclear reaction in nuclei situated in the area of fusion of the cylindrical layer. (Amlacher)

The nuclei of infected tumor tissue gave a normal Feulgen reaction (*Figure 43*). Together with the insular constrictions of epithelial tissue, in the eel there is to be seen a primary cutaneous invagination which becomes constricted inwards and is finally reduced to an epithelial ring. It may even be that this tumor formation is due to such rings.

One may say that in the vast majority of the papillomas the epithelial cells and, to a lesser extent the cylindrical cells of the epidermis are involved. The dermis provides the connective tissue which provides material for the formation of blood capillaries, and for this reason the hypodermis plays no part in the formation of this type of tumor. The neoformation is covered by epidermal cells.

These papillomas consist of mature homologous tissue and should be thought of as being fibro-epithelial tumors. Their growth is slow, and is neither destructive nor infiltrating, in spite of which metastasis is still possible.

THERAPY, PROPHYLAXIS AND HYGIENE: no therapeutic treatment of papillomatosis is possible, and even if it were such a procedure would only be feasibly practical in a small number of diseased fish. In spite of numerous experimental investigations which have failed to provide proof of an infectious etiology of this disease, this must of necessity be admitted in view of the evident contagious nature of the condition. The disease does not affect mankind (according to the data which have thus far been accumulated by fish pathologists), but it is better to destroy the fish so as to prevent their transmitting the infection to other species. Lühmann and Mann observed eels with papillomatosis, for which reason we may assume that the disease occurs in German waters. Diseased eels should never be returned to the water, but destroyed as quickly as possible.

Lymphocystis

This disease occurs chiefly in the sea, although its presence has also been recorded in marine and freshwater aquaria. In marine aquaria it affects coral fish, and in freshwater ones the Paradise fish (*Macropodus opercularis*). In North America, lymphocystis is found in wild populations of Centrarchidae and *Stizostedion*.

CLINICAL PICTURE AND SYMPTOMS: the diseased fish show raspberry-like growths (in flatfish for example) or small isolated pearl-shaped nodules in different parts of the body (*Figure 44*). Mortalities due to this disease have been observed in marine aquaria.

TECHNIQUE OF INVESTIGATION: fixation of tissues may be carried out using formalin, Stieve's or Carnoy's fluid. Sections are made from paraffin blocks. For special studies of the virus, it is customary to use the usual techniques of electron microscopy. However, Wolf, Grovell and Mulsberger (1966) have succeeded in cultivating the virus in Centrarchid cell cultures.

ETIOLOGY; MORPHOLOGY AND TAXONOMY OF THE CAUSATIVE AGENT; COURSE OF THE DISEASE: the causative agent of lymphocystis disease is a pox virus, as shown successfully for the first time by Weissenberg, it has been demonstrated under the electron microscope by Walker (1963) and Walker and Weissenberg (1965). The disease is contagious and may be transmitted experimentally from one fish to another and by cell free filtrate (Weissenberg, 1951; Wolf 1962). The first nodules are observed some two months after infection. The size of the virus is 180mu to 220 mu. The virus is filtrable, glycerol-sensitive, and preservable by lyophilization, simple desiccation, and by freezing at —20° C. or lower. It occurs only in the cytoplasm of infected cells; occasionally occurs in crystalline array.

For a list of affected fish, see Nigrelli and Ruggieri (1965).

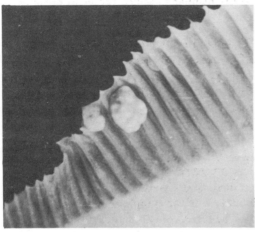

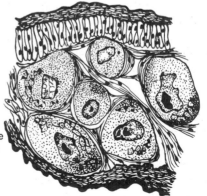

Figure 44. Lymphocystis warts (Anwand) and diagram through a lymphocystis growth; reticular inclusion bodies may be seen within the hypertophied cells and the hyaline capsule are clearly visible around the cell at the lower left. (Modified after Weissenberg)

HISTOPATHOLOGY AND HISTOCHEMISTRY: histologically the lymphocystic growths are composed of hypertrophied fibroblasts (giant cells). In the red mullet (*Mullus surmuletus* L.) the giant cells reach 340 microns in size according to Alexandrowicz (1951). These cells have a normal nucleus with nucleolus, but are differentiated from normal connective tissue cells by the presence of a special cellular inclusion (reticular body) and by a characteristic limiting membrane (*Figure 44*). According to Benisch (1937) the reticular body surrounds the virus, which develops from small granules. Weissenberg (1921) states that the giant cells require up to nine months in order to reach their final size, while at the same time the reticular body grows and occupies almost all of the cell. The giant cells degenerate in time and the inclusion body undergoes modifications which make it difficult to see. This may be the manner in which the virus acquires its capacity to infect new cells.

According to Walker (1963, 1965), the giant cells of lymphocystis warts are characterized by Feulgen positive cytoplasmic inclusions, myriads of polyhedral virus particles massed in the cytoplasm, and thick limiting capsules. The capsule is hyaline and it may be 10mu thick on a 500mu cell (*Stizostedion, Lepomis*). The capsule is strongly stained by alcian blue and is metachromatic. The lymphocystis cell is unique among virus infected cells in its extreme but slow terminal growth. It is not quickly destroyed by viral propagation. It is not stimulated to neoplasia. The lymphocystis giant cell shows a rich inclusion pattern of cytoplasmic DNA. Lymphocystis disease is virus transmitted, and electron microscopy shows that mature virus particles are found only in the cytoplasm, not in the nucleus. The inference seems clear that the DNA containing inclusion substance is a reduplicating pool of viral DNA. The large isohedral lymphocystis virus is of the DNA type (see Walker 1965). It is assumed then, that most of the viral DNA is synthesized in the cytoplasmic inclusions. The question as to whether there had to be any period of nuclear residence by the infecting DNA, is almost academic. Probably all viral DNA is synthesized in the cytoplasmic inclusions.

THERAPY, PROPHYLAXIS AND HYGIENE: it is impossible to treat the diseased fish. Since the disease is contagious, and infected fish caught by the fishermen should not be thrown back into the sea, but rather brought to port and either burned or buried. In aquarium practice the healthy fish are removed and placed in a new aquarium tank. They cannot be considered to be perfectly safe until at least two months have transpired. Contaminated aquaria must be emptied and disinfected with hydrochloric acid. It is only in aquaria that prophylactic measures can be adopted, and these include the two months quarantine period mentioned above.

Infectious pancreatic necrosis (IPN)

This disease was described by M'Gonigle (1940), as acute catarrhal enteritis. The newer name infectious pancreatic necrosis was given on the basis of histopathological investigations and the establishment of its infectious character. It is an acute disease of very young salmonid fishes, causing mortalities as high as 80 per cent.

CLINICAL PICTURE AND SYMPTOMS: As a symptom of infectious pancreas necrosis whirling has been described; for correct diagnosis careful microscopic examination is necessary. Sudden increase in mortality among young trout which have only recently begun to feed is often the first indication of trouble. Some fish will swim in a horizontal plane, but follow a spiral pattern—the "whirling" symptom; this is common among the larger, older fingerlings. At times fish will exhibit a frenzied swimming suggestive of severe pain; this will alternate with periods of quiescence when the fish comes to rest on the bottom. Internally a thick, clear or slightly whitish mucus material fills the stomach and anterior intestine, which is distended and food is typically absent. The spleen and liver may be almost colorless.

INVESTIGATION TECHNIQUES: preparation of bacteria-free (filtered) inocula of the pathogenic agent and inoculation of cell cultures with the infectious agent produce CPE (Wolf, Dunbar, Snieszko 1960, Wolf, Dunbar, Pyle, 1961, Wolf, Quimby, Bradford 1963).

ETIOLOGY, MORPHOLOGY AND BIOLOGY OF THE CAUSATIVE AGENT. Filtered inocula (bacteria-free) prepared from typically diseased fishes produce cytopathic degeneration in cell culture. Ability of inocula to produce degeneration in established tissue cultures is destroyed by heating at 60°C. for 1 hour and definitely reduced by treatment with ether. Initial inocula can be diluted at least a thousandfold and still produce degeneration. The effect of degeneration can be transferred in cell culture passage. These facts indicate the probability that a virus causes infectious pancreatic necrosis. The source and the reservoir of infection is unknown. Circumstantial evidence indicates possibility of egg transmission (Wolf, Quimby, Bradford 1963). Virus presence was demonstrated in egg fluids, egg homogeniates contained much less virus. The presence of virus within the eggs was not established. Under experimental conditions it was possible to infect healthy fish by placing them in water from diseased fish (but separated by a screen). Transmission was also effected by adding infected material with the food. Brook trout are particularly susceptible, the disease has also been identified symptomatically in cutthroat, rainbow and brown trout and in Atlantic salmon.

100

HISTOPATHOLOGY AND HISTOCHEMISTRY: histological examination shows severe necrosis of the pancreas and hyaline degeneration of the striated (skeletal) musculature. Microscopic lesions do not show microorganisms; the lesions are almost identical to those of Colsackie virus in mice.

THERAPY, PROPHYLAXIS, HYGIENE: fish which have been fed brine shrimp, have tended to be more severely affected than those which had been fed liver. The addition of fresh fish to the diet (M'Gonigle 1940) resulted in an aggravated condition. The disease has been reported from Alberta, the Canadian maritime provinces and the United States. Control of infectious pancreatic necrosis is not apt to be found in chemotherapy. Effective control must come about by prevention and perhaps to a degree through propagation of resistant strains of trout. When the source of infection is determined and the means by which the disease is transmitted is known and when the hatchery history indicates high mortality from infectious pancreatic necrosis the safest procedure would be to kill all fish in the infected troughs and thoroughly disinfect them and all equipment. Infectious pancreatic necrosis should be considered one of the most contagious diseases of trout. Under experimental conditions it was possible to prevent the spread of this disease from one trough to another by strict sanitation. Carrier fish can be identified by virological examination of fecal samples or peritoneal washings.

Sockeye salmon virus disease*

CLINICAL PICTURE AND SYMPTOMS: mortality is sudden and can be over 90%. The fish appear normal until shortly before death. The fish become lethargic, and dark. Abdominal swelling and hemorrhages at the base of fins are found. Pale gills and anemia is noted. The gastro-intestinal tract is fluid filled.

TECHNIQUE OF INVESTIGATION: histological sections are prepared in the usual manner. Suspect material is passed through a bacteria retaining filter and the filtrate inoculated into FHM or RTG 2 cells.

ETIOLOGY; MORPHOLOGY AND TAXONOMY OF THE CAUSATIVE AGENT; COURSE OF THE DISEASE: the agent does not pass a 100mu filter. It is inactivated at 60° C. in 15 minutes, by two cycles of freezing and loses infectivity when preserved in glycerol. Lyophilization preserves infectivity. It is not sensitive to ether, chloroform or alcohol and retains infectivity from pH 4 to pH 10.

---

* Recent information indicates that sockeye and chinook salmon virus diseases may be caused by the same virus (Amend, Yasutake and Mead, 1969). The virus also infects rainbow trout. Infectious Hematopoietic Necrosis (IHN) is proposed as the name for all three syndromes since the hematopoietic tissue is the primary target.

HISTOPATHOLOGY AND HISTOCHEMISTRY: the kidney is the primary organ showing pathology. Hematopoeitic tissues seem to show the greatest damage. Pathological changes occur also in the liver, spleen and pancreas. Cytoplasmic inclusions can be found in the pancreas.

THERAPY, PROPHYLAXIS AND HYGIENE: there is no known treatment. Infection probably results from exposure to carrier fish in the hatchery or water supply.

Chinook salmon virus disease

CLINICAL PICTURE AND SYMPTOMS: the fish turn dark and show exophthalmia. A subdermal lesion develops behind the head and appears as a reddened area. Hemorrhages at the base of the fins and pale gills are frequent. The guts are usually empty.

TECHNIQUE OF INVESTIGATION: as for Sockeye salmon virus disease.

ETIOLOGY; MORPHOLOGY AND TAXONOMY OF THE CAUSATIVE AGENT; COURSE OF THE DISEASE: the mortality is sudden and reaches 50–80%. Undisturbed, the fish tend to drift towards the outlet.

HISTOPATHOLOGY AND HISTOCHEMISTRY: the subdermal lesion is found to be an area of vascular damage. Hematopoeitic tissues are the primary targets. Renal tubules and the pancrease are also attacked. Necrosis is also found in the interrenal gland, liver and stomach.

THERAPY, PROPHYLAXIS AND HYGIENE: as for sockeye salmon virus disease.

BACTERIA

Bacteria are unicellular organisms with a simple cellular organization. In shape they may be round, cylindrical, bacillary or spiral. The cell membrane lacks both cellulose and chitin, and may swell up like gelatine and form a capsule or a mucus coat. Bacteria do not possess nuclei or chromatin, although they do have nucleic acid distributed throughout the cytoplasm, or joined together in small nodules called nucleoids (chromosome equivalent). Vacuoles may be formed in the cytoplasm. Many bacteria are motile by means of flagella, the distribution of which may be as follows:

  (i) monotrichous: (one polar flagellum, or if there are two they are bipolar);

 (ii) lophotrichous: (a tuft of two or more flagella, which may be mono- or bipolar);

(iii) peritrichous (or holotrichous): (the flagella cover all of the cell).

Many bacteria produce pigment: chromogenic bacteria—which diffuse their pigment into the surrounding medium and themselves remain colorless; and chromophorous bacteria—which possess their own color but lack chromatophores.

102

Bacteria reproduce by transverse division, forming a wall perpendicular to the longitudinal axis. This feature gives rise to the name Schizomycetes. Under certain conditions they produce refringent endospores within the cell, and these spores are liberated by a bursting of the cell wall or by a swelling of the membrane. The endospores are resistant to desiccation, cold, heat, and cellular toxins. On germinating they give rise to a new vegetative form, i.e. a new bacterium.

Piscine tuberculosis (tuberculosis piscium)

Tuberculosis is the most dangerous disease of aquarium fish, but to date it has been insufficiently studied. Since the external symptoms either closely resemble or are identical to those described for ichthyophonosis, it is quite easy to make an incorrect diagnosis if the presence of the causative agent is not detected in smears.

Bataillon, Dubard & Terre (1897) were the first workers to describe fish tuberculosis. They found acid-fast bacilli in a tumor present in the visceral cavity of a carp. They were also able to isolate the bacterium in pure culture and successfully reproduced the condition by means of the inoculation of other cold-blooded animals. In 1902 Terre again observed the same disease in carp. Bertarelli & Bocchia (1910) inoculated the bacilli of avian tuberculosis into goldfish (*Carassius auratus*). Von Betegh (1910) also mentioned the presence of acid-fast bacilli in fish. Maie (1922) performed experimental inoculations with goldfish. Aronson (1926) observed acid-fast bacilli in the spleen and liver of marine fish from the Philadelphia aquarium. Schreitmüller & Lederer (1930) encountered tubercular tumor-like formations in veiltails and Indian climbing perch (*Anabas testudineus*) from the Aquarium of the Frankfurt Zoological Gardens. The eyes, intestine and liver were seen to be affected. Of greater importance were the experiments of Jahnel (1940) on spontaneous infection of fish by acid-fast bacilli. Baker and Hagen (1942), Nigrelli (1943), Besse (1949), Reichenbach-Klinke (1953, 54), Amlacher (1959) and Bandlow (1959) observed further cases of this disease.

CLINICAL PICTURE AND SYMPTOMS: fish tuberculosis quite frequently leads to mass mortalities, particularly in tanks and large commercial installations. The external symptoms are as follows:

(a) internal emaciation, so marked that the fish appears to have a hollow belly;

(b) loss of weight which is apparent by their thin backs;

(c) loss of appetite;

(d) loss of color and paleness;

(e) scale defects and desquamation; superficial open ulcers; fin rot;

(f) deformities of the mandibles and the vertebral column;

(g) exophthalmos, falling out of the eyes (*Figure 45*);

103

(*h*) apathy and disturbance of swimming;

(*i*) nodules on and in the internal organs.

The fish behave in a listless manner, and commonly bang themselves against a corner of the tank. Frequently they are seen to be swimming obliquely, with the caudal fin retracted and the belly hanging down (when the swim bladder is affected).

On the surface of the internal organs may be seen soft nodules or lesions of a dirty grayish color, and of a pin-head size (*Figure 46*). In opposition to that which has been stated by many authors, it is uncommon to observe external nodular formations. The diseased swim bladder is white and full of a serous fluid. According to Besse, the presence of a colorless ascitic fluid may also be detected in the abdominal cavity.

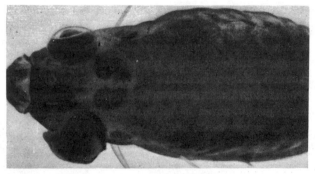

Figure 45. Tuberculous exophthalmos. (Amlacher)

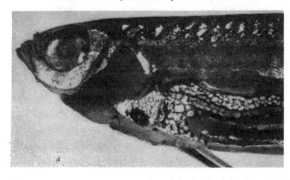

Figure 46. Spontaneous tuberculosis in *Daniomalabaricus*, showing numerous tubercles in the intestinal organs. (Jahnel)

TECHNIQUE OF INVESTIGATION: only live fish are of value for investigation. Smears obtained by squashing portions of the intestine, spleen, liver, kidney, heart and eye chamber are examined under a magnification of × 80–600. In the event that a brownish-yellow necrosis is present, it is advisable to make smears directly from the organs, particularly from the spleen and liver; these are stained by the Ziehl-Neelsen method, and observed under the oil immersion objective. For further studies on certain organs, the material is fixed in aqueous formalin (1 part of 40% formalin to 4 parts of water) or in Stieve's fluid. To stain bacteria in sections, the method indicated above should be followed.

According to Jahnel, a bacteriological investigation should be performed with fish killed by means of an electric current. The dead fish are placed for a short time in alcoholic formalin or in 70% alcohol, and immediately passed through a flame to dry the surface. With flamed instruments the lateral wall of the body is removed, material is taken from the liver, spleen and kidney with a spatula, and streaked onto tubes of Petragnani's medium. The tubes are incubated at 18–20° C. (approximately the normal room temperature). After 14 days the colonies are just visible to the naked eye. After a further week the little colonies join together and later form a moist clear yellow layer; this coloration becomes first lemon yellow and then orange-yellow (in old cultures). the same picture occurs with colonies on other media containing egg yolk. The addition of glycerine favors growth. The optimum temperature lies between 18–25° C., but some also grow well at temperatures of up to 30° C. No growth occurs at 37° C. In my own investigations (Amlacher 1967) good growth was obtained on my own mediums (*Figure 47*).

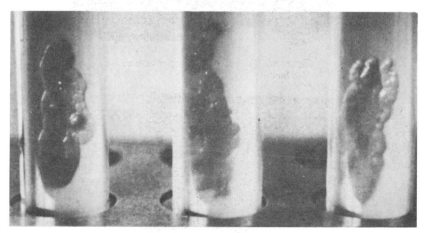

Figure 47. Subcultures of *Mycobacterium piscium*. (Amlacher)

Besse (1949) used different culture media, among which those of Petragnani, Lowenstein, Laporte and Jensen gave the best results. According to Besse the fish tuberculosis bacillus grows at temperatures between 12–33° C., with an optimum of 25° C. The same author believes that growth may occur up to 37° C. The colonies first begin to become visible after 7–8 days (Besse) and at the end of 15 days they reach a diameter of 0.5 mm., and 1 mm. after 21 days. Month old colonies have a granular appearance, and their color ranges from cream to orange-yellow. Besse confirmed that the most rapid growth takes place on Petragnani's medium.

A concentration method described by Conroy (1966) is based on that described by Petroff for human tubercle bacilli. A portion of the organ is removed and digested with 4% sodium hydroxide solution for 30–40 minutes at 25° C. The liquefied material is then centrifuged at 3000 rpm. for 30 minutes, and the supernatant removed by means of a sterile Pasteur pipette. Following the addition of a drop of a suitable indicator, the whole is neutralized with 6% hydrochloric acid. After this the material is carefully washed several times with sterile distilled water, centrifuging each time at 3000 r.p.m., and the deposit finally streaked onto a suitable culture medium. It may also be smeared onto slides for microscopical examination. This method has also been found useful in screening suspected carriers in quarantine, the fish being placed in chemically clean containers floating in the aquarium, and any feces dropped by the individual fish are collected with a pipette and submitted to the concentration method described. In this way it is possible to eliminate asymptomatic carriers from a population.

ETIOLOGY; MORPHOLOGY AND TAXONOMY OF THE CAUSATIVE AGENT; COURSE OF THE DISEASE: the probable agent of fish tuberculosis is *Mycobacterium piscium* Bergey et al (*Figure 48*). (*Mycobacterium piscium* is the name given to the organism isolated by Bataillon, Dubard and Terre from a carp. Other species of mycobacteria isolated from fish include *Myco. marinum*, *Myco. anabanti*, *Myco. platypoecilus*, *Myco fortuitum* and *Myco. salmoniphilum*. The present confusion in the taxonomy of the acid-fast bacteria tends to discourage the giving of a specific name to cultures isolated from fish, and such organisms should therefore be referred to as acid-fast bacilli resembling mycobacteria, until such time as they have been exhaustively examined by a specialist in mycobacterial taxonomy.) Almost all species of freshwater fish may be attacked, as much in cold water as in tropical water. *Myco. piscium* is an aerobic Gram positive, non-motile, acid-fast rod, with a very variable length (2–12 microns). The optimal growth temperature is 25° C., and the highest lethal temperature is 37° C.

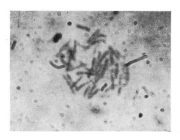

Figure 48. Distribution of acid-fast bacilli in the form of a cluster, from the spleen of *Nannacara anomala*. (Amlacher)

Jahnel (1940) observed the following cell size of the acid-fast bacilli from different species of tropical fish:

FISH SPECIES	LENGTH OF BACILLI IN MICRONS
Brachydanio albolineatus Blyth	2–3
Danio malabaricus Jordan	2–3
Gymnocorymbus ternetzi Boulenger	3–3.5
Haplochromis multicolor Hilgendorf	4–5
Aphyocharax rubropinnis Pappenheim	4–10

Besse observed the following sizes:

FISH SPECIES	LENGTH OF BACILLI IN MICRONS
Macropodus opercularis	1.5
Betta splendens Regan	1–1.2
Danio malabaricus Jordan	1.5–3.5
cyprinids	1

Reichenbach-Klinke (1954) obtained the following results:

FISH SPECIES	LENGTH OF BACILLI IN MICRONS
Cichlasoma meeki Brind	3–5
Hyphessobrycon innesi Myers	5–7
Tanichthys albonubes Linnaeus	5–7
Apistogramma ramirezi Myers & Harry	5–7
Symphysodon discus Heckel	6–8
Pterophyllum scalare C. & V.	6–10
Lebistes reticulatus Peters	6–10
Trichogaster leeri Bleeker	6–12
Barbus conchonius Hamilton-Buchanan	10–12

My own personal investigations (Amlacher, 1959) gave:

FISH SPECIES	LENGTH OF BACILLI IN MICRONS
Nannacara anomala Regan	1.7–2.8
Hyphessobrycon callistus Durbin	1.7–2.8
Hyphessobrycon callistus Durbin	1.3–4.4
Macropodus opercularis	2.2–3.3

My colleague Bandlow (1959) observed the following measurements:

FISH SPECIES	LENGTH OF BACILLI IN MICRONS
Nannacara anomala Regan	1.3–4.5
Barbus conchonius Hamilton-Buchanan	1.5–4.5
Brachydanio rerio Hamilton-Buchanan	1.5–3.2
Tanichthys albonubes Lin-Shu-Jen	1.8–3.3
Xiphophorus helleri Heckel	2.5–4
Hemigrammus ocellifer Steindachner	1.3–3.5
Hyphessobrycon serpae Durbin	1.5–2.3
Aequidens curviceps Ahl	2.1–4
Haplochromis multicolor Hilgendorf	2.3–3.5

With regards to the length of these organisms, our investigations up to the present are in agreement with those of Jahnel, Besse, and Bandlow, but I have no doubt that bacilli may be encountered which have a greater length.

The disease is passed from one fish to another, in all probability, with the bottom material.

Within the last few years, evidence has accumulated to the effect that tuberculosis may be transmitted by the intra-ovarian route in certain viviparous fishes (Nigrelli and Vogel, 1963). That this is so has been definitely demonstrated by Conroy (1966) in Mexican platys, where it seems that the embryos acquire the infection through ingestion of the intra-ovarian fluid from the infected ovary of the mother. The spread of tuberculosis in hatchery raised salmonids was due to the incorporation of diseased salmon viscera in the feed (Wood and Ordal 1958; Ross, Earp and Wood, 1959).

Sick fish are inclined to show listlessness prior to the appearance of the first external symptoms, or even in the absence of these latter. The disease may occur as an epizootic in such a manner that a lot of fish die suddenly without displaying any clear and well defined external symptoms; however in the majority of cases its course is slow and the symptoms vary in accordance with the nature of the organs affected. With great frequency the belly is found to be swollen and hollow, and there are hemorrhagic ulcers and scale defects. Besse observed opacity of the cornea in the eye, and blackening of the body. In severe cases Bandlow found fish with a fallen belly, this occurring as a result of a severe infection of the swim bladder.

Besse (1949) differentiated the following types of fish tuberculosis:
(a) tuberculosis of the Paradise fish group;
(b) ascites of the fighting fish group;
(c) exophthalmos in *Brachydanio*;
(d) nodule formation in the cyprinids;
(e) emaciation in the poecilids.

According to Besse, of 288 tropical fish examined, 243 of them were infected with acid-fast bacilli, i.e. an 80% positive result. In the opinion of the author, certain families such as the anabantids and the characins have a special predisposition towards this disease. These two groups are followed in turn by the Melanotaenidae, Cyprinodontidae, tropical cyprinids, Poecilidae, Cichlidae and Centrarchidae, in that order. The species *Hyphessobrycon flammeus* and *Pristella riddlei* are, according to Besse, particularly susceptible species.

It should be noted in this context that acid-fast bacteria identified as *Nocardia asteroides* have been isolated from cases of "tuberculosis" in tropical fish (Conroy, 1964). Nocardiosis has since been described as a disease of rainbow trout (Snieszko, Bullock, Dunbar and Pettijohn, 1965; Ghittino and Penna, 1968), and the whole question of nocardial infections in fish has recently been reviewed by Heuchsmann-Brunner (1965).

Jahnel, Besse, and Reichenbach-Klinke were able to transmit tuberculosis experimentally to healthy fish using pure cultures, and produced typical symptoms of the disease. Transmission of acid-fast bacteria which we isolated from *Gymnocorymbus ternetzi* and cultivated in *Cyprinus carpio* succeeded without difficulty (Amlacher 1967).

The following species of fish are considered to be predisposed to tuberculosis, in accordance with work carried out up to the present time.

Table 5
Tuberculosis Disposed Species

FAMILY	SPECIES	AUTHOR
Anabantidae	*Macropodus opercularis*	Besse
	Betta splendens	Besse
	Ctenops vittatus	Besse
	Colisa lalia	Besse
	Colisa labiosa	Amlacher
	Trichogaster trichopterus	Besse
	Trichogaster leeri	Reichenbach-Klinke
Characinidae	*Hyphessobrycon flammeus*	Besse
	Hyphessobrycon gracilis	Besse
	Hyphessobrycon ornatus	Amlacher
	Hyphessobrycon innesi	Besse
	Hyphessobrycon callistus	Amlacher
	Hyphessobrycon serpae	Bandlow
	Hasemania marginata	Amlacher
	Hemigrammus unilineatus	Besse
	Hemigrammus ocellifer	Bandlow
	Hemigrammus caudovittatus	Amlacher
	Aphyocharax rubropinnis	Jahnel
	Gymnocorymbus ternetzi	Jahnel
	Pristella riddlei	Besse
Cyprinodontidae	*Rivulus cylindraceus*	Besse
	Aplocheilus latipes	Besse
	Panchax panchax	Besse
	Aphyosemion australe	Besse
Cyprinidae	*Tanichthys albonubes*	Reichenbach-Klinke
	Rasbora heteromorpha	Besse
	Danio malabaricus	Jahnel
	Brachydanio rerio	Besse
	Brachydanio albolineatus	Jahnel
	Puntius conchonius	Amlacher
	Puntius nigrofasciatus	Amlacher
	Barbus conchonius	Besse
	Cyprinus carpio	
	Carassius auratus	
	Tinca vulgaris	Besse
	Tanichthys albonubes	Amlacher
Poecilidae	*Xiphophorus helleri*	Besse
	Lebistes reticulatus	Besse
	Belonesox belizanus	Amlacher
	Mollienisia sphenops	Amlacher
	Cnesterodon decemmaculatus	Amlacher
	Platypoecilus maculatus	Besse
Melanotaenidae	*Melanotaenia nigrans*	Besse

Cichlidae	Hemichromis bimaculatus	Besse
	Aequidens curviceps	Bandlow
	Aequidens maroni	Amlacher
	Pterophyllum scalare	Besse
	Apistogramma ramirezi	Reichenbach-Klinke
	Cichlasoma meeki	Reichenbach-Klinke
	Cichlasoma biocellatum	Amlacher
	Haplochromis multicolor	Jahnel
	Symphysodon discus	Reichenbach-Klinke
	Nannacara anomala	Amlacher
Centrarchidae	Eupomotis gibbosus	Besse
flatfish	Hippoglossus vulgaris	Sutherland
(Heterosomata)		
coral fish	Abudefduf mauritii	Aronson
	Centropristes striatus	Aronson
	Micropogon undulatus	Aronson
Pantodontidae	Pantodon buchholzi	Amlacher

(For a complete list of susceptible cold-blooded vertebrates see Nigrelli and Vogel 1963):

HISTOPATHOLOGY AND HISTOCHEMISTRY: in stained smears from the internal organs, the bacterium responsible for fish tuberculosis is generally-to be found in groups of two or three, as a "V", or in groups somewhat resembling nests (*Figure 49*).

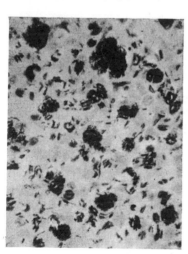

Figure 49. Massive agglomeration of tubercle bacilli, isolated and in clumps, from the swimbladder of *Nannacara anomala*. (Bandlow)

The spontaneous formation, as well as the experimental, of tuberculous granulomas is a proliferative process, in which reticulogenic macrophages take part (*Figure 50*). The resulting epitheloid cell tubercle necrotizes in the center, the necrosis proceeds toward the periphery. In the center of the necrotic tubercle, lies nuclear detritus. The necrotic center is bordered by several concentrated layers of necrotizing epitheloid cells

110

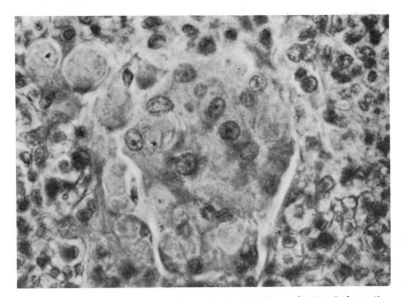

Figure 50. Proliferating macrophages in the initial stage of tubercle formation. (Amlacher)

Figure 51. Tubercles showing various stages of central necrosis. (Amlacher)

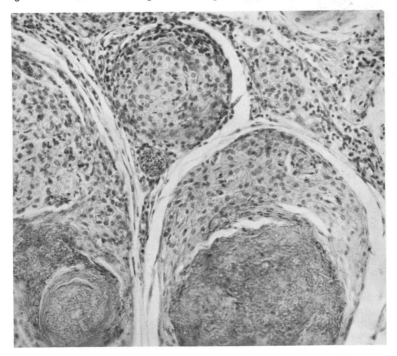

(*Figure 51*). The tubercles are set off from the intact organ tissue by connective tissue. Giant cells have not been observed with spontaneous originating granulomas, in the experimental they occasionally appear. Older tubercles are usually completely necrotic, the necrotic material bordered directly by the connective tissue shell of the tubercle. The tubercles are PAS positive. Iron containing macrophages are particularly involved in the spleen. In addition to submiliary and miliary tubercles, the formation of conglomerate tubercles is frequent, and extension can destroy entire organs (*Figure 52*). Inside the tubercle, acid-fast bacilli are

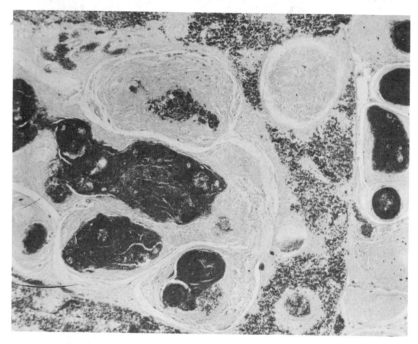

Figure 52. Fusion of tubercles, forming large conglomerate lesions.

regularly demonstrated especially after experimental infections (*Figures 53, 54*). Melanin accumulation in the tubercles show new formation of argyrophilic lattice fibers. The size of the tubercle is between about 60mu and 2000mu, the experimental initial stages of which have been described. Occasionally, the tubercle formation is accompanied by an inflammatory process, with which we find eosinophilic granulocytes. Late stages of the tuberculosis disease are marked by cirrhotic changes (*Figure 55*). It affects all organs: liver (*Figure 56*), spleen, kidney (*Figure 57*), heart, in-

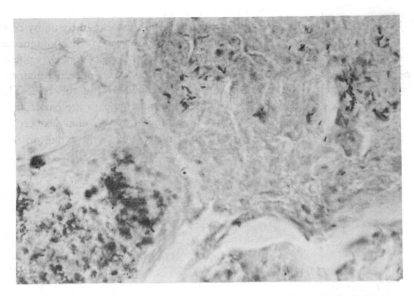

Figure 53. Tubercles from experimental infection exhibiting high concentration of acid-fast organisms. Oil immersion. (Amlacher)

Figure 54. Tubercles exhibiting numerous acid-fast organisms. (Amlacher)

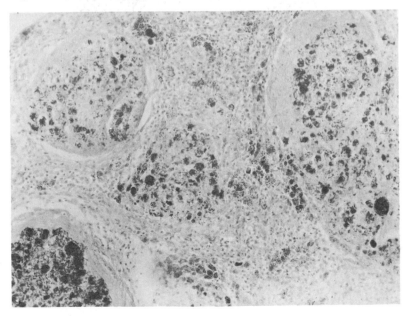

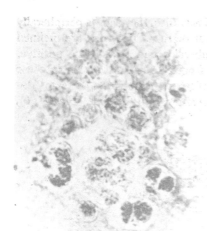

Figure 55. Spleen of *Nannacara anomala* with masses of necrotizing tubercle bacilli and incipient connective tissue encapsulation. (Original)

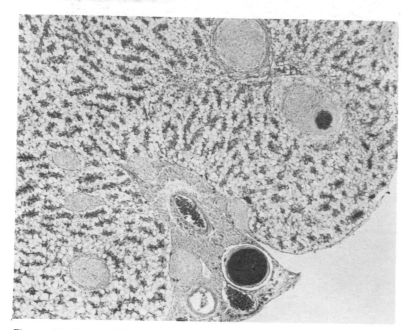

Figure 56. Liver with tubercles in various stages of development. (Amlacher)

testinal tract (*Figure 58*), gills, musculature, skin, eyes and skeleton. Occasionally, concurrent formation of edema occurs. Blood vessels can be closed by tubercles which grow into their lumen (*Figure 59*). Necrosis of the tubules is characteristic for the kidney. Rarely is the disease course septic. The granulomas of inoculated tuberculosis (*Figure 60*) are basically similar to those of spontaneous tuberculosis. Also, they show a peripherally progressing central necrosis with nuclear detritus. They also are inclined toward formation of conglomerate tubercles and react PAS positive. Occasionally, indications of giant cell formation are to be seen in these granulomas. Likewise, new formation of lattice fibers are to be seen. Also with inoculated tuberculosis, vessel alterations are frequent (*Figure 59*), likewise necrosis of the kidney tubules.

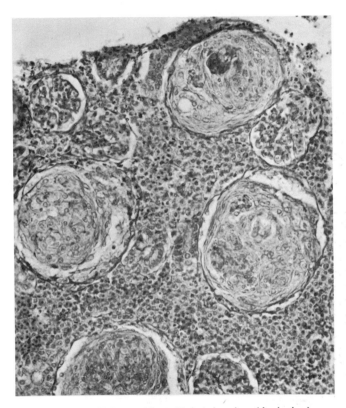

Figure 57. Kidney with multiple tubercles. (Amlacher)

Bandlow (1959) submitted the tubercle bacilli to Konrich's test, and from this observed that they did not decolorize after 24 hours treatment with sodium sulfite solution. The same author confirms the results of von Bergens (1922), according to whom the bacilli responsible for tuberculosis in cold-blooded animals are also resistant to the sulfite; they behave in other words like the remaining types of tubercle bacilli, and cannot be differentiated histochemically by Konrich's method.

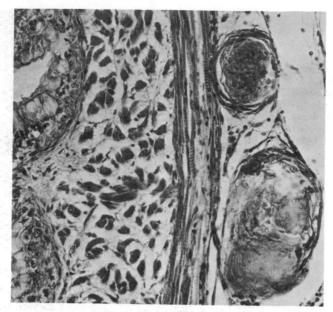

Figure 58. Intestinal blood vessels occluded by tubercle formation. (Amlacher)

Figure 59. Liver with plugged blood vessel (lower center) caused by tubercle formation. (Amlacher)

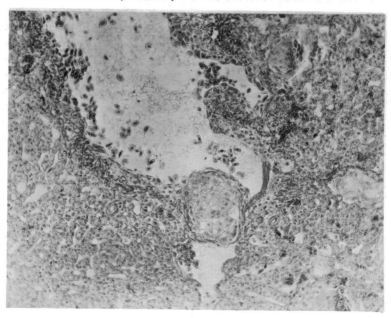

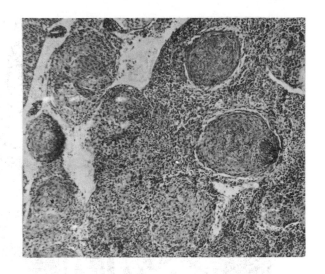

Figure 60. Experimental fish tuberculosis showing similarity of tubercles with those of the spontaneous disease. (Amlacher)

THERAPY, PROPHYLAXIS AND HYGIENE: Conroy (1966) reported 0.01% Kanamycin in the feed was effective. For a review of the subject see Conroy (1967). It may be stated on a basis of the research work carried out up to the present that tuberculosis is one of the results of a defective hygiene in the tank or pond, as occurs with human tuberculosis, where poor housing facilities and accommodation results in a higher incidence of the disease. The same thing occurs in cattle which are badly stabled. This is a good point at which to again remind the reader of my strongest recommendation: the minimum quantity of water per fish should never be less than 5 liters, and aquarium hygiene is most important in helping to prevent outbreaks of this infection. I know of aquarists who have had outstanding success simply by following to the spirit of the letter this piece of golden advice. As a prophylactic measure it is important not to stock the water too densely either with alevins or with adult fish. Attention must also be paid to general cleanliness, and contact between separate tanks must be studiously avoided on all occasions. Mixed tanks always constitute permanent foci of infection for fish tuberculosis.

Bacterial hemorrhagic septicemia; (Infectious abdominal dropsy or ascites: myo-entero-hepatic syndrome)

Infectious abdominal dropsy has been known for a long time and was studied by Schäperclaus (1930), who in his work made reference to historical sources. The disease was described scientifically by this same worker (Schäperclaus, 1928), in whose paper a picture of the possible causative organism first appeared. This infection owes its name to one of the predominant symptoms observed at the time, namely ascites and swelling of the body in the ventral region. The different types of symptoms displayed by fish infected with the disease has meant that it has also become known by many other names such as "Red Pest" and hemorrhagic septicemia. Numerous investigations carried out, particularly by Lajmann and Spolianskaia (1949), Herzog (1950), Schäperclaus (1956a, 1957), Wunder and Dombrowski (1953), Kopp (1951), Zöbe (1952), Flemming (1954, 58), Amlacher (1957d, 1958c), Offhaus, Brunner and Riedmüller (1955), and Bank (1960) have helped to complete our knowledge of the disease, especially with reference to its histopathology and physiology. The concept of infectious abdominal dropsy serves little other purpose than that of characterizing one single symptom of the disease, but since this terminology has acquired a certain popularity there is little doubt that it will continue to be used to describe this infection.

The disease is typical of the cyprinids (*Figures 61 and 64*). The losses among one-year-old carp (C_1) are between 20–40%. Dropsy is rather exceptional among tropical aquarium fish, and even when it does occur it appears more likely to be the sequel to some other infectious disease such as tuberculosis (*Figures 62 and 63*).

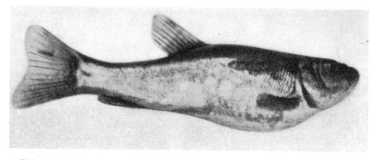

Figure 61. Tench with bacterial hemorrhagic septicemia. (Original)

CLINICAL PICTURE AND SYMPTOMS: from our experience of fish farming we know that there are two types of external symptoms which can be differentiated on sight; these are:

(*a*) typical dropsy (*Figure 64*);

(*b*) the ulcerative type (this shows scale defects on rare occasions) (*Figure 65*).

These two principal forms are related to each other by "transition forms" according to Schäperclaus (1954b) and Amlacher (1958c), and when the syndrome is well marked both types of symptoms may occur simultaneously. Amlacher (1959a) has distinguished three forms of infectious abdominal dropsy which are characterized as follows:

118

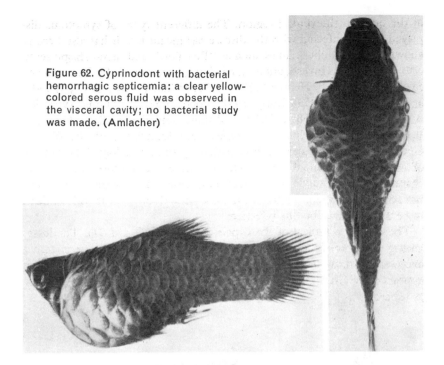

Figure 62. Cyprinodont with bacterial hemorrhagic septicemia: a clear yellow-colored serous fluid was observed in the visceral cavity; no bacterial study was made. (Amlacher)

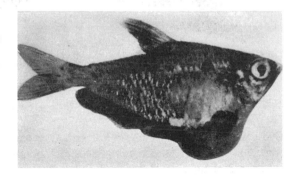

Figure 63. *Hyphessobrycon callistus* with ascitic cyst in the abdominal cavity, probably the result of a severe tuberculosis of the internal organs. (Amlacher)

(i) chronic ulcerative form. Ulcers in the skin and musculature.

The color of the ulcers, particularly when they are tending to heal up, is from the outside inwards: black, white, red. At times these are losses of the scales and fins, and very infrequently skeletal deformities. The internal organs remain normal in size in the majority of cases. The liver may appear to be normal but in certain instances it is hyperemic, due to capillary blood extasis and hyperemia of the portal branches. The hepatic glycogen reaction is positive and the blood sugar normal (with an average

119

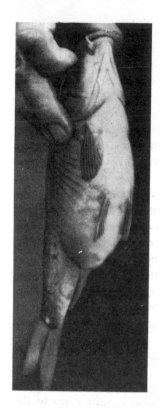

Figure 64. Carp with bacterial hemorrhagic septicemia (ascitic form) and anal prolapse. (Schäperclaus)

Figure 65. Carp with bacterial hemorrhagic septicemia (ulcerative form). (Schäperclaus)

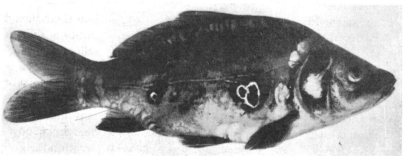

value of 60 mgm/100 ml.). There is no fluid in the visceral cavity. The occurrence of small amounts of fluid, in spring, may be a symptom of a slight edema produced by hunger. Most probably there is no destruction of the blood, or at least a very slight one. This form may pass to the subacute and to the acute forms respectively (see *Table 8*).

(ii) acute ascitic form (ascites *sensu stricto*): Exophthalmos or sunken eyes. The anus is inflamed and prolapsed. There is a foul-smelling yellowish or bloody-watery fluid in the abdominal cavity, or a gelatinous mass formed by the clotting of the ascitic fluid. In other instances this fluid is watery, clear in color and odorless. The intestine may be inflamed and hyperemic, and as thin as paper. The liver is yellow, dark yellow, gray-yellow, gray-green or pea green; at times with white or yellowish-colored blotches, and at other times with punctiform hyperemia (petechiae). Quite often the kidney is of a soft pasty consistency, and the spleen swollen. Scale defects, fin rot and ulcerations may be secondarily associated with the above symptoms. The hepatic glycogen is negative, and the blood sugar about 30 mgm./100 ml. (at times it may be as low as 14 mgm./100 ml.). The bilirubin level is raised to approximately double the normal figure (80 mgm./100 ml.). The total serum protein may be as low as 1.5 mgm./100 ml. Weltmann's band is cut short. This test is the band of serum coagulation when blood serum is placed into tubes containing different concentrations of calcium chloride. The band is interpreted as the number of tubes which coagulate as a result of a colloidal lability shown by the test serum. It is a proof or test of hepatic function. A widening and a narrowing of the band represents a greater and a lesser number of tubes showing coagulation respectively. The cadmium sulfate turbidity test gives rise to a strong turbidity. The disease occurs during the spring, producing numerous and heavy losses, and almost always as a mass mortality.

(iii) latent form: This form is not easy to diagnose with much degree of certainty. According to the experience we have obtained up to the present we may further sub-divide it as follows:

(a) sub-acute form: externally there are no symptoms, or if there should be any such there is nothing more than a small quantity of fluid in the visceral cavity. The liver is of a deep green, yellow or normal color. Very little ascitic fluid is present. The hepatic glycogen is positive, weakly positive or negative. The blood sugar is normal or slightly sub-normal. Weltmann's band is extended.

(b) dry form: no external symptoms. There is never any fluid in the visceral cavity, although there is a strongly perceptible ascitic odor. The liver is usually normal, but practically always with adhesions to the visceral cavity. The hepatic glycogen is weakly positive or negative. The blood sugar level is not known.

In the ulcerative form of the disease the carp usually behave in a normal manner. The sick ones are generally quite easy to recognize by their feeble and listless swimming, and by the fact that they tend to keep themselves near to the sides of the tank. It is common to encounter pieces of free and inflamed intestinal mucus in the water, often in the form of the intestine itself. Fish which are suffering from the sub-acute form of the

121

disease behave in exactly the same manner as those suffering from the acute form.

TECHNIQUE OF INVESTIGATION: if the external clinical picture is not sufficient to enable a concrete diagnosis to be made, the fish is submitted to an autopsy. On carrying out the autopsy, the liver gives useful data as was shown by Amlacher (1958c). The hepatic lesions may have the following interpretations:

(a) green coloration: destruction of the liver cells by biliary stasis;

(b) yellow coloration: adipose (fatty) dystrophy of the liver cells;

(c) blotches (the liver has a speckled aspect); zones of necrosis distributed throughout the liver tissues;

(d) a coloration ranging from rust red to blue; stasis due to inflammation of the blood vessels.

To complete the diagnosis, small portions of the liver are fixed in Stieve's fluid or in alcoholic formalin (alcohol 2: formalin 1), and the glycogen content is determined. Bauer's reaction for polysaccharides is very precise:

(a) fixation in one of the following fixatives: Stieve's, Carnoy's, alcoholic formalin;

(b) deparaffinization in xylol, absolute alcohol, celloidin (1–2 minutes in alcohol-ether, 2–3 minutes in etheric alcohol solution of 2% celloidin, 3 minutes in 80% alcohol);

(c) immersion in a freshly prepared 4% chromic acid solution for an hour (in the dark);

(d) wash in running water for 5 minutes;

(e) immersion in sulfurous acid—fuchsin for 10–15 minutes;

(f) wash in tap water for 10 minutes;

(g) 80–90% alcohol, absolute alcohol, remove the celloidin (from the absolute alcohol pass the sections for 3–5 minutes into ether-alcohol), absolute alcohol, xylol and balsam.

It is advisable not to stain the nuclei. To obtain sections the best fixative is Stieve's fluid. In order to finally establish a correct diagnosis it is necessary to certify the presence of the causative agent, in which instance material from the fish should be cultured onto agar, gelatine, or in broth.

ETIOLOGY; MORPHOLOGY AND TAXONOMY OF THE CAUSATIVE AGENT; COURSE OF THE DISEASE: The etiological agent of infectious abdominal dropsy is an aquatic bacterium, *Aeromonas liquefaciens typus* (or *forma*) *ascitae* Schäperclaus (*Figure 66*). In addition to this, the much less pathogenic *Aeromonas liquefaciens forma typica* Zimmermann also lives in open waters. On the other hand Pieskov, Goncharov and Tomaseč cited a virus as being responsible for this disease. Tomaseč (1965) and Fijan (1965) reported that infection experiments with cell-free filtrates were successful and they observed cytopathogenic effects also in cultures of kidney cells of the carp.

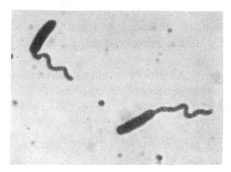

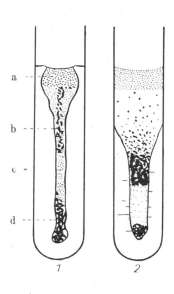

Figure 66. Aeromonas *liquefaciens* forma ascitae, Schäperclaus strain. (Schäperclaus)

Figure 67. Gelatin stab cultures of *Aeromonas liquefaciens* (18°C. cultures after ten days):
(1) *forma ascitae* Schäperclaus, strain 1218.
(2) *forma typica* Zimmermann, Muggel strain.

Aeromonas liquefaciens forma ascitae has the following characteristics according to Schäperclaus: it is a Gram negative, asporogenous and monotrichous rod measuring 0.4–0.5 × 0.9 microns. It dies out when the rivers and streams in which it lives dry up, or under the action of quicklime. Heat above 50° C. is lethal within 1–2 hours. The organism stains with aniline dyes or with iron hematoxylin. Agar cultures are of a grayish-white coloration and are smooth. Gelatine is rapidly liquefied (*Figure 67*). Gelatine plate cultures have a feathery appearance on the external border (*Figure 68*). In the liquefied zone are to be seen accumulations of punctiform bacteria. Milk is clotted and then digested. Cultures in litmus-casein-sugar at 22°C. give the following results after 2–3 days (Schäperclaus).
give the following results after 2–3 days (Schäperclaus):

MEDIUM	RED COLOR	REACTION		DECOLORIZATION
		GAS	COAGULATION	
litmus casein glucose	+ +	− / + +	+ / + +	—
litmus casein lactose	− / +	—	—	—
litmus casein saccharose	+ +	− / + +	+ / + +	—
litmus casein mannitol	+ +	− / + +	+ / + +	—
litmus casein maltose	+ +	− / + +	+ / + +	—

Broth cultures become intensely turbid at 22° C. and form a tenuous pellicle. Nitrates are reduced to nitrites. *A. liquefaciens* is a facultative

123

anerobe. 4 cc. of an agar culture of *A. liquefaciens forma typica* distributed in boiled water and injected intra-peritoneally into a 300–800 gm. carp maintained in water at a temperature of 16° C. produce symptoms of the disease in 24–48 hours, and in certain cases cause death towards the end of 6 days.

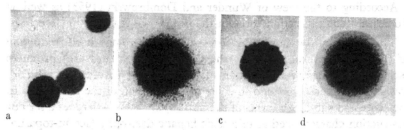

Figure 68. Gelatin plate culture of *Aeromonas liquefaciens forma ascitae*, strain 1218: after 30 hours at 21°C. (a) 0.05–0.2 mm. diameter; after 3 days (b) 0.3 mm. diameter; with ring formation (c) 0.3 mm. diameter, still without liquefaction of the medium; (d) 0.5 mm. diameter, beginning of liquefaction. (Schäperclaus)

Aeromonas subrubra is associated with *A. liquefaciens forma ascitae*. The former is of the same size, is non-pathogenic and has a completely different physiological behavior. This makes the obtaining of pure cultures of *A. liquefaciens forma ascitae* very difficult, and for this reason to obtain them at all one must start off with a single cell. Another bacterium associated with *A. liquefaciens* is *Pseudomonas fluorescens*, and this is pathogenic.

A. liquefaciens forma ascitae shows many biotypes which are differentiated by their different virulence and certain other peculiarities. This would explain the varied clinical picture seen in dropsy (ulcers, ascites), together with the susceptibility of the carp to strange types of bacteria (see epidemio-biological equilibrium). The bacteria causing infectious abdominal dropsy reach the intestinal tract together with mud from the tank. Since carp hardly feed at all during the winter period and there is no continual passage of chyme which eliminates the bacteria, these latter are concentrated in the intestine according to Schäperclaus. At the same time, as shown by Kopp (1951), hunger causes lesions in the intestinal mucosa and this favors the passage of bacteria into the bloodstream. This is what gives rise to inflammation of the intestinal wall and the transport of toxins to the liver via the intestinal and portal blood vessels. In this way the liver, which is in reality a gland functioning as a detoxicating center, is severely lesioned chiefly as a result of the action of hepatotropic bacteria. These same bacteria may also end up in other places such as the skin and muscles, to which they are transported by blood and lymph vessels. These dermotropic and myotropic types of *A. liquefaciens* give rise to small "bladders" in the integument, and ulcers in the musculature respectively. Ulceration is also induced by parasitic infestations, as shown by Dombrowski (1953) in particular. According to this worker the biting action of leeches (*Piscicola*) and carp lice (*Argulus*) could be a factor contributing to ulceration.

According to the view of Wunder and Dombrowski (1953) as well as Tomaseč (1965), infection through the skin is the real path of infection.

The lesions of the hepatic blood vessels and the blood itself (reduction of the albumin level and thus the colloid osmotic pressure) produces ascites. Inflammatory obstruction of the bile duct may produce biliary stasis (deep green color) and in consequence a lesion of the liver cells. In the acute and sub-acute forms of the disease, the liver undergoes a serious destruction characterized as of a toxic hepatic dystrophy (see histopathology and histochemistry).

My own investigations have lead me to the following conclusion: infectious abdominal dropsy occurs as two principal well known types, ascitic dropsy and ulcerative dropsy, respectively. Any one of these two forms may develop into the other, and each is clearly apparent by the type of symptom produced. There is no other external symptom which determines the course of the disease, except in the case of the acute form. The nature of the disease may be investigated by means of Bauer's histochemical reaction for glycogen. I showed that the amount of glycogen is diminished, without any doubt whatsoever, as the liver cells are progressively being destroyed, and that the ulcerative form may appear without any of the internal organs (particularly the liver) being involved. In this case the hepatic glycogen reaction is positive, as is the same in healthy fish. The appearance of small amounts of ascitic fluid in the visceral cavity, in the ascitic form, tends to indicate an initial reduction of the glycogen level. This reduction is much more pronounced in the sub-acute form. Finally, in carp suffering from the acute form of the disease, we find a negative glycogen reaction, the same as in fish having a deep green colored liver. However carp infected experimentally by the intra-peritoneal route gave a positive reaction, proof that the death of such animals is apparently due to a septicemia.

As was made quite clear by Dombrowski (1953), Flemming (1954), and by Amlacher (1956a, 1957d), the blood is also affected. The erythrocytes are progressively destroyed, and the leucocytes increase in number almost some 50% above the normal figure. The nucleus and cytoplasm are vacuolated. The hemoglobin is reduced to below 5.3 gm./100 ml. (Dombrowski). The hematological results on healthy and diseased 2-year-old carp are shown in table 6 (data according to Dombrowski):

TABLE 6: Numbers and percentage of blood elements and hemoglobin in healthy and dropsied carp.

	HEALTHY FISH	DISEASED FISH
number of erythrocytes	1,500,000/cmm.	23–950,000/cmm.
number of granulocytes	75–90,000/cmm.	90–135,000/cmm.
erythrocytes/granulocytes	17–20:1	8–15:1
percentage leucocytes:		
lymphocytes	89%	58%
granulocytes	11%	12–48%
degenerated granulocytes	—	0–24%
hemoglobin	9.6 gm.%	2–5.3 gm.%

The blood plasma of healthy and acutely dropsied carp has the composition shown in table 7 (according to Dombrowski, Flemming and Amlacher):

TABLE 7: Data on the blood composition of healthy carp and others infected with infectious abdominal dropsy.

COMPONENTS	HEALTHY	DISEASED	AUTHOR
total albumin	1.9–3.95 gm.%	0.4–2.75 gm.%	Dombrowski
albumin	0.86–1.04 gm.%	0.07–0.11 gm.%	Flemming
globulin	1.48–1.98 gm.%	0.23–0.49 gm.%	Flemming
uric acid	0.56–2.64 mg.%	0.83–3.1 mg.%	Dombrowski
total cholesterol	32.6–204 mg.%	15.6–98 mg.%	Dombrowski
bilirubin	0.13–0.45 mg.%	0.43–0.85 mg.%	Amlacher
glucose	40–90 mg.%	14–53 mg.%	Amlacher

According to Flemming (1958), Weltmann's band shows coagulation in tubes number 3 or 4. In fish suffering from dropsy the level of coagulation is raised, and may be found in tube number 1 and above. On the other hand carp with retention icterus have a low coagulation point in Weltmann's test, and may produce coagulation in those tubes above number 4. This indicates the presence of cirrhogenic factors in the liver, as was subsequently demonstrated histologically by Amlacher.

HISTOPATHOLOGY AND HISTOCHEMISTRY: the blood undergoes morphological changes, with destruction and disintegration of the erythrocytes. The granulocytes (*Figures 69, 70 and 71*) show characteristic vacuolization in the nucleus and ·cytoplasm (Dombrowski, 1953; Flemming, 1954).

According to Wunder (1953), in the ulcerative form the following cutaneous and muscular changes are observed: the blood vessels break after an initial capillary hyperemia; the erythrocytes are released into the surrounding connective tissue, and the serous fluid liberated in this process penetrates into the interstitial tissue and the skin. The erythrocytes may penetrate the epidermis under pressure and produce lesions therein, or even cause parts of it to fall away. In the places most seriously affected by this process the edges of the lesions undergo a gelatinous swelling and may become edematous. On the other hand an accumulation of fluid may take place near or under the epidermis, which gives rise to the formation of boils and pustules. Histologically these boils are spaces in the

Figure 69. Blood of bream (experimentally infected by the intra-peritoneal
route with *Aeromonas liquefaciens*)
showing strongly vacuolized granulo
cyte. (Flemming)

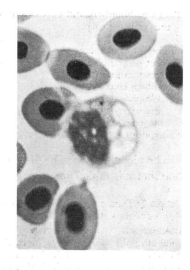

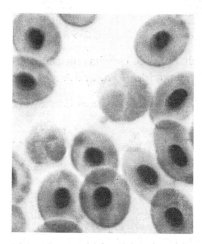

Figure 70. Blood of naturally infected
bream, showing initial vacuolar degeneration of the granulocytes. (Flemming)

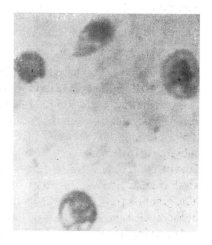

Figure 71. Blood of an acutely infected
bream, showing intense deformation
of the different blood cells: pointed
erythrocytes and two vacuolated granulocytes. (Flemming)

dermal connective tissue (chorion) or even of the epidermis (very rare).
The fluid of this edema contains serous components and isolated erythrocytes. The leucocytes, isolated or in groups, are rather more abundant.
The rupture of one of these bladder-like boils produces an open cutaneous
wound and, consequently, an ulcer where the skin is totally destroyed
down into the muscular layer. The melanophores become distributed
throughout the dermis in the vicinity of the necrotized area, and produce
a superficial black ring followed by a white one in the affected connective
tissues of the distended dermis, and finally in the muscle itself. The
muscular fibers also undergo changes. The crater of the ulcer contains

127

leucocytes towards the exterior, and leucocytes and lymphocytes in the interior. Scarring occurs from the edge of the ulcer inwards, so that at the same time that the ulcer is closed, a great quantity of melanin penetrates the newly formed tissue.

The intestine shows destruction of the mucosa, exudative inflammation of the propria, sub-mucosa, and muscularis mucosae. In the last named of these, edema may be produced which give rise to a transparent paper-like appearance of the intestine.

According to Amlacher (1958c) the liver shows the following pathological changes in carp suffering from the ulcerative form of the disease. The hepatic vessels appear to be intact as a rule, although they are usually full of blood (especially the porta). The veins are generally empty and almost all of the blood capillaries are hyperemic. The cells, nuclei and nucleoli remain intact and unaltered. The section as a whole appears perfectly normal, with the exception of the hyperemia observed in the capillaries. The glycogen level is normal, and Bauer's reaction is positive. When ascitic symptoms accompany the chronic ulcerative form, the histological picture is changed: the vessels show no visible lesions, as is the case with the chronic form; the veins are almost always empty, and are generally obstructed by connective tissue; the capillaries are dilated, at times full and at other times empty. The decisive factor is that which refers to the liver parenchyma. In this is observed first of all a marked cellular necrosis which is normally observed only in cases of acute ascites; it is nevertheless true that this type of cellular necrosis is seen only during the initial phase of the infection as a whole. Isolated histiocytes are found in the liver tissue. Small circumscribed areas of cirrhosis may be seen, these having their origin in the connective tissue blocking the veins and capillaries. The cellular necrosis is recognized by a fatty dissolution of the cell wall in practice, as well as by a partial disappearance of the nucleus and a shift in the glycogen content to give a weakly positive reaction.

In the sub-acute form are to be observed: fragmentation of the liver tissue, a similar lysis of the cell walls, and circumscribed cirrhosis. The capillaries are distended, and frequently fail to stain at all. The numerous histiocytes demonstrate the presence of a defensive reaction by the connective tissue. In 18 tests performed with 2-year-old carp the glycogen test was positive on seven occasions and negative on two of them. In fish suffering from the chronic form with ascitic symptoms, or from the sub-acute, form, it is seen that the liver parenchyma undergoes a progressive degeneration due to the cirrhotic elements which reach their maximum development in the event of a super-acute ascites. The liver shows a picture typical of an acute toxic degeneration of the tissue (*Figures 72 and 73*). The nuclei of the liver cells are still easy to stain, although the cells themselves are undergoing degeneration. The swollen capillaries resemble the histopathological picture shown by the so-called yellow liver atrophy in man. A marked cirrhosis accompanies these lesions (*Figures 74, 75, 76, 77 and 78*). The porta and the veins are seriously lesioned in the majority of cases and their cells become somewhat bladder-like. From the center, connective tissue tails, of a cirrhotic nature, penetrate into the surrounding

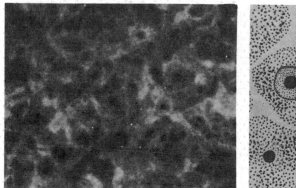 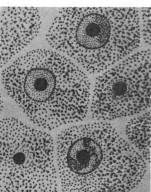

Figure 72. Toxic liver dystrophy in acute dropsy of carp, showing degeneration of the cell walls and cytoplasm, yet the nuclei and nucleoli are scarcely affected. (Amlacher)

Figure 73. Schematic representation of figure 72 condition. (Amlacher)

Figure 74. Acute bacterial hemorrhagic septicemia in carp, showing vacuolar degeneration of the liver parenchyma and to the right and below, incipient cirrhosis. (Amlacher)

Figure 75. Schematic representation of figure 74. (Amlacher)

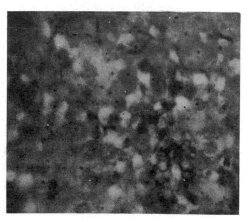 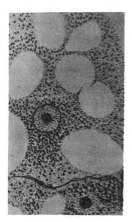

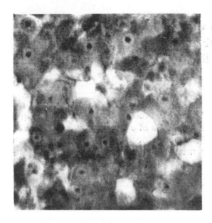 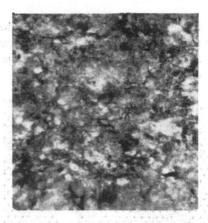

Figure 76. Acute bacterial hemorrhagic septicemia in carp, showing lacunar edemata in the diseased liver tissue. (Original)

Figure 77. Acute bacterial hemorrhagic septicemia in carp, showing very advanced cirrhosis of the hepatic connective tissue. (Amlacher)

Figure 78. Diagrams from figure 77: (a) breaking up of the liver parenchyma, cellular necrosis, and different degrees of caryolysis; (b) cirrhosis of the necrotized liver parenchyma, in which only the degenerating nuclei are visible, and showing that histiocytes have invaded the connective tissue network. (Amlacher)

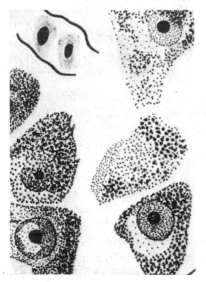 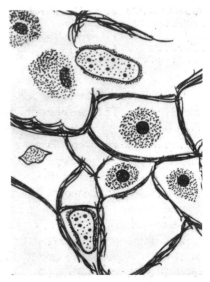

tissue. It is very common to find the vascular space occluded by connective tissue. *Figure 79* shows a vein with infiltration of rounded cells. In the space between the intestine and the liver, other inflammatory occlusions are produced (*Figure 80*).

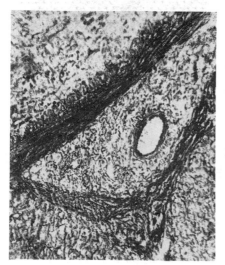

Figure 79. Acute bacterial hemorrhagic septicemia of a carp, showing a heavily inflamed blood vessel with the lumen almost closed; to the right, the neighboring bile duct is joined to the vessel as a result of the inflammation. (Amlacher)

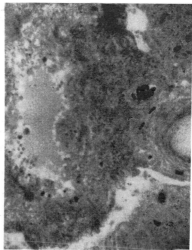

Figure 80. Acute bacterial hemorrhagic septicemia of a carp, showing connective tissue with large fibers in the space between the intestine and the liver, the result of inflammation. (Amlacher)

The contents of the blood vessels vary, and these may in fact be completely empty. They are of disordered distribution in the advanced cellular degeneration and blood capillary disorganization phase. Connective filaments lead out from their walls, indicating a scar process. Necrosis of the hepatic cells develops in three phases: it commences with a general dissolution of the cell walls (*Figures 72 and 73*) and partial karyolysis (initial phase), but it may also begin with a vacuolar degeneration (*Figures 74 and 75*) and with incipient lesions of capillary cicatrization. In this phase the cellular limits are not visible; the cytoplasm looks like a homogenous surface with degenerated nuclei and fat globules. In the majority of cases the degenerative cellular fragmentation predominates so the cells as well as the cell walls, and as much the cells as the bordering capillaries are distributed in a disorderly fashion (*Figure 78a*). The zones which in paraffin sections appear to be free from tissues, between cellular fragments, are edematous lakes. The cells show diverse grades of disintegration which are made more manifest by a destruction of nuclei and nucleoli (second phase, *Figure 78a*). Finally, the marked increase in the connective tissue eliminates any cellular detritus by means of a cirrhotic scarring process (third phase, *Figures 77 and 78b*). Tissue macrophages, or histiocytes, take part in this cleansing operation. The processes which have been described above are confirmed histochemically by a negative glycogen reaction. In the space between the intestine and the liver there are also modifications manifested by the presence of occlusions and hepato-intestinal adhesions. These points of adherence are united by a large fibrous tissue which fails to stain blue with specific connective tissue stains (*Figure 80*). Green colored livers due to biliary stasis show an intense cellular necrosis, fatty vacuolization, degenerative fragmentation, capillary hemorrhages with little blood, empty blood vessels, and cirrhosis. The glycogen reaction is negative.

Very occasionally there are lesions in the pancreas: a fatty or a fragmentary degenerative process, where the cells show displacement towards one pole of the secretion granules.

Experimentally infected carp give a positive glycogen reaction and show a distinct histopathological picture (*Figures 81 and 82*). *Table 8* gives a synopsis of the histochemical glycogen analyses carried out by Amlacher (1958). In this, the amount of glycogen is expressed as strongly positive, positive, weakly positive and negative. This table confirms the existence of three forms of dropsy (chronic, acute and sub-acute) and also indicates that transition forms of the disease do in fact occur.

TABLE 8: Qualitative glycogen data—normal and diseased livers in different types of bacterial hemorrhagic septicemia (microscopical examination).

DEGREE OF INFECTION	NUMBER OF CASES				
	NORMAL		DOUBTFUL	PATHOLOGICAL	TOTAL
	strong +	+	weakly (+)	negative	
fed normally	7	16	1	0	24
chronic ulcerative form	4	5	1	0	10
chronic, little ascites	0	1	3	2	6
sub-acute, no ascites	0	7	9	2	18
sub-acute, with ascites	0	0	5	6	11
acute, much ascites	0	0	2	9	11
green liver	0	1	0	4	5
experimentally infected	3	5	3	0	11
	14	35	24	23	96

THERAPY, PROPHYLAXIS AND HYGIENE: the susceptibility of a fish to bacterial hemorrhagic septicemia, and indeed to infectious diseases in general, depends on three factors:

(*a*) resistance (hereditary susceptibility);

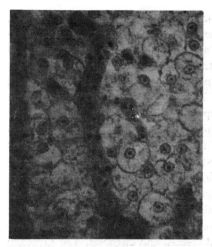 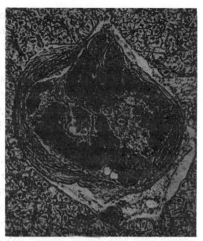

Figure 81. Carp experimentally infected with *Aeromonas liquefaciens*, showing hyperemia of the liver, with cells and cell nuclei intact, and capillaries gorged with erythrocytes. (Amlacher)

Figure 82. Carp experimentally infected with *Aeromonas liquefaciens*, showing connective membrane of large fibers around the degenerated portal vein covered with pancreatic tissue, the result of an inflammatory process between the liver and the vascular network. (Amlacher)

(*b*) immunity (defensive mechanism acquired by survival in the presence of the disease);

(*c*) hygiene (feeding, water quality, etc.).

The joint action of these three factors decides the course of the infection. In the future, more attention must be given to the hygienic aspects of carp farming, particularly in intensive fish farming operations, and also to hibernation. Furthermore, the part played by contaminated hatcheries as foci of infection must be carefully and studiously taken into account. Winter tanks, wherein carp from contaminated hatcheries pass the winter period, can easily turn into permanent foci of infection for other fish. These fish acquire an immunity against the causative agent of bacterial hemorrhagic septicemia, especially if they suffer a light infection at the end of winter. This immunity may be increased in adult fish by means of a re-infection. The tests on agglutination titers carried out by Mann in 2-year-old carp showed that in many cases no agglutinins could be detected in the blood during autumn, but that these increased up until April of the following year. Even when from the agglutination titer it is not possible to tell whether there is any immunity or not, it does suggest that the carp would in fact react to an eventful infection which appeared in February, mobilizing their defenses and with a certain degree of immunity.

But should this infection occur later on or in the spring, when the water is warmer and the fish has not been able to produce antibodies, then it cannot do so in such a short time and consequently an epizootic of dropsy takes place.

From what has just been said it may be deduced that the immunity acquired against the bacterium must not be placed in danger by populating the tanks with fish of a different origin.

Results obtained from paper electrophoretic examinations show that carp which have a suitable amount of total proteins and these serum proteins are in an optimal relationship with each other, do not become diseased, even when maintained in tanks wherein the disease is rampant. On the other hand, carp whose serum proteins do not show such a favorable relationship are very susceptible to bacterial hemorrhagic septicemia, even when they are maintained in optimum conditions.

Preventive treatment is accomplished by the use of chloromycetin or streptomycin (Schäperclaus, 1955; *Figures 83 and 84*). These antibiotics should not be considered as a panacea, since hygiene still retains its value.

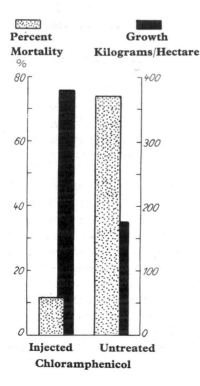

Figure 83. Comparative histogram of two carp hatcheries wherein the fish in one (left) were treated with injections of chloramphenicol whereas those in the other (right) were untreated: stippling shows the percentage of deaths and black shows growth expressed as kilograms/hectare. (Slightly modified from Schäperclaus)

When dropsy makes its appearance, any dead fish should be collected, counted, and buried. Those which have been ill are never put into hibernation together with healthy fish. After the fish have been removed, any foci of infection are carefully disinfected with quicklime or calcium cyanamide, and are left dry throughout the winter period.

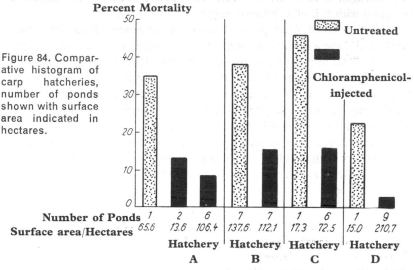

Figure 84. Comparative histogram of carp hatcheries, number of ponds shown with surface area indicated in hectares.

Number of Ponds	1	2	6	7	7	1	6	1	9
Surface area/Hectares	65,6	13,6	106,4	137,6	112,1	17,3	72,5	15,0	210,7
	Hatchery A		Hatchery B		Hatchery C		Hatchery D		

All therapeutic measures previously described are at the same time preventive measures, but once again we must insist upon the necessity for a good overall hygiene to prevent recurrence of the disease. Great care must be taken to avoid traumatic injuries during transportation and selection, as well as to avoid unsuitable water (lack of oxygen, sudden overheating etc.). An excessive population and overfeeding (for example, never try to force feed the fish), coupled with an overfertilized water all favor the appearance of bacterial hemorrhagic septicemia.

As a prophylactic measure it is recommended that wintering be carried out in large tanks, particularly when it is remembered that the fish may start to eat at temperatures below 9° C. This possibility is not allowed for in narrow winter tanks; the fish suffer hunger, and their resistance is lowered (as has been shown by electrophoresis of the blood proteins by Offhaus, Brunner and Reidmüller, 1955; and by Flemming, 1958). On the other hand in large tanks the fish are able to move from one side to another when the climate is somewhat more benign, and thus they encounter food even in the middle of the winter. The destruction of dangerous fish (small tench, pope, *Leucaspius delineatus*) which play a part as carriers of dropsy, as well as leeches and carp lice, are also included together with the preventive measures.

"Red Pest" of freshwater eels

This disease is also produced by a pathogenic variety of *Aeromonas liquefaciens*. It has been known since 1928 in the waters of central Europe, and occurs among eels of different sizes independently of the season of the year. The losses sustained may vary considerably, being higher in autumn and lowest of all in spring.

CLINICAL PICTURE AND SYMPTOMS: the body of the diseased eels shows red blotches, and occasionally spots of the same color, especially in the ventral and anal parts. The fins may also be reddish in color. The lesions of the skin are whitish blotches which become ulcerated and come to show a partially pink border which is formed by the necrotized dermis, and a center in which the muscle tissue is exposed and reddened by inflammation. Ulcer formation is especially confined to the cephalic region (as in the case of ulcerative form of bacterial hemorrhagic septicemia); firstly boils are formed, of a size which varies between that of a small pea to that of an acorn, and these burst open and may cicatrize or persist as ulcers (*Figure 85*). This disease may also continue without any external symptoms being produced, and in this case the eels swim with slow irregular movements, and come to the surface shortly before death in a slightly curved position.

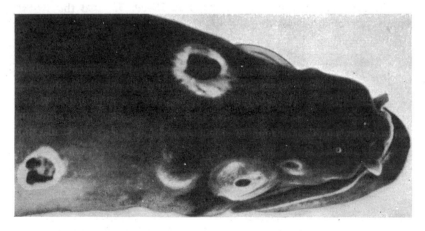

Figure 85. Diseased freshwater eel with ulcers on the head and the formation of a boil just behind the right eye. (Schäperclaus)

TECHNIQUE FOR INVESTIGATION: for bacteriological analyses of the boils, these are cauterized at the surface with a red hot knife, and material is taken from the center with a flamed platinum loop. At the same time the kidney and liver (or muscle tissue) may be cultured as described in the section on techniques given at the beginning of this book. In the case of recently dead eels, blood from the aorta should also be cultured. Any material taken is streaked onto agar slopes. Cultures are likewise made onto gelatin plates. Following this the usual morphological and physiological examinations of the bacteria are completed (gelatin liquefaction, glucose utilization, salinity requirements etc.).

For the fixation of pathological material Stieve's fluid or formalin is used.

ETIOLOGY; MORPHOLOGY AND TAXONOMY OF THE CAUSATIVE AGENT; COURSE OF THE DISEASE: the cause of freshwater eel pest is *Aeromonas liquefaciens forma sarcowiensis*, which according to Schäperclaus has the same characteristics as *Aer. liquefaciens forma ascitae*. It is capable of living in a medium having a concentration of 0.0 0.75% sodium chloride, and dies out at a concentration of 4.5% and above. Its form varies from coccoid to bacillary. It measures 0.8–2.0 × 0.5 microns. The cells are monotrichous, and the flagellum is 3–4 times longer than the cell itself. No spores or capsules are produced. The organism is extremely motile, and the cells stain with iron hematoxylin and with the usual aniline dyes. They are Gram negative. Growth on agar is always of a grayish color, and according to Schäperclaus the medium gives a strong fluorescence when viewed under ultra-violet light*. Stab cultures in gelatin produce a funnel-shaped liquefaction. Gelatin plate cultures show liquefaction at 18–20° C., and the darker colonies come to be distributed progressively throughout the zone of liquefaction. In glucose medium at 18–20° C. the organism produces acid and gas within 2–3 days, according to Schäperclaus.

The disease is probably propagated during the migrations of the eels. In closed waters, the infection made its appearance, above all, following stocking with eels from the lower Elbe river. Its dissemination takes place, in all probability, by direct contact, and its course is dependent upon the climatic conditions and certain other unknown factors. The disease attacks isolated individuals, but may also give rise to mass mortalities—in which instance it produces bacteremia. Its duration lasts for several months. Should the action of the bacteria be limited to the integument and musculature alone, the fish tends to cure itself.

HISTOPATHOLOGY AND HISTOCHEMISTRY: the ulcers produced in freshwater eel pest contain a serous liquid with atrophied leucocytes and erythrocytes in a proportion of 3:2 (Schäperclaus). A section through the ulcer reveals a hollow space situated in a zone limited by the hypodermic connective tissue and the dermis, but this may also be situated exclusively in the hypodermis. The hollow area is full of pus. The tissue with which

---

* The presence of fluorescence in a culture under ultra-violet light is now taken as being characteristic of the fluorescent pseudomonad group only (e.g., *Ps. fluorescens, Ps. putida*).

this purulent cavity is limited is seen to be necrotized. The dermis shows intense hemorrhage in the proximity of the ulcers, for which reason these are seen macroscopically as having a red border, a condition similar to that observed in the boils. Between the connective fibers, which also contain bacteria and hemorrhagic zones, are to be seen edematous lacunae. The greatest lesions occur in the heart. These are intensely hemorrhagic in the cardiac wall, and bacteria may be shown in sections without any difficulty.

THERAPY, PROPHYLAXIS AND HYGIENE: it is difficult to successfully combat this disease. When it makes its appearance those eels which can be used should be removed as quickly as possible, since they die off very quickly in tanks. There is no danger of this disease being infectious to man. Any dead eels should be immediately buried. Theoretically it is possible to attempt chloromycetin therapy. No special preventive measures can be taken; the only sensible piece of advice is that of not trying to carry out any super-intensive exploitation of eels in the hatchery.

"Red Spot" of freshwater fish

This disease has been observed in numerous species of freshwater fish, and particularly in pike, North Sea salmon, cyprinids, perch and pikeperch. Since the year 1920 it has caused great losses among small salmon and bream.

CLINICAL PICTURE AND SYMPTOMS: the diseased fish show cutaneous blotches which may be round, oval or elongated in shape, of a whitish coloration, and in some places loss of epithelium and scales may be observed (*Figure 86*). On the head, particularly in pike, muscular necrosis appears in addition to the ordinary skin lesions. Such necrosis is especially common in the maxillary and ocular regions of the head. Similar ulcers are also to be found at the bases of the fins. According to Layman, the spots on the pike have a pinkish-colored border, and measure some 5–20 cm. in diameter. This clinical picture is similar to that found in the cyprinids. The blotches originate following edema and scale defects. After the necrosis of the skin which follows this process, the muscle tissue becomes exposed and surrounded by a white zone of dermis which is undergoing necrotization. On autopsy, roach and bream may show an ascitic fluid. Furthermore, especially in the bream, hyperemia of the hepatic and intestinal blood vessels is common.

TECHNIQUE OF INVESTIGATION: the same techniques as have been desscribed above may be used.

ETIOLOGY; MORPHOLOGY AND TAXONOMY OF THE CAUSATIVE AGENT; COURSE OF THE DISEASE: Schäperclaus believes that *Aeromonas liquefaciens forma pellis* is responsible for this disease. On the other hand however, *Pseudo-*

monas fluorescens, Proteus vulgaris and physical factors (for example, cold) have also been suggested as possible causes of this particular condition. Finally the hypothesis of a viral infection cannot be completely discarded (Schäperclaus, 1930).

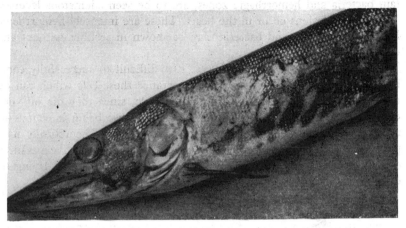

Figure 86. Pike infected with Red Spot. (Matthels)

The disease makes its appearance in pike during the spawning period or immediately afterwards. There is probably a relation between the physiological susceptibility of the pike at this time and the appearance of the disease; cases of such an infection in pike have nevertheless also been observed at other times throughout the year. In the remaining species of fish the disease usually appears in spring or early summer. The losses may greatly affect the biological yield of lakes, and mortalities of 40–60% have been registered in certain instances. In the initial phase of the blotch formation, some scales are lost and there is a localized scale protrusion in the zone immediately surrounding this (colateral edema according to Schäperclaus), reddening, and inflammation. Destruction of the dermis increases the size of the blotches until the muscle, surrounded by a dermal ring, becomes necrotized, white, and exposed. The formation of blotches extends slowly to cover the whole body, and these may be subject to a secondary mycotic infection. Schäperclaus (1930) pointed out that in roach and bream an ascites occurred in addition to a serious destruction of the muscle tissue in the cephalic region. The hemoglobin concentration was normal except for cases in which the fish also showed symptoms of ascites. The heart, liver and kidney do not have lesions, with the sole exception of a little localized hyperemia. Schäperclaus (1930) observed marked hyperemia of the intestinal and hepatic blood vessels.

139

HISTOPATHOLOGY AND HISTOCHEMISTRY: histologically a destruction of the dermis is noted in sections. The inflammation extends through the muscular and connective tissue to penetrate deeply. The muscular fibers do not suffer any appreciable lesions, but in some cases may show necrosis. Seresevskaja found hemorrhages of the liver and kidney.

THERAPY, PROPHYLAXIS AND HYGIENE: *mutatis mutandi* the same measures may be applied to this disease as for the "Red Pest" of freshwater eels.

"Red Pest" of saltwater eels (red bubonic plague or pestis rubra anguillarum)

Bergman (1909) first described the causative agent of this disease as a vibrio and called it "Red Pest"; however, Canestrini first isolated the organism in 1893 from cases among eels in Italy, and called it *Bacillus anguillarum*–Schäperclaus (1927c, 34b) described the disease in migratory eels from the Rügen area. These eels, to quote from Schäperclaus, in contradistinction to the native eels which have lived for some time in the Baltic, had not yet acquired any immunity against the causative agent of the disease. However in 1931 the local eels also became infected, and one of the greatest mass mortalities of fish ever known took place in that area. According to the data collected by Meyer (1933), in Vilm island more than a thousand dead eels were collected daily from a stretch of 1 km. of coast.

CLINICAL PICTURE AND SYMPTOMS: Schäperclaus (1934b) describes the following symptoms as being characteristic of the "Red Pest" of salt-water eels:

(*a*) no external symptoms; the fish swim listlessly at the surface of the water; spasmodic twitching of the body shortly prior to death;

(*b*) red marks on the lateral and ventral zones of the body, at times only the edges of the fins and the anus are reddened;

(*c*) pinkish-colored inflammation of the musculature in the thoracic region, especially in eels of about 38 cm. in length (this same symptom is seen in pike infected with *Vibrio anguillarum*); muscular spasms in the anal region which may lead to contraction of the anus;

(*d*) boils or red ulcers, surrounded at times by hyaline masses of cutaneous tissue.

Autopsy reveals hemorrhages in the liver. Asymptomatic cases of this disease are the most frequent, but these nevertheless give rise to the greatest losses of fish.

TECHNIQUE OF INVESTIGATION: Material is cultured from the liver, kidney or musculature of freshly killed eels, and whenever possible from the aorta as well. This material is streaked onto agar slopes containing a concentration of sodium chloride sufficient to support the growth of *Vibrio anguillarum*. Furthermore, plates of gelatin should be streaked, and a morphological and physiological study of the bacterium made (gelatin stab, glucose medium, salinity requirements etc.). The bacteria are stained with methylene blue, Loeffler's stain, alcoholic gentian violet or phenicated gentian violet. Tissues are fixed in Stieve's fluid or in formalin.

ETIOLOGY; MORPHOLOGY AND TAXONOMY OF THE CAUSATIVE AGENT; COURSE OF THE DISEASE: the causative agent of "Red Pest" in saltwater eels is *Vibrio anguillarum* Bergman. Schäperclaus (1954b) describes this organism as follows:

Comma-like form, somewhat S-shaped; monotrichous, having a polar flagellum; Gram negative, asporogenous and non-encapsulated; it measures 1.5×0.5 microns; it liquefies gelatin; agar colonies are at first water clear, and later become grayish-yellow; it does not form gas, but produces acid from glucose and maltose; no hydrogen sulfide is formed; it is both halophilic and hemolytic. Optimum growth occurs at a sodium chloride concentration of 1.5–3.5%. With a concentration of sodium chloride lower than 0.07% and greater than 8.5%, it dies out. No growth occurs at 6° C. Temperatures of 37 and 45° C. are lethal. Two physiological types may be distinguished (Schäperclaus, 1934b):

Type A: acid from saccharose and mannitol, indole formed;

Type B: no acid from saccharose and mannitol, no indole formation.

The way in which the infection occurs is still unknown. The disease develops according to the form in which it appears: when external symptoms are absent (frequently as a result of a bacteremia) the course of the disease is catastrophic and is accompanied by a mass mortality; when there are ulcerations the course is less violent and fewer deaths are produced. Experimentally infected eels (Schäperclaus, 1927c) die within 3–6 days showing symptoms of red blotches.

Vibrio anguillarum is also known to cause widespread infections in marine fish such as plaice, cod, turbot, brill, lemon sole, and others (Anderson and Conroy, 1968). Outbreaks of disease caused by vibrios have been described in trout and salmon (Cisar and Fryer, 1969). A further vibrio disease caused by an organism known as *Vibrio ichthyodermis* has been described and a halophilic vibrio was found to be responsible for a disease in cultured "ayu" (*Plecoglossus altivelis*) in Japan.

HISTOPATHOLOGY AND HISTOCHEMISTRY: according to Schäperclaus (1927c) it is possible to find the following types of lesion: the reddened cutaneous zones show dermal hemorrhages in sections. Neither the hypodermis nor the muscular tissue show any pathological changes. The walls of the dermal blood vessels are destroyed and in their surrounds there occurs an accumulation of cells. The hemorrhages are very pronounced, especially in the region of the scale pockets.

141

The liver is also characterized by the presence of parietal lesions of the large vessels, together with capillary hyperemia.

THERAPY, PROPHYLAXIS AND HYGIENE: it is not possible to either combat or cure this disease. Sick and suspect eels are collected together in cold freshwater. Nets are frequently changed to prevent an accumulation of infected eels when they die in masses, because the bacteria contaminate the water and may come to attack healthy fish. Frequently changes of the fishing areas helps to prevent the continual passage of *Vibrio anguillarum* through different fish and thus increase its virulence. Diseased and suspect eels should not be kept for longer than three days. Empty containers, in the event that they should have held sea water, are dried in the sun to destroy the bacteria; it is only after having completed this operation that they may be used to hold other eels.

Other species of fish infected by *V. anguillarum* have been treated with sulfonamides and nitrofurans.

Vibriosis or pike pest

Immediately following upon the appearance of saltwater eel pest in the vicinity of Rügen, a similar disease appeared which caused just as many deaths among the pike as the former had done among the eels. Previously this disease was known as pike pest, but currently it is better known as pike vibriosis. The disease appeared in 1925 in the Breeg and Breetz bays during the month of April at the time of spawning, but Schäperclaus (1928b) has similarly observed its occurrence in May and June. A total of 25% of the pike were diseased.

CLINICAL PICTURE AND SYMPTOMS: the first symptoms of this infection are small red spots or petechiae on the throat, under the opercula, and in the ventral and cardiac region, and just immediately anterior to the pelvic fins.

Later on a loss of skin is to be seen, around which is observed a reddish coloration of the dermis and muscle tissue. The muscle itself may be exposed. Cephalic ulcers have also been seen. On autopsy hyperemia of the intestine and liver, reddening of the rectum, and hemorrhages and necrosis of the liver are observed. The kidney is normal, but occasionally small necrotic patches may be detected in it. The hemoglobin concentration is in the region of approximately 9.5 gm./100 ml.

TECHNIQUE OF INVESTIGATION: as for saltwater eel disease.

ETIOLOGY; MORPHOLOGY AND TAXONOMY OF THE CAUSATIVE AGENT; COURSE OF THE DISEASE: the causative agent of pike vibriosis is *Vibrio anguillarum* Bergman (see saltwater eel disease). The course of the disease is slow, long, and almost invariably asymptomatic.

HISTOPATHOLOGY AND HISTOCHEMISTRY: the skin shows areas of total destruction of the loose dermis, while the dense dermis remains intact.

In the hypodermis are to be seen inflammations which may involve the musculature. The intestine, and above all the rectum, show pronounced vascular hyperemia, probably caused by a thrombosis. Between the circular muscle fibers and the longitudinal ones, and between the muscularis mucosae and the serosa are hemorrhages and inflammatory foci which may occasionally even reach the longitudinal muscle layer itself. The kidney is generally free from lesions. Schäperclaus (1928b) observed accumulations of pigment and local necrosis in the renal tubules. The liver at times is hyperemic, and shows necrotic patches. The peritoneum and the swim bladder may likewise be hyperemic.

THERAPY, PROPHYLAXIS AND HYGIENE: the statements and recommendations given above for saltwater eel "Red Pest" apply equally well to this disease.

For a fuller consideration of vibrio infections in marine and freshwater fish, the paper by Rucker (1959) should be consulted.

Furunculosis

Furunculosis of salmonids has been known for many years, and was the first bacterial disease to have been scientifically described (in 1894). Its name is derived from the appearance of ulcers on the skin, but even these bear little resemblance to those produced during outbreaks of furunculosis in human beings.

McCraw (1952) and Herman (1968) have reviewed the furunculosis literature from 1868 to 1966.

CLINICAL PICTURE AND SYMPTOMS: the symptoms typical of this disease are boils and ulcers (*Figure 87*) which are found isolated or in groups, chiefly in the dorsal region. These ulcers are tinged with blood. The bigger ones contain a sticky, dark reddish pus. Ulcers may be absent, and in such an event autopsy shows an intestinal inflammation, principally in the pyloric and rectal regions. The swim bladder is hyperemic; small spots and hemorrhages are found in the liver. Similar hemorrhages are encountered at times on the inner side of the opercula, in the eyes, and on the fins. In the event of a bacteremia these symptoms are usually lacking and the blood is filled with bacteria. As in bacterial hemorrhagic septicemia and VHS, several forms of furunculosis may be differentiated:

(*a*) ulcerative form (slow course);

(*b*) asymptomatic form (acute course);

(*c*) intestinal form (enteritis and anal prolapse).

Furunculosis attacks salmonids, above all, principally fish of 2 years or more. Young alevins may also be infected, but in these the disease is not severe and persists more as a latent form which confers a type of immunity to the fish. The disease has been observed in fish of at least nine families. Furunculosis is a notifiable disease in Great Britain (Diseases of Fish Act, 1937).

TECHNIQUE OF INVESTIGATION: the surface of the boils is sterilized with a heated blade. With a platinum loop, duly sterilized, material is taken from the interior of the ulcer. Latent infections are investigated by making cultures of the kidney on agar slopes or on alkaline gelatin. Plehn recommended Fehlmann's agar. The composition of this medium is as follows: 1000 gm. of meat (or fish), 1000 cc. of water—heated for two hours and then filtered; 40 gm. of agar; 10 gm. of sodium chloride; 10 gm. of glucose (not absolutely essential); 20 gm. of peptone and 100 gm. of glycerine. Gelatine stab cultures are very characteristic.

(a)

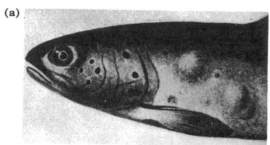

Figure 87. Furunculosis in trout: (a) boils; (b) ulcers. (Plehn)

(b)

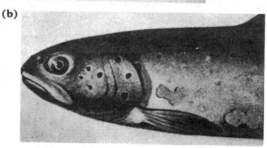

A specific furunculosis agar has been placed on the market by Difco Laboratories Inc., which favors the presumptive identification of *Aeromonas salmonicida* by the characteristic production of a dark pigmentation. Griffin's test is also a rapid means whereby a presumptive diagnosis of *A. salmonicida* may be made, and is based upon the black coloration given by colonies of this organism when flooded with 1% aqueous para-phenylene-diamine solution. Blake and Anderson (1930) described a complement fixation test for the serological diagnosis of furunculosis, and Rabb, Cornick and McDermott (1964) have more recently developed a macroscopic slide agglutination test with the same object in view.

144

The autopsy and histopathological procedures are carried out as has been previously described in this book.

ETIOLOGY; MORPHOLOGY AND TAXONOMY OF THE CAUSATIVE AGENT; COURSE OF THE DISEASE: the causative agent of furunculosis is *Aeromonas salmonicida* Emmerich and Weibel. It measures 0.8×0.5 microns, is non-motile, non-flagellated, and Gram negative. According to Schäperclaus its behavior in culture is as follows: agar colonies at 20° C. become dark and even black in color within 2–3 days, due to the formation of melanin in the presence of oxygen. Gelatin stab cultures give a very characteristic liquefaction in the form of a funnel within 2–3 days, accompanied by abundant sediment formation. Litmus-casein-sugar solutions at 20° C. give the following coloration:

glucose: cherry red;
fructose: blue;
lactose: violet;
mannitol: pinkish violet;
maltose: pale red.

A. salmonicida grows at an optimum temperature of 20–30° C. and dies at 37° C. It is ubiquitous and may be found in water and in mud, often in very large numbers.

The appearance of the disease is favored by poor living conditions for the fish. Infection occurs within a few hours through small lesions of the skin or through the intestinal tract. Death may occur some 3–4 days later. The numbers of fish lost reaches a peak between the fourth and the ninth day after the first appearance of the outbreak. Those fish which have boils and ulcers are slow in movement after some 8–14 days; they become separated from the other fish and remain in one corner of the tank usually allowing themselves to be picked up in the hands. Death takes place within two to three weeks in such cases. The boils may become cured leaving a scar. *A. salmonicida* dies out in pure water after a few days; for this reason water contaminated with organic residues are especially favorable to the development of this organism. Higher temperatures (15–18° C.) may greatly contribute to the reactivation of latent infections.

HISTOPATHOLOGY AND HISTOCHEMISTRY: the ulcers develop from small sub-cutaneous foci, and grow by means of infiltration during which they produce lesions in the musculature. As a result of the extension of the infectious foci boil-like growths in the skin are produced which subsequently burst open and necrotize. The contents of the boil—pus mixed with tissue remains—are released into the water. The point of inflammation may be recognized by an accumulation of melanophores.

Klontz, Yasutake and Ross (1966) reported that *A. salmonicida* produces an extracellular leucocytolytic substance that destroys the inflammatory reaction of fish. This phenomenon accounts for the lack of inflammatory reaction to the disease noted by earlier workers.

THERAPY, PROPHYLAXIS AND HYGIENE: as in all other infectious diseases, removal and destruction of dead and gravely infected fish is suggested. These should preferably be either burned or buried. Fish which are suspected of having furunculosis are isolated in special tanks, taking care to ensure that these are fed with an independent supply of water which should be cold and clean. All hatchery utensils are disinfected continually with an aqueous solution of potassium permanganate (1 gm. in 50 liters of water). Priasol (cresol derivative) solution also serves this purpose quite well. The empty tanks must be disinfected with quicklime, which is also placed onto the sides and the walls. It is also important to ensure that the basic requirements of the fish are adequately met with, above all with regards to a rational and vitamin-rich food. In the transportation of the fish and the emptying of tanks, care must be exercised to ensure that the oxygen supply is sufficient and that handling is performed with the greatest possible care. Foreign material should on no account be allowed to enter the tank, and the water supply must at all times be maintained free of organic impurities.

Sulfonamides (sulfamerazine, sulfaguanidine, sulfadiazine, sulfamethazine, sulfisoxazole) given orally with the food at a rate of 10 grams per 100 pounds of fish per day are useful for therapy (Snieszko and Hoffman, 1963). Among antibiotics, chloramphenicol and oxytetracycline are the best; dosage, 2.5–3.5 grams per 100 pounds of fish per day (Snieszko and Hoffman, 1963). Leaman (1965) reported excellent results in preventing furunculosis in returning Atlantic salmon by giving 10 mg. chloramphenicol/lb. fish *i.p.*

Klontz (1966) has developed an oral vaccine based on the saline-soluble leucocytolytic extract of *A. salmonicida*. It has shown good results in most field tests.

Bacterial tail rot

One disease which is frequently observed, especially in young fish, is bacterial fin rot. This was described for the first time by Schäperclaus (1950a), who studied it in black mollies.

The first symptoms of the disease are ill defined and may pass without notice. Generally there is a slight cloudiness of the outer edges of the fins. On the advance of the infection the symptoms become more apparent. The size of the fins is reduced as a result of a progressive death of their tissues. With the subsequent loss of the fin rays there finally remains little more than a stump of the fin. From these stumps Schäperclaus isolated bacteria of the genera *Pseudomonas* and *Aeromonas* more specifically *Aeromonas liquefaciens* and *Ps. fluorescens*. Schäperclaus also suspected that the black molly shows a hereditary disposition towards the disease; on the other hand it should be taken into account that the disease also affects many other species of fish, freshwater and marine, held under artificial conditions. Schäperclaus (1950a), Rankin (1953), and Reichenbach-Klinke all state that bacterial fin rot is a contagious disease. Sterba (1956) and most other workers are of the opinion that ecological factors favor the appearance of this particular infection. This latter author has had occasion to observe that the disease becomes apparent in breeding tanks, especially when the water has not been partially changed. Maintenance of the fish in cold water also predisposed the fish to fin rot, as was observed particularly in the angel fish (*Pterophyllum scalare*).

The control of fin rot is not always successful according to Schäperclaus, as for instance an effective painting of the open wounds invariably damages the fish tissues. He recommends long baths in acriflavine (1 gm./100 liters) or in sulfonamide (Albucid or Globucid, 1 gm./10 liters). According to Rankin (1953), phenoxethol is active against the causative agent of fin rot at the following concentration: 10 cc. of a 1% stock solution are added for each liter of aquarium water. Sterba states that careful treatment of old fish and the raising of the water temperature have a curative effect. When such symptoms occur following a change of water, Sterba recommends that a fourth part of the old clean water be added to the tank. Recent work by Mattheis (1961) gave rise to a complete cure within 6 days, by using 60 mgm./liter of chloromycetin in the form of an extended duration bath.

Bacterial fin rot has been shown to respond readily to kanamycin therapy Conroy (1963). The antibiotic is administered as an intra-peritoneal injection, calculating the dose as 2 mgm./100 gm. fish body weight. The disease is treated in fish farming practice by malachite green dips, and by disinfection of the tanks and raceways with chlorine. Some workers have achieved good results by prophylactic dips in copper sulfate 1:2000.

Columnaris disease

CLINICAL PICTURE AND SYMPTOMS: columnaris is a common and very widespread disease of freshwater fish, and gives rise to characteristic symptoms which in aquarium fish are sometimes known as "cotton wool disease" or "mouth fungus." The latter is not strictly correct, since this infection is due to bacteria rather than to fungi. Typically the diseased fish show the presence of gray-white spots on the head and fins, although the gills and lateral sides of the body may also be affected. Gradually these lesions become ulcerated, and in the case of the fins the rays are frayed and exposed. In fish which do not possess scales, a reddish-colored periphery is usually observed around the lesion (*Figures* A and B).

TECHNIQUE OF INVESTIGATION: to diagnose a case of columnaris, a scraping is taken from the infected area of the fish and examined microscopically as a hanging drop preparation. The bacteria may be seen as long, thin, rod-shaped organisms, which show characteristic slow gliding movements. They are not truly motile, as they do not possess flagella. Typically these bacteria become attached to the slide at one end, while the other end pivots around in a manner suggestive of the movements of a leech. A most important feature of these organisms from the point of view of diagnosis is the fact that they are reported to form aggregates not unlike columns, and the name columnaris has been derived from this peculiarity (*Figure C*). It may be seen to occur around a scale or other small object in the preparation. Cultures may be taken from the diseased areas and streaked onto Ordal's columnaris medium (Bullock, 1961), which is incubated at 18°C. for several days.

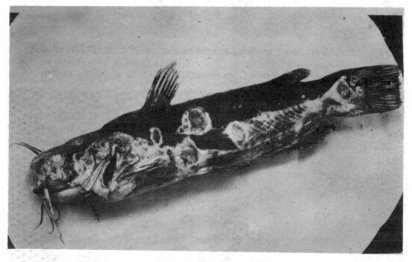

Figure A. Columnaris disease, bullhead (*Ictalurus*). (Davis photo)

ETIOLOGY; MORPHOLOGY AND TAXONOMY OF THE CAUSATIVE AGENT; COURSE OF THE DISEASE: columnaris is a serious infection, and may be transmitted from fish to fish by contaminated nets, through the water etc. The resistance of the fish to this disease is reduced as the temperature of the water increases. Both warm-water and cold-water species of fish are subject to

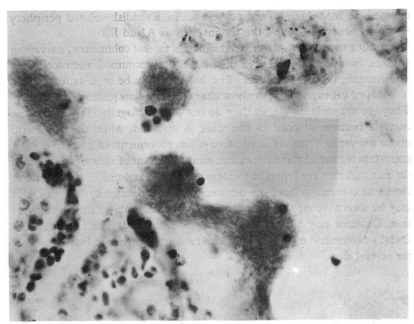

Figure B. Gill section showing *Chondrococcus columnaris*. (Davis photo)

Figure C. Gills infected with *Chondrococcus columnaris*. (Davis photo)

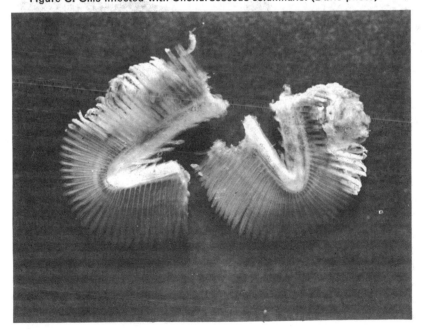

columnaris, although it has recently been suggested that there is a true cold-water form of the disease which attacks salmon and trout, and a warm-water form which affects aquarium fish and other warmer water species. The disease may reach epizootic proportions in hot and dry weather.

The causative organism of this infection is a myxobacterium, *Chondrococcus columnaris* (*Cytophaga columnaris*). The individual cells measure 0.5×5–10 microns, and display the gliding movements of the myxobacteria as mentioned above. The bacterium is Gram negative. On special medium they form microcysts.

Columnaris has been declared a notifiable disease in Great Britain, by an amendment of the Diseases of Fish Act (1937).

HISTOPATHOLOGY AND HISTOCHEMISTRY: the effects of columnaris are first felt on the body surface. The bacteria usually enter the body by means of small abrasions on the skin, and gain access to the epidemis and dermis, wherein they multiply rapidly. The dermal capillaries become swollen and finally rupture, filling the interstitial areas with blood. The bacteria then begin to attack the muscle fibers, and when the destruction of the skin is complete it is quite common to observe loss of the scales.

THERAPY, PROPHYLAXIS AND HYGIENE: cases of "cotton wool disease" in aquarium fish may be treated by dipping them in 1:2000 copper sulfate solution for 1–2 minutes. Chloromycetin at a level of 5–10 ppm. in the water has also given good results in the treatment of columnaris disease. Dipping in 1:15,000 malachite green solution for up to 30 seconds is recommended as a prophylactic measure, following handling etc. Acriflavine dips at a concentration of 2 mgm./gallon have also been reported to be a useful prophylactic procedure, but in this case the aquarium must first be freed from plants and sand. The treatment of columnaris in salmonid fish has been attempted by the addition of sulfa drugs to the food, but the results of these experiments leave much to be desired. Oxytetracycline (75 mg./kg. fish/day) has been reported very effective.

Coldwater disease (Peduncle disease)

CLINICAL PICTURE AND SYMPTOMS: Coldwater disease derives its name from the fact that it attacks fish in water below 10° C. The typical lesion starts as a small whitish or bluish spot behind the dorsal fin. From this, erosion occurs until a crater is present in the muscle. In severe cases, the entire caudal area may be lost leaving exposed vertebrae. The skin of sac-fry is attacked in such a manner that yolk material is lost. This results in death of the sac-fry with little damage to other tissues.

TECHNIQUE OF INVESTIGATION: diagnosis is similar to that of columnaris disease. The coldwater organism is somewhat smaller and does not aggregate like columnaris organisms.

ETIOLOGY; MORPHOLOGY AND TAXONOMY OF THE CAUSATIVE AGENT; COURSE OF THE DISEASE: loss of sac-fry may reach 50%. The further advanced the fry are the less the loss. The optimum temperature is between 4 and 10° C. and is usually not seen above 10° C.

The agent is a myxobacterium, *Cytophaga psychrophila*. It is similar to *Chondrococcus columnaris* but does not form microcysts on special medium.

THERAPY, PROPHYLAXIS AND HYGIENE: sulfamethazine, sulfisoxazole; 100 mg./kg./day for 10–20 days. Observe the usual practices of disinfection of equipment and avoid exposure of uninfected fish to "wild" fish or known carriers.

Bacterial gill disease

CLINICAL PICTURE AND SYMPTOMS: the first indication of bacterial gill disease is loss of appetite. Fish tend to ride high in the water and orient themselves into the flow of water. They appear lethargic and may be pale. Hematocrit values increase initially, rising to 50–60% in fingerling fish. If the affected fish are not treated after the first symptoms are noted, the mortality increases rapidly, and 50% or more of the fish may be dead in 24 to 48 hours.

Figure D. Gross appearance of bacterial gill disease. (Davis photo)

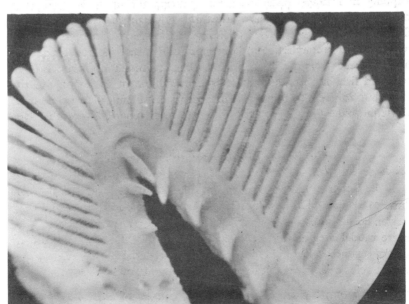

TECHNIQUE OF INVESTIGATION: in severe cases, gross examination of the gill will show excessive mucous secretion and characteristic clubbing and fusion of the filaments (*Figure D*). A wet mount or stained smear from such a gill will show the presence of numerous filamentous bacteria on the surface of the epithelium. They may be attached by one end with the other moving freely but slowly. Histological sections show epithelial hyperplasia (*Figure E*) and gram negative bacteria on the gill surface (*Figure F*).

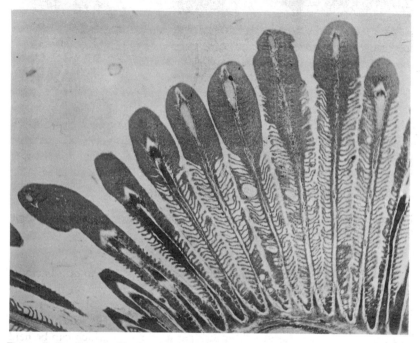

Figure E. Section of gill, showing hyperplasia with fusion of lamellae caused by bacterial gill disease. (Davis photo)

ETIOLOGY; MORPHOLOGY AND TAXONOMY OF THE CAUSATIVE AGENT; COURSE OF THE DISEASE: bacterial gill disease is associated with the presence of large numbers of myxobacteria (5–10mu × 0.5mu) on the gill epithelium and overcrowding in the raceways or ponds. Bacterial gill disease appears to be caused by a group of bacteria rather than a single type as in other myxobacterial infections (e.g., columnaris). Serological tests show that a variety of types may be responsible for outbreaks, although one type will usually predominate in a particular case. Serology also shows that the myxobacteria of gill disease are different from those of columnaris disease and coldwater disease.

152

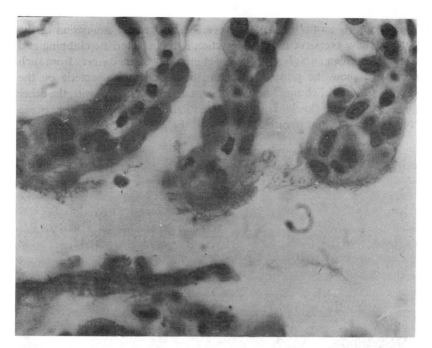

Figure F. Section of a gill, showing clumps of Myxobacteria as found in gill disease. (Davis photo)

Bacterial gill disease, as the name implies, is considered to be a bacterial infection. However, the environment has a great influence on the occurrence of the disease. Wood (1968) is able to predict outbreaks of the disease in chinook salmon on the basis of stocking loads. Each type of holding facility has some weight of fish per unit of flow which can be held without difficulty. Exceeding this weight results in an outbreak of bacterial gill disease. Herman (1970) observed that trout receiving a nutritionally poor diet were very susceptible to bacterial gill disease.

HISTOPATHOLOGY AND HISTOCHEMISTRY: bacterial gill disease is one of several diseases which cause hyperplasia of the respiratory 'epithelium (Wood and Yasutake, 1957).

It is most like nutritional gill disease caused by a deficiency of pantothenic acid. The pattern of hyperplasia will usually distinguish the two. With bacterial gill disease (*Figure E*), the hyperplasia begins at the distal end of the lamellae. Fusion of the ends may result in "holes." Hyperplasia and lamellar fusion is greatest at the distal ends of the filaments, but such areas are found the entire length of the filaments. Hyperplasia caused by pantothenic acid deficiency begins at the base of the lamellae and progresses outward. Lamellar fusion starts at the distal end of the filament and extends evenly to the proximal end. No holes or islands of hyperplasia are seen.

THERAPY, PROPHYLAXIS AND HYGIENE: the two major factors in preventing bacterial gill disease are maintenance of water quality and avoiding overcrowding. Water sources with high turbidity or wild fish are dangerous. If recirculation is necessary, the water must be reconditioned to remove waste products and reduce any bacterial buildup. Good sanitation practices are required.

Organic mercurial compounds have been among the most effective chemicals for controlling bacterial gill disease. Only one, ethyl mercury phosphate (Timsan), is now available. It is used as a bath at 1–2 ppm, as it comes from the package, for 1 hour. The high toxicity of mercurials to both fish and man and the high retention in the tissues make the use of the mercurials questionable.

Quaternary ammonium compounds are the most widely used chemicals for control of bacterial gill disease today. Roccal, Hyamine 1622, and Hyamine 3500 are the more common. A bath of 1–2 ppm active ingredient for 1 hour is most effective. Hard water reduces both the toxicity and the effectiveness of these compounds to some extent.

Diquat, a herbicide, has recently been shown to be effective in the control of bacterial gill disease. It is used at 2–4 ppm of the active agent for 1 hour.

For control of an outbreak, the treatments are continued daily until the fish are behaving normally. The same dose rates are used for prophylactic treatments but at 7 to 14 day intervals.

Bacterial kidney disease

CLINICAL PICTURE AND SYMPTOMS: kidney disease is of considerable economic importance in salmon and trout farming operations in North America. Externally it may often be impossible to detect any obvious symptoms, although in some fish there may be a few ill-defined lesions on the sides of the body. These lesions contain pus along with blood cells and bacteria. Of the internal organs, the kidney in particular is the seat of an infection, and may be seen to be covered with grayish-white necrotic zones filled with purulent material. Occasionally the liver may be pale, and the spleen swollen (Bell, 1961). The appearance of the kidney has given its name to this disease. It occurs in an acute and in a chronic form, either of these apparently making its appearance in relation to the prevailing water temperature. In the chronic form a false membrane over the kidney and certain other internal organs may be seen. A similar if not identical disease is found in Europe. Here it is known especially from Scotland, where it is called Dee disease (Smith, 1964).

154

TECHNIQUE OF INVESTIGATION: the diagnosis of kidney disease rests almost entirely on the finding of the causative organism in smears of the kidney, and possibly of the spleen. An attempt may be made to culture the organism onto Ordal and Earp's medium (tryptone 10 gm.; beef extract 3 gm.; sodium chloride 5 gm.; yeast extract 0.5 gm.; cysteine hydrochloride 0.1 gm.; agar 15 gm.; distilled water 1 liter. 200 ml. of sterile human blood are added per liter to this basal medium immediately prior to use). The plates are incubated at 18° C., and growth should occur within 7–10 days. The bacterium appears as small Gram positive diplobacilli in smears of the kidney, and may occur either intra- or extra-cellularly. The finding of such bacteria is usually sufficient to establish a presumptive diagnosis as kidney disease. Care must be taken not to mistake pigment granules in the kidney for bacteria.

ETIOLOGY; MORPHOLOGY AND TAXONOMY OF THE CAUSATIVE ORGANISM; COURSE OF THE DISEASE: the etiological agent of kidney disease has been shown to be a small non-motile Gram positive diplobacillus, measuring 0.4 × 0.8 microns. It is believed to be a species of *Corynebacterium*.

The exact mode of transmission is unknown as yet, although it has been suggested that the organism may be carried with the eggs.

THERAPY, PROPHYLAXIS AND HYGIENE; strict quarantine measures must be enforced to prevent the entry of carriers of this disease into water supplies, hatcheries and fish farms previously free from it. Any diseased fish must be destroyed, and preferably burned or buried in quicklime. On no occasion should the viscera be used to feed healthy fish. Rigid precautions must be taken to ensure complete sterilization of all hatchery equipment such as nets and waders.

No fully effective therapeutic measures are known at the present time. Wolf and Dunbar (1959) tested 34 agents against kidney disease and found erythromycin (100 mg./kg./21 days) the most effective. Sulfa drugs are sometimes effective in acute outbreaks but seem to be of little value in chronic cases. However, they are sometimes used for prophylactic treatments (40 mg./kg. day) with adequate results.

Ulcer disease

CLINICAL PICTURE AND SYMPTOMS: ulcer disease is another economically important disease of trout in certain parts of North America. Typically it produces ulcers or shallow open sores and lesions on the body surface, and these are usually of a reddish color. To the superficial observer ulcer disease may easily be confused with furunculosis (see above). The fins may also be attacked, and in this case the disease gives rise to symptoms not unlike those of fin rot, with destruction of the soft inter-ray tissue and fraying of the fin rays themselves. The ulcers on the body surface generally start as pimples, whitish in color, similar to those produced in certain fungal infections. With the further development of the infection the lesions show a tendency to grow together and give rise to a large irregular lesion. It is common to find the mouth and jaws eroded away.

TECHNIQUE OF INVESTIGATION: the only sure way in which to establish a diagnosis is to culture the causative organism. This is often necessary in order to differentiate ulcer disease from furunculosis, even though the two infections quite frequently occur concurrently in the same fish, the latter tending to mask the former. Material from the ulcers, kidney and blood is streaked onto a specific culture medium known as Leetown medium No. 8 (Bullock, 1961). This medium is rather difficult to prepare in practice, and in most instances is obtained in small quantities by requesting it from a fish pathology laboratory. The bacterium which causes ulcer disease is extremely fastidious in its growth requirements.

ETIOLOGY; MORPHOLOGY AND TAXONOMY OF THE CAUSATIVE AGENT; COURSE OF THE DISEASE: the etiological agent of ulcer disease is a short non-motile gram negative rod, *Haemophilus piscium*. This is asporogenous, and occurs singly, in pairs, or in short chains. For a full description of this, see the work of Snieszko, Griffin and Friddle (1950).

H. piscium appears to be transmitted to fish with contaminated water or food. The presence of carriers is also of the utmost importance, since the ulcers and the feces of infected fish serve as continual foci of infection for other fish. The incubation period of ulcer disease may vary from 1–2 weeks. Snieszko (1952) has published an all-embracing description of its importance in fish farming practice. Ulcer disease seems to be confined to North America.

THERAPY, PROPHYLAXIS AND HYGIENE: prophylaxis is an important factor in the control of ulcer disease in hatcheries. The strictest quarantine and disinfection schedules should be adopted and maintained in force. All fish eggs and hatchery utensils must be disinfected.

Treatment of the disease may be accomplished by the administration of chloromycetin or terramycin with the food, at a concentration of 2.5–3.5 gm. pure antibiotic/100 lb. fish per day. This treatment should be continued until the outbreak has ended.

Chapter 6

DISEASES CAUSED BY DINOFLAGELLATES

Other thallophytes apart from bacteria are known as fish pathogens, and among these are the dinoflagellates. The causative agents of coral fish disease and of pillulariasis are both dinoflagellates. *Oodinium ocellatum* was described by Brown (1934) as a pathogen present in marine aquaria. Schäperclaus (1951) discovered *Oodinium pillularis* to be present among freshwater fish.

Coral fish disease

CLINICAL PICTURE AND SYMPTOMS: on occasions a slight cloudiness of the skin may be present. Under the microscope small dark spheres (*Figure 88*) may be recognized in smears from the skin and the gills. Hemorrhagic inflammation and necrosis are present in the gills.

TECHNIQUE OF INVESTIGATION: smears of the skin and gills, or gill filaments, are examined. Gill filaments preserved in formalin or alcohol are particularly suitable for study. The examination should be made using a ×80 and a ×600 magnification.

ETIOLOGY; MORPHOLOGY AND TAXONOMY OF THE CAUSATIVE AGENT; COURSE OF THE DISEASE: the causative agent of coral fish disease is *Oodinium ocellatum* Brown. Its shape is rounded or slightly oval (*Figure 89*). *Oodinum* is a dinoflagellate pertaining to the Peridineae. Its size, according to Schäperclaus, varies from 20–70 microns; according to my own measurements it may be from 50–100 microns. The cell is limited by a perfectly visible cell wall or membrane. In the interior of the cell is found a round or oval nucleus, which in the majority of cases is not readily visible because *Oodinium* appears dark and opaque in smears. In stained smears it is noted that the nucleus is surrounded by numerous starch granules which obscure it from direct observation. The protoplasm is seen to be filled with droplets of an alveolar granule appearance in fixed preparations. The parasite is non-motile in smears. The biological life cycle of *Oodinium ocellatum* is similar to that of *O. pillularis*, and is shown in *Figure 90*. Coral fish disease makes its appearance in tropical marine aquaria where the temperature is between 20–25° C. Epizootics caused by this organism have been known to occur in large public aquaria since the year 1934.

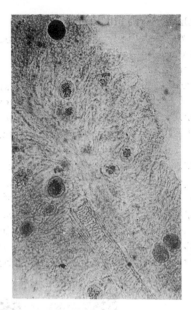

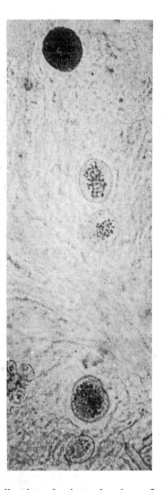

Figure 88. *Oodinium ocellatum* in the gill of *Pterois russelli*. (Original)

Figure 89. Parasites (*Oodinium ocellatum*) of differing sizes in gill of *Pterois russelli*. (Original)

The disease eventually spreads in the tank following the introduction of freshly imported fish (for example from Bermuda and the East Indies). In Berlin and Hamburg cases of mortalities have frequently been seen in the tanks of public aquaria, following their repopulation with freshly arrived specimens. Schäperclaus observed deaths in the Berlin aquarium, especially in *Procheilus percula, Dascyllus aruanus, Psettus argenteus, Chaetodon capistratus,* and *Balistes vetula.* I myself had an opportunity to demonstrate the presence of the infection in the Berlin Aquarium from the following fish species: *Pterois radiata, Pterois russeli, Scatophagus argus, Balistapus rectangularis, Heniochus acuminatus,* and *Chaetodontoplus mesoleucas.* Furthermore, the existence of the disease in *Platax vespertilio* and *Platax orbicularis* has been shown. Research on the biology of *Oodinuim ocellatum* allows the differentiation of three phases:

158

(*a*) a non-motile parasitic phase on the gills and skin;

(*b*) a cystic stage outside the fish body, following loosening of the parasite, and in which numerous intra-cystic divisions occur;

(*c*) a dispersive phase (the so-called dinospores).

Numerous dinospores are released from the cyst, and these swim freely by means of flagella. At 25° C. in three days, some 259 dinospores are formed, each one of which measures from 9–15 microns in length. The dinospores search out a new host fish, to which they immediately become attached.

HISTOPATHOLOGY AND HISTOCHEMISTRY: the action of the parasite becomes manifest by necrosis of the gill epithelium. I observed that *Oodinium ocellatum* penetrates the sub-epithelial connective tissues of the gills (*Figure 91*), in the same way as was described by Reichenbach-Klinke (1956a) for *O. pillularis*; an observation which had already been made previously by Schäperclaus (1954b). This leads to small spherical whitish-colored masses on the gill epithelium, which at first seem to be nodules.

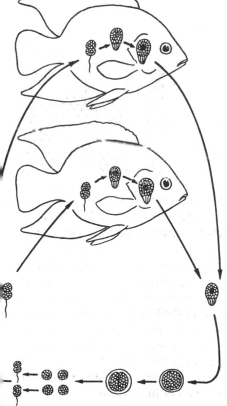

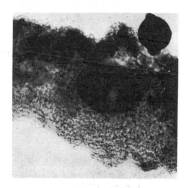

Figure 91. Two of the different stages of *Oodinium ocellatum*; one above the other, in the branchial epithelium. (Original)

Figure 90. Stages in the growth and development of *Oodinium*: the dinospores freed from the cysts on the substratum infest fishes, grow, and become adult; the mature parasites then fall to the bottom and form cysts. (Amlacher)

These observations have not been fully confirmed, and this type of lesion may also be due to other parasites.

THERAPY, PROPHYLAXIS AND HYGIENE: acriflavine baths (1 gm./100 liters water) for 2–12 hours are recommended. Prolonged baths in antibiotic solutions such as aureomycin have also been made use of in this connection. Copper sulfate has recently been used with a great measure of success as a prophylactic in the Berlin Aquarium.

Dempster (1956) used the following solution of copper sulfate against *Oodinium limneticum*: stock solution 1 gm./liter; for use add 2 ml. of this stock solution to each liter of water. I would personally recommend that the copper sulfate concentration be increased to 1.5 gm./liter. With this latter quantity (to be even more precise 1.6 gm./liter), encouraging results have been obtained in the Berlin Aquarium. Any recent arrivals from abroad should always be kept under observation, and in quarantine.

Velvet disease

CLINICAL PICTURE AND SYMPTOMS: diseased fish lose their normal coloration on the skin, and in advanced cases the skin may assume the appearance of a dark grayish or even yellowish layer (from which the British name "velvet disease" is derived). At times the skin even peels away in strips. The fish rub themselves against stones and other stationary objects and become thin. The spawn shows a complete lack of normal embryological development. The fish die sporadically over a period of several weeks.

TECHNIQUE OF INVESTIGATION: in living fish the investigation is made by means of a microscopical examination at a magnification of ×120 and ×200. Strips of skin and pieces of gill filaments and fins are examined. Dead fish are useless for the detection of this parasite, although those which have been sacrificed just prior to their natural death and are immediately placed in formalin may also be used for diagnosis.

ETIOLOGY; MORPHOLOGY AND TAXONOMY OF THE CAUSATIVE AGENT; COURSE OF THE DISEASE: *Oodinium pillularis* Schäperclaus was discovered and described scientifically by that worker in 1951, from *Colisa lalia*. Apart from *Colisa*, it attacks *Macropodus, Hyphessobrycon, Tanichthys, Nannostomus, Platypoecilus, Aphyosemion, Rasbora, Xiphophorus, Panchax* and the barbs. It also attacks goldfish and young carp, according to Schäperclaus. In shape *O. pillularis* ranges from oval-round to pyriform. The nonmotile parasite, adhering to the skin and gills, has a chitinous layer which terminates in a point at one end of the body, giving the organism the appearance of a bottle-neck (*Figure 92*). The parasites stick to the fish by means of this extremity, and through it they produce barely visible rhizoidal protoplasmic ramifications which penetrate in between the host cells. *O. pillularis* has a large oval nucleus in its interior, but does not possess the starch granules surrounding the nucleus as is characteristic of *O. ocellatum*. The protoplasm has the appearance of being filled with little droplets and granules. According to Schäperclaus the size of *O. pillularis* is from 50–70 microns, but fluctuations between 30–140 microns have been observed. My own measurements of this parasite would give its length as 30–100 microns. The life cycle and infectivity of this organism are exactly the same as in the case of *O. ocellatum*. On completing their growth, the parasites separate themselves from the fish and within a few minutes form a ball in the bottom of the water, in which the palmelloid phase takes place according to Hirschmann and Partsch (1953), who have studied and most carefully described this process. At this time the parasite undergoes a multiple division which gives rise to 32–64 daughter cells. These leave

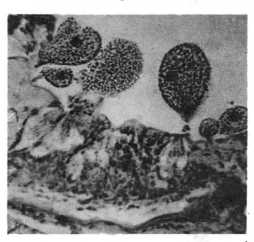

Figure 92. *Oodinium pillularis* lodged in the skin of *Colisa lalia*. (Schäperclaus)

the cyst, round off, and within 2 minutes are converted into flagellated dinospores with an annular ring and an eye spot. They then attack another fish, and should they not do so within 12–14 hours, they die. Since the adult parasites are grouped together in large numbers on the skin, they produce crateriform concentrations in which new dinospores preferentially install themselves, having now lost their flagella on invading the host. The course of the disease is very slow.

HISTOPATHOLOGY AHD HISTOCHEMISTRY: Reichenbach-Klinke (1954) demonstrated that *Oodinium pillularis* is capable of causing thickening of the opercula and surrounding tissue in tropical freshwater fish such as *Neolebias ansorgi* Boulenger. As will already have been seen, *O. pillularis* penetrates into the sub-cutaneous connective tissue and produces inflammatory reactions. In connective tissue, the parasite appears as rounded bodies, but in the majority of cases prolongations of the oral tube are also to be observed. Their average diameter is from 50–70 microns. They also attack the gill tissue.

THERAPY, PROPHYLAXIS AND HYGIENE: for the treatment of velvet disease in fish, a prolonged bath in acriflavine is recommended in conjunction with an increase in the temperature of the water to approximately 30° C. It is convenient to remove plants and bottom material from the tanks, which latter should be kept dark.

Copper sulfate treatment may be experimented with as was recommended for *Oodinium ocellatum* above. However, little concrete data have thus far been obtained with regards to the treatment of velvet disease. In aquaria it may be introduced together with live fish or food from pools and marshes which are themselves populated with wild fish. Recently imported fish must be placed in quarantine prior to being released onto the wholesale market.

Miscellaneous

Other dinoflagellates are of considerable importance in fish pathology, particularly that which concerns marine fish. *Gymnodinium brevis* has been cited as the cause of an important epizootic which occurs in the Gulf of Mexico, and which is known as the "Florida Red Tide." A similar occurrence is often seen in freshwater environments, and is caused by *Prymnesum* sp. Other important marine dinoflagellates responsible for fish mortalities are *Gonyaulax* and *Noctiluca* spp. As far as has been determined up to the present, such organisms secrete an ichthyotoxin which affects the nervous system of the fish.

Chapter 7

MYCOSIS (FUNGAL DISEASES)

Within the true Fungi, members of the Phycomycetes (algoid fungi) are those which cause the more important mycotic diseases of fish. The thallus of the lower Phycomycetes is mononucleate and of a microscopic size; in the taxonomically higher varieties, the thallus is multinucleate, ramified, and well developed. As a general rule the thallus of the higher Phycomycetes is siphonated, or, in other words, non-septate.

Ichthyosporidium (Ichthyophonus)

Hofer described this fungus in 1893 as the cause of whirling disease in trout and believed it to be a zooparasite. In 1905 Chaullery and Mesnil found two parasites in marine fish, *Ichthyosporidium gasterophilum* and *I. phymogenes*, and it was their belief that they were haplosporidians. Robertson (1908, 1909) found it in the flounder (*Pleuronectes flesus*), in sea trout, and in *Gadus aeglefinus*. In 1910 Laveran and Pettit, and Plehn and Mulsow, decided that the parasite was in fact a fungus. Plehn and Mulsow called it *Ichthyophonus hoferi* in honor of Hofer. Neresheimer and Clodi (1914) clarified its biology. Daniel (1933) and Fish (1934a) made additional studies. Of the more recent papers, mention will be made of those by Dorier and Degrange (1961), and Amlacher (1965). Sindermann (1954) cultured the organism under artificial conditions, and contributed greatly to the clarification of its biology. Basing himself on the identity of the organism as a Phycomycete given by Chaullery and Mesnil on the one hand, and by Plehn and Mulsow on the other, Pettit recommended the name *Ichthyosporidium hoferi* Plehn and Mulsow. Reichenbach-Klinke and Sindermann (1954, 1956) also use this name, but other authors still maintain the name *Ichthyophonus hoferi* P. and M. Schäperclaus (1953) has drawn attention to the occurrence of an *Ichthyophonus* peculiar to aquarium fish, and suspected that in certain circumstances it could constitute a separate species not identical with the *Ichthyosporidium* of trout and marine fish. In our own studies (Amlacher 1965), we were able to show that the *Ichthyophonus* of aquarium fish described by Schäperclaus (1953b) is a symptom of fish tuberculosis.

CLINICAL PICTURE AND SYMPTOMS: according to Sindermann the most frequently occurring external symptom in the herring is a roughness of the scales which gives rise to an effect described as "sand paper" (*Figure 93*). This is observed chiefly in the latero-ventral region of the tail, and is produced by very small black granulations which are the result of a necrotizing inflammation of the dermis. The destruction of the epidermis in these points results in desquamation and the formation of tiny white-colored necrotic areas, produced by the growth of the fungus. With these lesions are associated either large isolated abcesses or smaller abcesses in groups, as well as hemorrhagic ulcers (*Figure 94*).

In the internal organs of the herring, one's attention is drawn to the intensity of the cardiac (*Figure 95*) and hepatic lesions (formation of white nodules). Similar nodules have also been found in trout (Neresheimer and Clodi, 1914; Darier and Degrange, 1961; Amlacher, 1965). The retraction of the connective tissue, especially in the heart and kidney, also produces a "sand paper" effect when these organs are touched. In diseased herring a curvature of the vertebral column may be produced as a result of muscular spasms. This symptom was described for the first time in salmonids by Neresheimer and Clodi. Herring show disordered swimming movements and a heavy mortality rate, whenever they are exposed to mechanical stimuli. Trout frequently show vacillating movements and abdominal tumefaction.

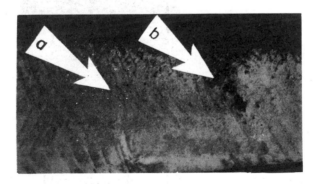

Figure 93. External lesions in a herring attacked by *Ichthyosporidium*: arrows (a) sandpaper effect involving numerous small, hard nodules; (b) ulcers resulting from proliferation of the fungus. (Sindermann)

According to Sindermann (1954) the following organs are attacked in the herring, and in an ever increasing degree of intensity as shown:

heart	strongly
lateral muscle	strongly
liver	regular
kidney	occasionally
spleen	rarely
gonads	rarely

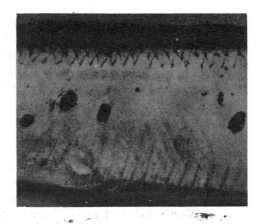

Figure 94. Swellings in the skin of a herring attacked by *Ichthyosporidium*. (Sindermann)

Figure 95. Cardiac muscle invaded by masses of *Ichthyosporidium hoferi*. (Sindermann)

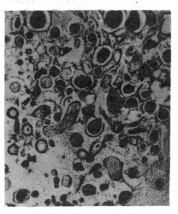

mesentery	rarely
digestive tract	rarely (above all the submucosa)
brain and spinal medulla	rarely
gill filaments	rarely (chiefly the branchial blood vessels)

TECHNIQUE OF INVESTIGATION: moribund fish are the most suitable for diagnosis. They are killed by a blow on the head, by an electric shock, or by cutting the neck. Preserved fish may be used, even though their study is somewhat more difficult to carry out. Squash preparations are made from the spleen, kidney, heart and liver, and where necessary from the brain. Often the scraping of fresh ulcers is sufficient to establish the presence of the fungus. Microscopical observation is best carried out at a magnification of ×45–120. Tissues are fixed in Stieve's fluid or in formalin and water (1:4). Cultures may be set up in gelatin peptone agar or in serum broth, For a differential diagnosis from sections it is important to stain with Giemsa, according to Neresheimer and Clodi, because with this particular stain the amoeboid forms are colored blue. Larger granulomas do not stain well, and hematoxylin-eosin is recommended for them. The parasites are very clearly visible in squash preparations of trout organs, where they appear as spheres from which arise smaller tubes, which in turn terminate as a spherical swelling. I once had the opportunity of observing microscopically the same form from the liver of marine fish in the port of Marseilles.

ETIOLOGY; MORPHOLOGY AND TAXONOMY OF THE CAUSATIVE AGENT; COURSE OF THE DISEASE: the fungus generally has a spherical or oval form, and shows numerous nuclei in the cytoplasm. Its size, according to Neresheimer and Clodi (1914), is between 6–20 microns in young plasmodia, and between 110–210 microns in the oldest and most mature ones. The diseased organ shows a layer of granulation tissue around the fungus. Sindermann (1954) cultivated it *in vitro*, as had been done by Plehn and Mulsow in 1911 and Forster in 1941. Sindermann was able to maintain the fungus alive in cultures for up to 14 months. It gave a very good growth in glycerine-peptone-agar containing 1% bovine serum (Sabouraud's medium with dextrose plus 1% bovine serum). This culture medium is streaked under aseptic conditions with material taken from the muscles and the heart of an infected herring. It grows between 3–20° C. (with an optimum of 10° C.). It always germinated within the culture medium, rarely on the surface and never under strictly aerobic conditions. Nonseptate hyphae were produced from the spores, and the fungal cytoplasm was concentrated at the extremities of the hyphae in the form of a solid mass. The claviform and terminal masses in the hyphae invariably produced new rounded or oval bulges due to a continuous growth of the cytoplasmic mass *(Figure 96)*, and they tie themselves up in a knot some 39 days after germination. Such formations are termed hyphal bodies and are produced by the hundred, but in old cultures this germination results in the formation of a terminal large quiescent or resting spore *(Figure 97)*. This latter type of spore rarely germinates in cultures. Endogenous division has not been observed in spores in culture media, but on certain occasions this must of necessity take place in the living tissues. The depth of the cultures ranges from 5–15 mm. Growth ceases within 30–60 days after this. The hyphae produced in culture are much bigger than those which occur in living tissue. The spores which are found in the blood measure from 10–90 microns; they are round and possess a cell wall or membrane. According to Sindermann they retain their infective nature for up to 6 months in sea water. The spore, according to this same worker, may form another heavy-walled spore on a hypha or may produce hyphal

166

Figure 96. Formation of hyphal bodies of *Ichthyosporidium* ten days after culturing in an artificial medium. (Sindermann)

Figure 96. Formation of hyphal bodies of *Ichthyosporidium* ten days after culturing in an artificial medium. (Sindermann)

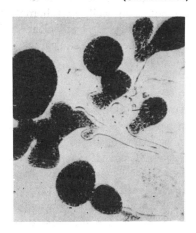

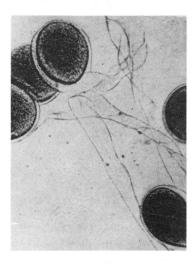

Figure 97. Formation of solitary quiescent spores of *Ichthyosporidium* thirty days after culturing in an artificial medium. (Sindermann)

bodies. The cytoplasm of the fungus is finely granular and of an alveolar structure (Neresheimer and Clodi). The cytoplasmic bodies and inclusions stain with nuclear stains. The amoeboid bodies, from 6–20 microns, contain some 5–12 nuclei which may agglomerate together.

According to Dorier and Degrange (1961), the development of *Ichthyosporidium* in salmonids occurs as follows (*Figure 98*):

After infection *per os*, amoeboblasts (D1, D2, D3) are freed from the latent cysts (A) in the digestive tract, or it comes to a filamentous (B) or plasmodial (C) germination of the parasites in the parasitized tissue. Amoeboid embryos become free in the intestine through rupture of the amoeboblast shell (E). They have one to two nuclei and penetrate through the intestinal mucosa to the blood stream. With the blood, they arrive in various organs (musculature, heart, liver, spleen, kidney). Here, new cysts (K1, K2) arise through endogenic division. From many cysts in parasitized tissue, plasmodia hatch (I1) or endospores (I2) are formed.

The infection takes place by means of spores and hyphae present in fish feces, in open ulcers, and probably on copepods, as was supposed by Sindermann (1954). The spores liberate amoeboid bodies which cross the intestinal mucosa and reach the bloodstream. Once here, they are distributed throughout the different organs by means of the blood. They particularly attack the heart (*Figure 99*), the spleen, the liver, and the

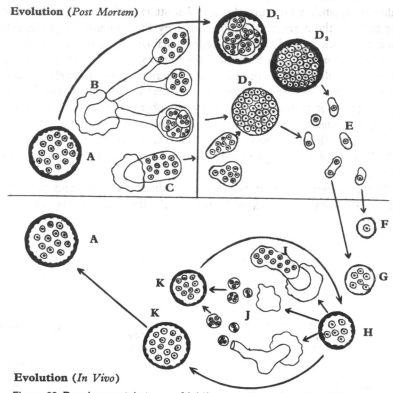

Figure 98. Developmental stages of *Ichthyosporidium*: A, cyst; B, filamentous germination; C, plasmodial germination; D, amoeboblasts; E, amoeboid embryos; F through K, formation of new cysts; I, plasmodium; J; endospores.

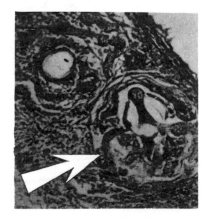

Figure 99. Germinating *Ichthyosporidium* in the heart muscle of the herring. (Sindermann)

kidney because the blood flows through these organs slowly and in considerable quantities; the muscles are also attacked. In *Figure 100* we see the cycle in the herring as demonstrated by Sindermann. In young fish such an attack may give rise to skeletal deformities, particularly of the vertebral column, due to muscular contractions. In the great majority of cases these deformed fish also have their internal organs intensely invaded by the fungus. The above-mentioned visceral organs encyst the fungus and surround it with connective tissue membranes. Reichenbach-Klinke (1954) described a number of experimental infections which were crowned with success; the results were obtained by feeding the fungus to aquarium fish. Similar proof was given by Sindermann on feeding the parasite to herring.

The numerous granulomas replace the healthy tissues and produce ascites or other tissue reactions ("sand paper" effect), and finally cause the fish to die.

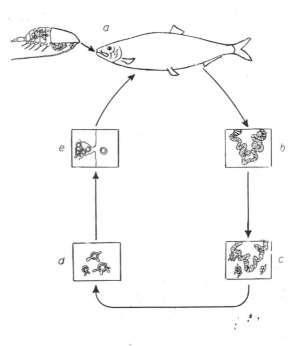

Figure 100. Life cycle of *Ichthyosporidium hoferi* in the herring: (a) ingestion of the fungus, carried by a copepod or contacted from the water; (b) the spores liberate amoeboid bodies which cross the intestinal mucosa; (c) the fungus penetrates the blood vessels of the sub-mucosa; (d) spores and hyphal bodies are disseminated throughout the body in the blood and give rise to focal lesions; (e) spores reach the exterior through lesions in living fish (new drawing, slightly modified, after Sindermann)

HISTOPATHOLOGY AND HISTOCHEMISTRY: according to Neresheimer and Clodi (1914) invasion of the tissues produces a chronic inflammation and, in the case of long-standing infection, granulomas. These lesions are typical in the heart. The muscles are infiltrated by round cells, they tend to disintegrate, and their overall appearance is one of cirrhosis. Externally the lesions give rise first of all to a thickening of the tissue affected, and finally to a cicatrization. By this means the relatively small fungus produces infiltration of round cells, necrosis and neoplasms in the connective tissues. The connective tissue encapsulates the parasite either singly or in groups. Inside these connective tissue capsules may be seen necrotic remains of the parasitized tissue (for example, of kidney or liver). In trout, contrary to that which is the case in summer, no outbreaks of this disease are observed during the winter period.

According to Dorier and Degrange (1961), the amoeboid embryos penetrating the tissues are phagacytized after 48 hours. The phagocytosis lasts up to 9 days and occurs in the adventitia of the vessels and in the gills. In the heart musculature a leucocyte wall is formed around the maturing cysts which is strengthened later with fibrocytes (*Figure 101*). The defense ring can become 40–70mu thick in 1–2 months. The enclosed cysts can necrotize. The granulomas can become up to 900mu and larger.

We found (Amlacher, 1965) sizes of *Ichthyosporidium* of 40–140mu in the liver, heart, spleen, and kidney. The smallest stages were 8mu–16mu in size. The nuclei of the plasmodiens were 1.6mu–3.5mu in size. The thickness of the cyst capsules, in most studies, amounted to 2.2mu–11mu. The shell of the cyst (capsule) is PAS positive (see color plate 1). The plasmodium contained glycogen and fat.

The numerous granulomas seriously damage the infected organs, which react with an infiltration of round cells and by encapsulating the parasite with connective tissue. When there are numerous granulomas, cirrhosis and necrotic atrophy are produced within the organs attacked. *Figure 102* shows a section through the body muscle of a herring with different stages of *Ichthyosporidium* infection. In extreme cases almost all of the organ is little more than granulation tissue; the normal tissue itself being replaced and atrophied. At times ascites and accumulation of serous fluid may be produced in the peritoneal cavity, this having arisen from the blood.

THERAPY, PROPHYLAXIS AND HYGIENE: experiments carried out up to the present time suggest that ichthyosporidiosis is incurable. As far as marine fisheries are concerned, the throwing back into the sea of infected fish is a practice worthy of the strongest prohibitions. Dead herring should be taken to the shore and buried there (Sindermann, 1954). In trout hatcheries where sea fish are added to the food, they should be carefully steamed

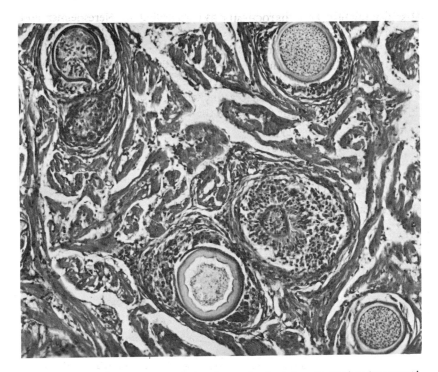

Figure 101. Atrophic processes In heart muscle of rainbow trout showing granulomas enclosing the *Ichthyosporidium* parasite. (after Amlacher)

Figure 102. Different stages of *Ichthyosporidium* infection in musculature of a herring; arrows—(a) hyphal bodies; (b) germinating spores; (c) quiescent sporos. (Sindermann)

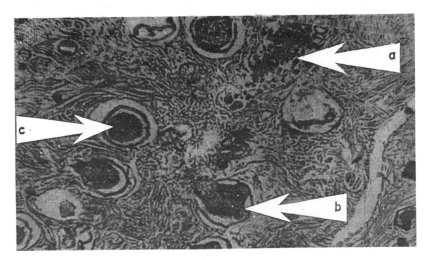

beforehand. Schäperclaus (1954) suspected that infected marine fish transmit the disease to trout farms. This has since been proven.

Branchiomycosis (gill rot)

Plehn (1912), Wundsch (1929), and Schäperclaus (1929) painstakingly studied and described mycotic gill rot. Scheuring and Walter (1926), as well as Scheuring and Gaschott (1928), made mention of sporadic cases. The frequency and the intensity of this disease are variable factors, and in the majority of fish hatcheries the disease is totally unknown. Between 1925–1927, Schäperclaus (1929) observed a total of 15 cases in all. In 1961, I myself observed a heavy mortality among one- and two-year-old carp in a tank wherein ducks had previously been living.

CLINICAL PICTURE AND SYMPTOMS: gill rot (fungal) is caused by two different fungi, and therefore appears as two separate varieties:

(a) gill rot of carp (also of tench, goldfish and sticklebacks);

(b) gill rot of pike and tench.

Both forms have been observed occurring simultaneously in tench. In carp gill rot, the diseased fish show ecchymoses or necrotic patches on the gills, together with false membrane formation made up of proliferation and adhesions of the gill epithelium. Repair processes may similarly be observed in the tissue. These later fall away. The fish begin to show signs of asphyxia, and lie gasping at the surface of the water. One-year-old fish are more susceptible to the disease than are two-year-old ones. They tend to refuse food, and are often observed at the water inlet of the tank.

In gill rot of pike, under the microscope may be seen tubular formations (even under a low magnification) with a dendritic branching (*Figure 103*), which develop in the gill filaments (Wundsch, 1929). The gills are pale and often grayish-white in color, although certain isolated parts retain their normal red coloration. The symptoms are very similar to those produced in gill rot of carp.

TECHNIQUE OF INVESTIGATION: fresh preparations from the gill filaments are examined microscopically at $\times 45$–120 magnification. To prepare sections, material may be fixed in Stieve's or Bouin's fluid, or in formalin. Staining is carried out with hematoxylin and eosin, iron hematoxylin, or by Mallory's trichrome method.

ETIOLOGY; MORPHOLOGY AND TAXONOMY OF THE CAUSATIVE AGENT; COURSE OF THE DISEASE: the causative agent of branchiomycosis in carp is the Phycomycete *Branchiomyces sanguinis* Plehn (*Figure 104*). Its non-septate hyphae measure from 8–30 microns in diameter, or 13.8–20.7 microns according to my own personal observations. The organism is localized in the blood vessel of the gill arch, gill filaments and respiratory filaments. The spores, 5–9 microns in diameter (6.9 microns according to my own measurements) originate in the plasmodium. Gill rot of pike is also caused by another Phycomycete, which is very similar in appearance to *Branchiomyces sanguinis*. It is *Branchiomyces demigrans* Wundsch (*Figure 105*). The hyphae have thicker walls (0.5–0.7 microns) than in *B. sanguinis*; and the fundamental difference between the two, as the name suggests, is that in *B. demigrans* the hyphae grow from the gills outwards. The width of the hyphae is from 13–14 microns, although in the final stages of growth they may measure up to 22–28 microns. The spores are 12–17 microns in diameter.

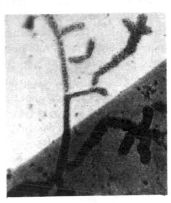

Figure 103. Greatly magnified free portion of *Branchiomyces demigrans* with typical branching and fruiting stages. (Wundsch)

Figure 104. *Branchiomyces sanguinis* in a gill lamella and in the respiratory folds. (Redrawn after Plehn)

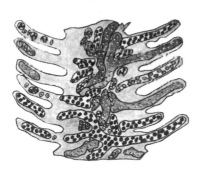

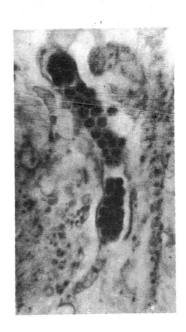

Figure 105. *Branchiomyces demigrans*, hyphae containing numerous spores as shown under high magnification. (Wundsch)

173

The presence of *Branchiomyces* gives rise to thrombosis of the branchial vessels, hemostasis, swelling of the veins, and in consequence necrosis of the affected parts of the gills. *B. demigrans* destroys the gill tissue in an extremely rapid manner due to its movement towards the exterior (*Figure 106*).

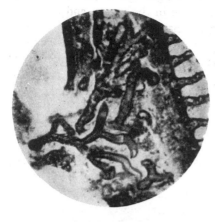

Figure 106. *Branchiomyces demigrans*, typical point of rupture and growth towards the exterior. (Wundsch)

Infection takes place by means of fungal spores which reach the water with necrotized gill tissue from other fish. Nothing at all is known of the way in which the primary infection occurs.

The disease appears in summer with no apparent relation to the prevailing temperature, although in the majority of cases following a period of heat. It is occasionally observed in May, with low water temperatures (14° C.). Its course is very rapid (2–4 days), so much so that the fish pathologist is usually unable to find any fungi at all within a few days of the disease having first made its appearance. Losses among two and three-year-old carp may reach from 30–50%.

According to Schäperclaus (1954) water rich in nutritive organic substances tends to favor the appearance of branchiomycosis, for which reason tanks and ponds that are frequently fertilized with organic fertilizers are particularly susceptible to outbreaks of the disease. Other factors favoring its appearance are waters rich in phytoplanktonic algae, a too dense population, and a temperature in excess of 20° C.

HISTOPATHOLOGY AND HISTOCHEMISTRY: it is seen that in the diseased gills, *Branchiomyces sanguinis* predominantly attacks the oxygen-rich efferent branchial arteries, from which it seems to be an oxyphilic organism. The attack takes place from without, on the small branchial filaments; the fungus grows in the efferent branchial artery and from here returns again to the filaments. The parasitized gills show epithelial proliferations in the area of the respiratory surface and adhesions on the neighboring branchial laminae. The blood capillaries are displaced by the fungus. When *B. demigrans* penetrates into the lumen of an efferent branchial artery, it produces angiectasia, and finally, after breaking the vascular wall and the wall of the gill lamina, breaks out as a mass of hyphae characteristic of *B. demigrans (Figure 106)*.

THERAPY, PROPHYLAXIS AND HYGIENE: the fight against gill rot can only be carried out by observing strict hygiene in the ponds, and by this is meant the avoidance of too much organic material such as might be caused by adding an excess of food on hot days. Any dead fish must be removed and destroyed. If the presence of this disease is suspected, the quantity of incoming water should be increased. In order to disinfect the tank, this should be drained, coated with quicklime or calcium cyanamide, and finally refilled with clean water.

Aphanomycosis (crab or crayfish pest)

Aphanomycosis, generally known as crab or crayfish pest, practically destroyed all the crayfish population in German rivers and lakes during the 19th century. Towards 1870 the disease progressively moved from France to Germany (1878–72) in an easterly direction; in the period 1891–96 it decimated the crayfish population of Russia, and it penetrated via the Ural mountains to eastern Siberia. In 1894 it was introduced into Lithuania; and Scandinavia, which for a long time had remained free from the disease, was invaded by aphanomycosis in 1929.

Shanor and Saslow (1944) reported it in fish.

CLINICAL PICTURE AND SYMPTOMS: symptoms are not always immediately visible, but as the disease progresses the crayfish show definite symptoms which may justify the suspicion that aphanomycosis is present. The crayfish tend to adopt a supine position and ceaselessly move their legs until they die. They probably lie on their backs because the fungus attacks and destroys the articular membranes; for this reason the diseased animals walk awkwardly, and lose their legs, and at times their claws. If a diseased crayfish is lifted up, its claws hang downwards as if they were paralyzed *(Figure 107)*. Later on it is possible to observe a generalized lassitude. If the chitinous membrane of the ventral abdominal surface or the articulated membranes of the legs are explored with a pair of fine-pointed forceps, it is often possible to find isolated areas destroyed by the fungus, and these areas are soft and readily yield to pressure; sometimes they possess a yellowish coloration. The anal region is another common place for the attack to take place.

TECHNIQUE OF INVESTIGATION: the suspected points of the articular membranes are cut away and examined microscopically. In positive cases, a fine network of hyphae is seen *(Figure 108)*.

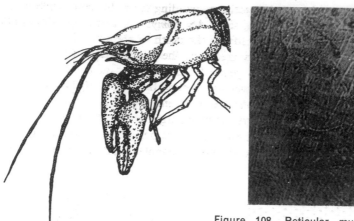

Figure 107. Hanging claws caused by paralysis in a crayfish suffering from aphamomycosis. (Original)

Figure 108. Reticular mycelium of *Aphanomyces astaci* in the inter-segment membrane of the ventral abdominal surface in *Astacus leptodactylus*. (Amlacher)

ETIOLOGY; MORPHOLOGY AND TAXONOMY OF THE CAUSATIVE AGENT; COURSE OF THE DISEASE: the causative agent of this disease remained completely unknown for a long time. Hofer believed it to be *Bacterium pestis astaci* until Schikora (1903) demonstrated that the Phycomycete *Aphanomyces astaci* was the cause. Schäperclaus, in 1935, gave definite proof to the effect that *Aphanomyces* produces this disease, and his results were subsequently confirmed by Nybelin (1935) and Mannsfield (1942). The name *Aphanomyces* means difficult to see. The hyphae cross through and destroy the chitinous carapace, which softens and becomes brittle in the points of greatest destruction (*Figure 108*). It also attacks the connective tissue and, above all, the nervous system; in exceptional cases it also invades the musculature. The nerve lesions are probably the decisive cause of death, even when the carapace lesions favor the occurrence of bacterial infections which perhaps play an important role in the fatal results of an attack of aphanomycosis. At a greater magnification ($\times 600$) we see that the hyphae frequently possess a markedly granular and colorless cytoplasm (*Figure 109*). The filaments have rounded ends, and their transparency makes them difficult to see. The net is formed by the hyphae when the ramifications of these are in close proximity to each other. The filaments measure from 4–8 microns in width. Propagation is carried out by means of vegetative spores of 8.1–9.5 microns in diameter, which have their origin in the filaments, or by sexual reproduction between male and female organs. Asexual reproduction takes place when the external conditions are unfavorable, and after the death of the host animal. It is for this very reason that a fine mycelium spreading from the joint membranes may be seen in dead crayfish, since *Aphanomyces* is a strict parasite and does not enjoy a saprophytic life on the death of the host. The infective powers of this fungus are very great, and the disease may reappear in the same place even after 10–20 years. Dr. Barthelmes (of the Institute of Ichthyology, Humboldt University, Berlin) has found *Aphanomyces* in *Diaptomus gracilis* and in *Asplanchna priodonta* (personal communication). THERAPY, PROPHYLAXIS AND HYGIENE: lethargic and dead crayfish must be removed from the water and buried. Where possible, a strict quarantine should be maintained on animals used to populate stretches of water and tanks.

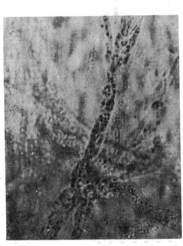

Figure 100. *Aphanomyces astaci*: greatly magnified hyphae showing densely granular cytoplasm and branching. (Amlacher)

Saprolegniasis and achlyasis

Fungi of the genera *Saprolegnia* and *Achlya* are also of importance in fish pathology, and these are sometimes known under the name of "fish fungi." In the majority of cases the infection has arisen from open wounds on the body of the fish, while on other occasions they may live on the decaying remains of food (for example, in *Daphnia, Figure 110*). According to Sterba, long-finned fish are those which seem to be most subject to the disease. In aquarium fish saprolegniasis almost universally appears as a result of a lowering of the temperature of the water. If the disease continues the fins become frayed, and this gives rise to bacterial invasion and infection. In fish which are raised for food, *Saprolegnia* appears above all in the tanks used for the hatchery operations. The mold attacks the skin, gills, mouth, fins and eyes. Also it is well known that fish eggs, especially dead ones (for example, in trout hatcheries) may become moldy. In severe cases *Saprolegnia* may actually penetrate into the muscle tissue.

Propagation takes place by means of spores, grouped together in the ends of the hyphae (*Figure 111*). These leave the host and swim freely in groups by means of two flagella. Following a transitory change of shape, they implant themselves upon the substrate and form a new siphonated tube. The control of these fungi is carried out by raising the temperature of the aquarium water and changing the fish into fresh water. Food fishes should not be scratched or damaged in any way, either on fishing or transporting them. A bath of potassium permanganate (1 gm./100 liters water) for 90 minutes has been shown to be a good therapeutic measure.

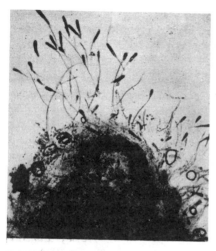

Figure 110. Fungus-covered abdomen of a *Daphnia*. (Original)

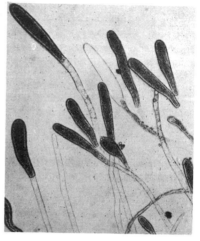

Figure 111. Detail from figure 110 showing the swollen and spore-filled tips of the hyphae. (Amlacher)

Chapter 8

PROTOZOAN DISEASES

Certain types of protozoans exist which are capable of causing serious diseases in fish (for example, *Ichthyophthirius*, *Trypanoplasma* and *Myxosoma*). Others become parasitic as a result of the presence of other diseases, or because of an overall weakness in the fish (*Costia*, *Chilodonella*, *Octomitus*). The following is a brief classification of the more important groups of parasitic protozoans: For a complete list of North American species see Hoffman (1967).

Super Class: MASTIGOPHORA (FLAGELLATA)
  fish pathogens: *Costia necatrix* Henneguy; *Octomitus truttae* (Duj.) Schmidt; *Trypanoplasma borelli* Lav. and Mes.; *Trypanoplasma tincae* Schäperclaus; *Trypanosoma* spp.

SPOROZOA
  Class Telosporea
    sub-class: Coccidia
      fish pathogens: *Eimeria truttae* Leger and Hesse; *Eimeria cyprini* Plehn; *Eimeria subepithelialis* Moroff and Fiebiger; *Eimeria anguillae* Leger and Hollande; and more than 28 other species from the internal organs of freshwater and marine fish
    Order: Hemosporidia
      fish pathogens: more than 23 species have been described, usually as parasites in the blood of marine fish
  sub-Phylum: Cnidospora
    Class: Myxosporidea
      Family: Unicapsulidae
        fish pathogens: 3 species, in the tissues and gall bladder of marine fish
      Family: Myxosomatidae
        fish pathogens: *Myxosoma cerebralis* Hofer and Plehn; and species in the gall bladder and different organs of freshwater and marine fish
      Family: Chloromyxidae
        fish pathogens: more than 20 species, in the gall bladder and different tissues of freshwater and marine fish

Family: Myxobolidae

fish pathogens: *Myxobolus*, *Thelohanellus*, *Henneguya*, *Hoferellus*. More than 32 species, most of them in freshwater fish; give rise to cysts and infiltrations in various organs

Family: Myxidiidae

fish pathogens: more than 30, the majority of them in the gall bladder of marine fish

Class: Microsporidea

Family: Nosematidae

fish pathogens: *Nosema* Naegeli (with 5 important species that parasitize different organs of marine fish); *Glugea* Thel. (12 important species, chiefly in marine fish); *Thelohania* (with *T. contejeani* Henneguy, causative agent of "porcelain disease" in crayfish); *Plistophora* (15 important species, among which is *P. hyphessobryconis* Schäperclaus, chiefly in muscles)

Family: Mrazekiidae

fish pathogens: 2 species

Class: Haplosporidia

fish pathogens: the genera pathogenic to fish include *Dermocystidium*, which produces cysts in the skin and on the gills

sub-Phylum: CILIATA (CILIOPHORA)

sub-Class: Holotrichia

fish pathogens: *Ichthyophthirius multifiliis* Fouquet; *Chilodonella cypirni* Moroff

sub-Class: Peritrichia

fish pathogens: *Trichodina domerguei* Wallengreen, very slightly pathogenic

FLAGELLATES (MASTIGOPHORA)

The Flagellates are the most ancient group of protozoans, and there is a gradual taxonomic transition between zooflagellates, phytoflagellates and algae. The cytoplasm is encased by a cell wall and there may be from one to various flagella. Locomotion takes place by means of a motor flagellum which emerges from one pole of the cell, being firmly united internally to a basal corpuscle, and is prolonged to the blepharoplast (kinetonucleus or locomotory center). The cell nucleus is situated near to the blepharoplast, and food vacuoles are to be seen. There is frequently a trailing flagellum. The undulating membrane also serves in a locomotory function. The flagella may be numerous (in *Octomitus* there are eight). Flagellates reproduce asexually by means of longitudinal divison.

Costiasis

This disease is widely distributed and is of frequent occurrence in winter tanks used for young trout and where fish are grouped together. The lack of food during hibernation or at the end of the growth period of carp weakens the fish and makes them more susceptible to costiasis. For this reason, coupled with the fact that the majority of cases occur secondarily, it is believed that *Costia necatrix* is a "debility parasite." Isolated parasites may be found in almost all healthy freshwater and marine fish and they have similarly been observed in aquaria.

CLINICAL PICTURE AND SYMPTOMS: a soft grayish-white film or sheet is observed on the surface of the body, and the more intensely affected parts are reddened and hemorrhagic. The fish frequently show awkward swimming movements, and their fins are held close to the body. They scrape themselves against stones and other solid objects. In year old carp, a great weakness and generalized debility is noted.

TECHNIQUE OF INVESTIGATION: the investigation is performed on fresh smears of the gills and skin. Preserved material is useless. Dead fish may be utilized on the condition that very little time has elapsed since their death. In smears examined at a ×120 magnification the parasites may be recognized by their characteristic way of making "S" movements. Methanol fixed smears may be stained with hematoxylin.

ETIOLOGY; MORPHOLOGY AND TAXONOMY OF THE CAUSATIVE AGENT; COURSE OF THE DISEASE: The disease is caused by a skin flagellate called *Costia necatrix* Henneguy. It has a bean-shaped form (i.e. reniform), and is constant in shape. Two locomotory flagella arise from the convex side of the body (*Figure 112*). The body measures from 10–12 microns in length, and from 6–8 microns in width. The nucleus is situated in the center of the cell. The parasite fixes itself by its posterior extreme to the superficial cells of the epidermis, adhering to it by means of a type of canal or sac which exercises a sucking action, and results in a destruction of the skin cells (*Figure 112d*). For this reason the parasites which are fixed to the skin have a pyriform appearance. When they are in this state, they may reproduce asexually by means of longitudinal division. Those individuals which are about to reproduce have four flagella (*Figure 112b*). Outside the fish the parasite becomes rounded off and dies in the majority of cases after 30–60 minutes (*Figure 112e*), which means that it cannot live except where the fish are tightly packed together. In aquarium fish, it particularly attacks the soft fins. *Costia* is seldom found in tropical aquarium tanks. Probably this is due to the fact that it does not like temperatures above 25° C., as was suggested by Sterba (1956). The parasite dies at 30° C.

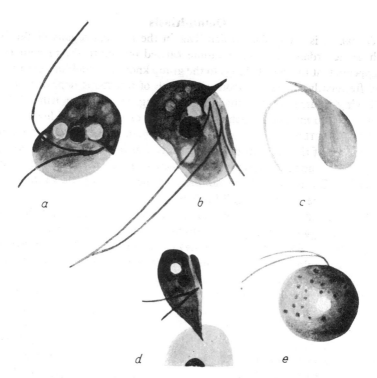

Figure 112. *Costia necatrix*: (a) normal bi-flagellate form; (b) tetra-flagellate (dividing) form; (c) lateral view; (d) parasite adhering to surface of skin; (e) parasite reduced to a ball. (Modified after Benisch)

HISTOPATHOLOGY AND HISTOCHEMISTRY: an intensive attack of costiasis produces necrosis of the epidermal cells. The dermis may be hyperemic, as has been noted by Schäperclaus.

THERAPY, PROPHYLAXIS AND HYGIENE: young trout or carp infected with costiasis are bathed for 20 minutes in a 1% sodium chloride solution, and are then placed in fresh tanks with abundant food. Formalin baths may also be applied (see Table 2). The parasites die in these baths. In aquarium practice, a longer bath in trypaflavine (1 gm./100 liters) kills the parasites within 2 days. The fish should, of course, be given their bath in a separate tank. A simple increase of the temperature to above 30° C. also kills *Costia*. It is convenient to free the skin parasites from breeding fish (spawners) by means of a short bath before passing them to the breeding tanks, so as to ensure that the spawn is not contaminated. The fish should never be placed too closely together, and pH fluctuations in the tank must be corrected since they damage the skin and favor infection by *Costia*.

Octomitiasis

Octomitus is a flagellate which lives in the internal organs of the host fish. In accordance with observations carried out up to the present time, it appears that this also belongs to the group known as "debility parasites", and frequently appears in trout as a result of infectious nephritis etc., or following an unsuitable or inadequate feeding. In aquarium fish it follows as a sequel to infections such as tuberculosis or ichthyosporidiosis.

CLINICAL PICTURE AND SYMPTOMS: affected young trout alevins remain at the bottom of the tanks near to the side, and as in diseased aquarium fish, they show sudden swimming movements. Emaciation is occasionally observed. On autopsy, large numbers of the parasites are found in the lower intestine and in the gall bladder.

TECHNIQUE OF INVESTIGATION: squash preparations are made from the rectum and gall bladder, and examination of these is made at a ×120 magnification. Only live fish are usable in the search for this parasite, and these should be killed by means of a cut in the neck. Preserved material and dead fish are of no use for this study.

ETIOLOGY; MORPHOLOGY AND TAXONOMY OF THE CAUSATIVE AGENT; COURSE OF THE DISEASE: *Octomitus truttae* (Duj.) Schmidt, the one found in trout, has an oval cellular body, and when fixed shows one nucleus (or, according to Reichenow, two nuclei). At the anterior pole there are two flagellar cords, each one made up of three individual flagella. The posterior pole bears two long terminal flagella (*Figure 113*). In the living parasite flagella are also observed just prior to death, when the protozoans diminish the velocity of their flagellar activity. The body is 10 microns long and 4.5 microns wide. In the same way as *Costia*, *Octomitus* moves in jumps by the movement of its flagella. Schäperclaus observed and described species of *Octomitus* in angel fish (*Pterophyllum scalare*), *Cichlasoma severum* and *Heterandria formosa*.

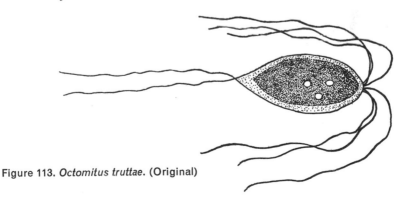

Figure 113. *Octomitus truttae*. (Original)

I myself was able to see them in angel fish kept in aquaria. They have also been found in viviparous cyprinodonts and in barbs, as well as in cichlids (*Cichlasoma severum*). The parasite lives in the intestine of the fish.

According to North American investigations (Davis), *Octomitus* may encyst, and besides this Davis has also described a rounded intra-cellular stage. (Reexamination of some of this material has revealed histological evidence of IPN. Thus, the intra-cellular stage recorded may have been the inclusions seen with IPN.) In *Symphysodon discus*, I was able to observe rounded forms together with the normal variety. These seemed to be smaller versions of the parasite. Nothing certain is so far known regarding the reproduction of these parasites.

HISTOPATHOLOGY AND HISTOCHEMISTRY: *Octomitus truttae* produces inflammations and changes in the epithelium of the gall bladder, which latter becomes thickened.

THERAPY, PROPHYLAXIS AND HYGIENE: apart from prophylaxis by means of a suitable feeding schedule which prevents the formation of intestinal lesions, there are really no well proven remedies, owing to the comparative rarity of the disease. American workers recommend the addition of 0.2% calomel to the food for 2 days, or 0.2% carbarsone for 4 days.

According to Bellet (1959) calomel (2 gm./kgm. food for 4 days) has given good results in the fight against *Octomitus truttae*. This drug requires a prescription, and may only be used under the strictest veterinary vigilance.

In collaboration with Dr. Steffens, I studied the therapeutic action of trypaflavine added to the diet for trout fingerlings. A 0.1% solution of trypaflavine was added to minced meat and given as a food. 25% of the diseased fish refused this fare, and after 17 days of observation the fish were sacrificed and autopsied. In the first experimental batch of controls 2 out of 19 were found to be infected, while the 19 treated fish were completely free from the parasite. In the second lot, there were 7 out of 14 control animals infected (50%), and 3 sick fish out of 18 treated fish (16.6%). A further non-treated control batch also gave a 50% rate of infection. Among the control fish there were some which showed evidence of a massive attack, while the positive cases among the treated fish were extremely mild in their intensity.

Octomitus symphysodoni nova species (?)

In 1959 I was able to make an interesting observation in *Symphysodon discus*. The fish refused food, and were examined some three weeks after having stopped eating. The first animal died shortly after receipt, and on autopsy it was seen that there was a disseminated macular necrosis and a deep yellow color with a blackish pigmentation in the liver and spleen. An intense necrosis accompanied by atrophy of the renal tubules was observed in the kidney. The fish had no parasites. The second fish, which was autopsied on the same day, presented signs of a heavy attack by an *Octomitus* sp. measuring 11.5×4.6 microns; the posterior flagella being 12 microns in length. They moved in a spiral fashion and either continued doing this or made a ball after 30 minutes in 40% alcohol. In partially clotted blood smears the parasite continued living for more than one hour.

Contrary to the case in *Octomitus truttae*, which parasitizes the gall bladder and intestine, this flagellate was found in the liver. It was so abundant that it rather gave the impression that the liver smear was actually moving. I also found the parasite in the still beating heart of the diseased fish, and it could be seen in large numbers in the gall bladder and rectum. The kidney presented symptoms of tubule necrosis, with small clusters of bacteria, but no parasites were seen. In another fish, I found large numbers of flagellates in the small intestine, and a few isolated ones in the spleen. Munchin (cited by Doflein-Reichenow) was the first to voice the suspicion that certain flagellates which live in the intestine may become blood parasites of their host. That this concept is a valid one is shown by the studies carried out with true intestinal flagellates (*Trichomonas, Eutrichomonas, Octomitus, Giardia*) parasitic to reptiles and amphibians. Lavier and Gaillard found *Octomitus* in the blood of a toad, without being able to observe it in the intestine. We see therefore that the types of observation mentioned above are not all that infrequent. Experimental infections of *Nannacara anomala*, in which pathological material was added to the aquarium, also gave a positive result after one month. In view of its occurrence in the blood, heart, liver, and spleen of *Symphysodon discus*, I propose that this parasite be called *Octomitus symphysodoni*.

Trypanoplasma (Cryptobia)

This disease is found, above all, in tench, particularly during the winter period when leeches are present. Its presence has also been described from carp, goldfish, and other species of fish in Europe. In the United States, cyprinids, salmonids and cottids are notably infected.

CLINICAL PICTURE AND SYMPTOMS: the tench have pale gills indicating anemia, deeply sunken eyes, and a certain degree of emaciation. They frequently remain in an oblique position, resting their heads on the bottom of the tank. From time to time they swim around on their own axis.

TECHNIQUE OF INVESTIGATION: the best preparations are made fresh from the kidney. Trypanoplasms are also found in the blood shortly after the animal has died, and they may be identified using a $\times 120$ magnification. Blood smears are made, fixed, and stained by the usual procedures (see blood analysis).

ETIOLOGY; MORPHOLOGY AND TAXONOMY OF THE CAUSATIVE AGENT; COURSE OF THE DISEASE: the causal agents of these diseases are flagellates of the genera *Trypanoplasma* and *Cryptobia*, of which the following species occur:

(a) *T. tincae* Schäperclaus: in tench; length 15 microns, width 3–4 microns, length of the flagella 15 microns;

(b) *T. cyprini* Plehn: in carp, goldfish, golden carp; length 20–25 microns;

(c) *C. borelli* Lav. and Mes.: length 20 microns, width 3–4 microns, length of the flagella 15 microns;

(d) *C. salmositica* Katz: salmonids, sculpins, cyprinids; length 6.0–25 microns, width 1.25–4.0 microns.

The trypanoplasm lives in the intestine of leeches, and these transmit them to fish by means of their bites. The parasite may be found in the blood of the fish seven days after infection (*Figure 114*). The disease may cause death with typical symptoms of anemia. Schäperclaus (1954) observed an insignificant decrease in the hemoglobin in diseased tench of 9.6–8.8 gm./100 ml., compared with 10.1 gm./100 ml. in healthy fish. The red blood cell count was 0.96–2.31 millions/cmm. in sick fish, and 1.7 millions/cmm. in healthy ones.

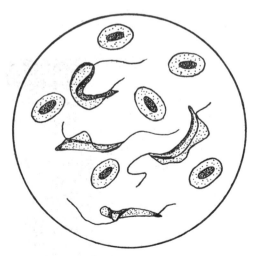

Figure 114. *Trypanoplasma tincae* in a blood smear. (Original)

HISTOPATHOLOGY AND HISTOCHEMISTRY: no detailed studies are available. THERAPY, PROPHYLAXIS AND HYGIENE: in view of the fact that only a small proportion of the fish seem to be affected, it is sufficient to remove these. Leeches should be destroyed, since these are vectors of the disease.

SPOROZOA

The Sporozoa live exclusively as parasites, and their nutrition is osmotic, which explains why food vacuoles are not found within their cytoplasm. The body is bordered by a strong membrane serving as a protection against the defensive mechanism of the host. Movement is virtually non-existent, and the greater majority of sporozoans are non-motile. Their life cycle is complex, and both sexual and asexual reproduction (metagenesis or alternating generations) occur within it. Among the animals which are infected, the one in which sexual reproduction takes place is called the final or definitive host, while that in which the sexual reproduction of the parasite occurs is known as the intermediate host. For selective staining of spores, the Ziehl-Neelsen or Giemsa methods are excellent.

Nodular coccidiosis in the intestine of carp

This particular disease is caused by *Eimeria subepithelialis* Morrof and Fiebiger, and appears in tanks which are used to hold young fish. The middle and lower intestines show small nodules about 2 mm. in diameter under the mucosa, which seem almost to be transparent through the muscle tissue. The diseased fish have sunken eyes and may be somewhat emaciated. *Eimeria subepithelialis* multiplies intra-cellularly by schizogony and sporogony. The occysts measure from 14–17 microns, and the spores 8–10 × 5–8 microns (*Figure 115*).

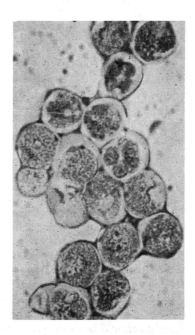

Figure 115. *Eimeria subepithelialis* oocysts containing oospores. (Original)

Enterococcidiosis in the carp

Enterococcidiosis appears principally in young and 1-year-old carp. The causative agent is *Eimeria cyprini* Plehn. Infection takes place following ingestion of the parasite together with the mud from the tank in summer and in autumn. Schizogony and sporogony occur inside the cells of the intestinal mucosa and in the closest part of the cells of the submucosa. The disease makes its appearance as a type of enteritis during March and April. Any infected carp may have sunken eyes, a general emaciation, and are often seen to be on their heads. When pressure is put onto the abdomen, a yellow colored fluid may pour out of the anus. On opening the intestine in severe cases there is a yellowish coloration due to the penetration of blood into the hollows produced by the sporozoans in the intestinal epithelium, and its progressive destruction (bilirubin). In this way are to be found the yellow bodies which have been described by Schäperclaus.

Analysis of the fish is made by scraping a small amount of the intestinal and mucosal contents with a spatula, placing this material in a drop of water, covering with a coverslip and examining microscopically.

Within the oocysts, there are usually four spores (5–8 microns) in the interior of which there are always two sporozoites. The parasite progresses all along the intestinal mucosa by means of successive schizogony. The vegetative forms of the organism are only visible after staining with carmine. Following enterococcidiosis it is common to encounter secondary infections such as that caused by *Aeromonas liquefaciens forma ascitae*.

As is the case with whirling disease (see below), any infected tanks should be disinfected with calcium cyanamide. Apart from this, the raising of young carp should always be carried out in tanks where there have never been any adult fish. A population which is too dense favors the appearance of outbreaks of enterococcidiosis.

Whirling disease

In the same way that plistophorosis is a plague among aquarium fish (particularly in neon tetras), so whirling disease in fish farming operations is a pestilence affecting young trout.

CLINICAL PICTURE AND SYMPTOMS: the diseased trout show as the first symptom rotatory movements and a black coloration in the caudal region of the body. Moving the surface of the water (for example, either with the foot or with a stick), the fish start this whirling movement when they swim. The movements are over an angle of 180° and also over 360°. The lesions of the vertebral column give rise to the dark coloration of the tail by irritation of the pigment fibers of the skin. This coloration usually commences level with the anus. Trout which overcome the disease show

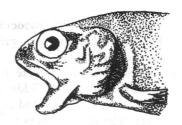

Figure 116. Retraction of the operculum and deformities of the mandible of a rainbow trout which has survived an attack of whirling disease. (Redrawn after Schäperclaus)

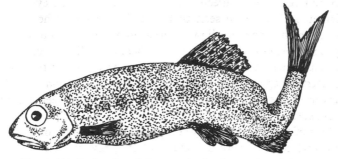

Figure 117. Deformity of the vertebral column of a rainbow trout having suffered from whirling disease. (Modified redrawing after Schäperclaus)

defective opercula (*Figure 116*), mandibular and vertebral deformities (*Figures 116, 117*), and depressions in the cranium particularly posterior to the eyes.

TECHNIQUE OF INVESTIGATION: with a sharp scalpel the cartilagionus tissue is cut away, especially from the otolith region. The shavings so obtained are placed into a drop of water, covered with a coverslip, and examined microscopically for spores. It is also advisable to stain a few smears, for example as is done with blood smears. Histological sections, stained with Giemsa stain, will show the infection before spores are formed as well as after.

ETIOLOGY; MORPHOLOGY AND TAXONOMY OF THE CAUSATIVE AGENT; COURSE OF THE DISEASE: the causative agent of whirling disease is *Myxosoma cerebralis* Hofer and Plehn (Family: Myxosomatidae), and the spores measure 6.5–7 × 7.5–8 microns (*Figure 118*). Infestation takes place by means of spores, which move up from the bottom of the tank. At a water temperature of 15° C., the first symptoms appear after 50 days. The course of the disease is as follows: the trophozoites leave their capsule when this breaks in the trout intestine; they cross the intestinal wall by amoeboid movements, and reach the cartilage of the head and vertebral column carried in the blood stream. Once the cartilage has been reached, the trophozoites penetrate it directly. They multiply and destroy among

189

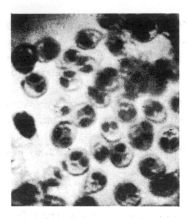

Figure 118. Spores of *Myxosoma cerebralis*. (Schäperclaus)

other things the semicircular canals of the organ of balance. The results of this in the fish include sensitivity to being touched and the typical whirling movement described above. A progressive ossification of the cartilaginous skeleton encapsulates the parasite in the bone cavities, inside which it sporulates. The whirling movements slowly subside in the infected trout, but such fish are extremely dangerous as carriers of the spores, a form of behavior which masks the disease in a latent form. Should these fish die, they contaminate anew the bottom of the tank with spores. Putz and Hoffman (1966) have shown that rainbow trout sac fry can become infected as early as 3 days post-hatching. Hoffman, Dunbar and Bradford (1962) discuss the disease in the United States.

HISTOPATHOLOGY AND HISTOCHEMISTRY: the action of the amoeboid forms of *Myxosoma* is probably not only mechanical but also toxic. This gives rise to destruction of the bone on the one hand, and to the formation of granulomas on the other. These granulomas in the organ of balance, and the exotoxins of the parasite must without doubt be contributing factors to the occurrence of the whirling movements and of the hypersensitivity of the fish to touch.

THERAPY, PROPHYLAXIS AND HYGIENE: there is no satisfactory medication for whirling disease. Trout which have had the disease should not be sold, since they constitute contaminated material and as such are carriers of spores. Apart from this, their growth is poor and stunted, and their maintenance is uneconomical. In fish hatcheries, only fresh stream water should be used where possible, since this is free from spores. No excuse can be made for taking water from any tanks to feed the hatchery as a whole. Prior to liberating the trout fingerlings, they should be given food for five weeks whenever it becomes impossible to separate the spawning and the rearing tanks into two entities. Notwithstanding, these separations must be carried out in due time, and in a systematic fashion. The rearing tanks are cleaned of fish (at the very latest in September), and left dry. In the majority of cases no spores can be formed any earlier than September (when the fingerlings measure some 8 cm. in length). Under no circumstances whatsoever should the tanks be repopulated with fingerlings, since these may well be carriers of the spores.

Contaminated tanks must be disinfected with grease-free calcium cyanamide (1 kg./square meter), the bottom being carefully and uniformly covered. All the tanks in the hatchery should be disinfected, for if this is not done the disease may spread from the non-disinfected tanks, as has been described by Tack (1951).

In using calcium cyanamide, no alcoholic beverage should be consumed for 6 days so as to avoid any possible toxic effects.

The importation of foreign stock of unknown history to a hatchery free of *Myxosoma* is to be avoided. Imports of salmonids into the United States must be certified free of *Myxosoma cerebralis*. This is true in several European countries also.

Nodular diseases (Sporozoasis tuberosa)

Nodular diseases are likewise caused by Sporozoans. They infect skin, gills, and internal organs. The nodules can be more than a millimeter in size, their shape varies with the agent, e.g. ball or rice kernel shaped. The nodules, which arise through a connective tissue reaction, are also called cysts, in which numerous spores or round or elliptical shape are found. The spores consist of two solid shell like halves which set on one another and often produce a growth at the edge. Internally, one finds the sporozoite (embryo) polar capsule (one usually but may be two) which contains a spirally coiled filament. These are extruded and serve for anchorage to the host tissue (*Figure 119*). One can cause the extrusion of the polar filaments by the addition of weak acid or alcohol. The treatment of the spores with iodine solution stains, brownish-yellow, the iodophilic vacuole found inside of the sporozoite. This is absent in many species. From the spores, the ameboid sporozoites hatch and penetrate the host cells. Of the Sporozoans causing nodular diseases, only the genera *Myxobolus* and *Henneguya* are noted here.

CLINICAL PICTURE AND SYMPTOMS: the infected fish (cyprinids, pike, ruffe, pike-perch) show round or rice shaped cysts on the gills with infections of *Myxobolus*. *Henneguya psorospermica* causes half round, white cysts on the gills of pike. On the skin of carp, *Myxobolus exiguus* Thelohan causes pin-head size cysts. In the dorsal part of the gill cavity of pike-perch, pea sized, white cysts occur (*Figure 120*). Their agent is *Myxobolus luciopercae*. TECHNIQUE OF INVESTIGATION: expressed cysts are examined microscopically in a drop of water at ×120. Smears of the cysts are fixed and stained.

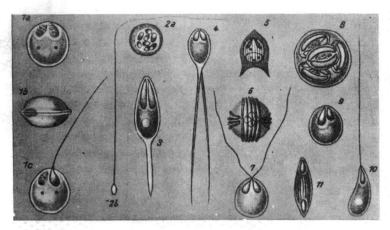

Figure 119. Spores: (1a) surface view of *Myxobolus*; (1b) side view of *Myxobolus*; (1c) *Myxobolus* with evaginated polar filament; (2a) sporoblast and spores of *Glugea anomala*; (2b) *Glugea anomala* spore with evaginated filament; (3) *Henneguya lobosa*; (4) *Henneguya psorospermica*; (5) *Hoferellus cyprini*; (6) *Chloromyxum*; (7) spore of *Myxosoma* with polar filament; (8) four spores of *Eimeria cyprini*, each with two sporozoites within the oocyst; (9) *Myxobolas dispar*; (10) *Myxobolus piriformis*; (11) *Myxidium*. (After Plehn)

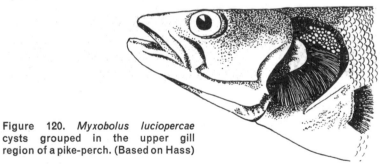

Figure 120. *Myxobolus luciopercae* cysts grouped in the upper gill region of a pike-perch. (Based on Hass)

ETIOLOGY; MORPHOLOGY AND TAXONOMY OF THE CAUSATIVE AGENT; COURSE OF THE DISEASE: the agents are, as already mentioned, *Myxobolus* and *Henneguya* species. The spores attach themselves to the host cells, discharge the sporozoites into the cell, where it divides, grows and produces a cyst after encapsulation by the connective tissue of the host (*Figure 121*). It forms macro and micro gametes which give rise to pansporoblasts by copulation. The size of the spores of *Myxobolus* (*Figure 122*) is 8–16×8–9 microns (*Myxobolus cyprini*); 8–11×7.4–9 microns (*Myxobolus luciopercae*); 10×12 microns (*Myxobolus pfeifferi*); 10–12×9–11 microns (*Myxobolus mulleri*); of *Henneguya* (*Figure 123*) 30–40×7–8 microns (*Henneguya psorospermica*); of *Thelohanellus*, 7–8×16–18 microns (*Thelohanellus piriformis*).

192

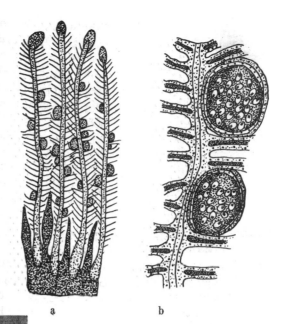

Figure 121. Sporozoan cysts: (a) In gill filaments; (b) internal spores as shown under high magnification (based on Hofer).

a   b

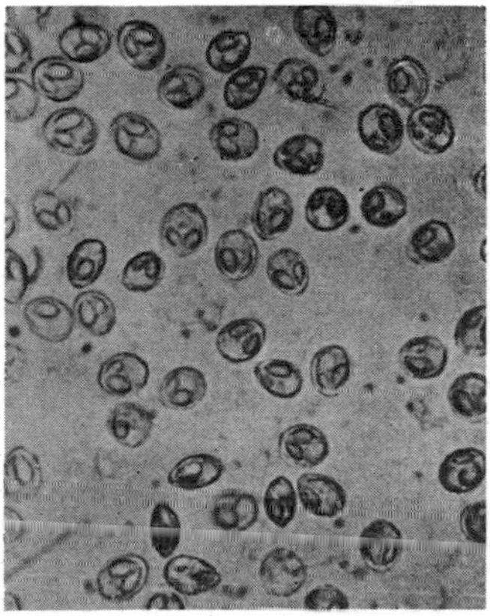

Figure 122. *Myxobolus* spores. (Original)

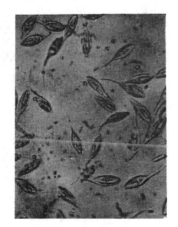

Figure 123. *Henneguya psorospermica* spores. (Original)

The diseased fish behave normally, even in the case of severe attacks which may involve more than half of the respiratory epithelium. No immediate mortalities are generally observed.

HISTOPATHOLOGY AND HISTOCHEMISTRY: the affected parts of the organs react to massive attacks by a connective tissue encapsulation, which forms a cyst (*Figure 121*). A complete lack or absence of reaction may also be observed on some occasions.

THERAPY, PROPHYLAXIS AND HYGIENE: no therapy is possible, and for this reason all infected fish should be destroyed or burned. Nodulosis is extremely rare in well looked after tanks.

Tubero-ulcerous myxoboliasis

This particular disease, which is the cause of great losses, has been known since the year 1870 among barbel of all age groups, and the causative agent is *Myxobolus pfefferi* Thelohan (*Plate 1*). The size of this parasite is 10×12 microns. At the beginning of the disease muscular changes are observed, and these take on a yellowish color and turn soft and gelatinous. Swellings appear chiefly in the muscles of the trunk, and impede movement. The skin loses its sheen, the scales fall away, and hemorrhages are produced at the points of desquamation. These swellings are hard at first, but later they soften and burst, releasing their contents into the water. Secondary bacterial infections follow, the fish become fatigued, they swim abnormally, and finally they die. The heaviest losses are experienced during the warmer months of the year, and diseased fish are not seen in winter. *Myxobolus pfefferi* also attacks the internal organs, forming swellings in the peritoneum, intestine, heart, liver, and kidney. This disease is to be found in those stretches of river which are populated by barbel. Certain species of *Henneguya* also give rise to a similar disease.

Plistophorosis (myolytic sporozoiasis)

CLINICAL PICTURE AND SYMPTOMS: the clinical picture of plistophorosis varies considerably, since there are no uniform symptoms. I was myself able to see those in which the pigmented line had become pale, but where there was no accompanying infectious agent present, while others appeared to be perfectly normal yet at the same time were seen to be intensely infected. In spite of all this, paleness of color, particularly of the bright horizontal line, should be considered as being symptomatic in neon tetras. The paleness usually starts as small spots, which eventually lead to a complete decolorization. Thieme (1956) called this condition "whiteness." Lateral inflexions (scoliosis) have also been observed. Later on difficulties of equilibrium occur which are noted particularly because the fish does not swim in a horizontal position, but rather in an oblique one, and with the head uppermost. The fish attempt to return to their normal position by swimming backwards. Thieme observed that neon tetras infected with plistophorosis swim uninterruptedly all night long, without ever assuming the usual sleeping position a few centimeters from the bottom. A further symptom described by Thieme is that the neon tetras tend to remain away from others of the same shoal or group. Emaciation and a sunken abdomen may be considered as symptoms of plistophorosis as well as tuberculosis.

TECHNIQUE OF INVESTIGATION: the investigation may be carried out both with fresh and with formalin preserved material. Parasites localized in the muscles are usually found in points which appear soft when touched with a mounted needle. This detail is not always foolproof, as I have often had cause to show. Squash preparations are made of the body muscles, and on microscopical examination the parasites may easily be recognized.

ETIOLOGY; MORPHOLOGY AND TAXONOMY OF THE CAUSATIVE AGENT; COURSE OF THE DISEASE: the life cycle of *Plistophora hyphessobryconis* Schäperclaus has not yet been fully investigated. Schäperclaus (1914) described the parasite for the first time from a neon tetra, and this has unfortunately degenerated into the popular name of "neon tetra disease" in place of plistophorosis. Today it is known that *Plistophora* also affects other species of fish, among which are included the following:

Characidae: *Hyphessobrycon innesi*
                    Hyphessobrycon gracilis
                    Hyphessobrycon flammeus
                    Hemigrammus ocellifer
Cyprinidae: *Brachydanio rerio*

It is for this reason that the term plistophorosis is to be preferred to that of "neon tetra disease." While we do not have any concrete information concerning the life cycle of *Plistophora hyphessobryconis*, we may admit the following evolutionary cycle by analogy to *P. mülleri*, which lives in the abdominal muscles of water fleas (*Daphnia* spp.).

It invades the muscles of the trunk, in which we find pansporoblasts, rounded formations occurring in groups of 3–30, or in nests (*Figure 124*). The pansporoblasts measure 28–30 microns; they are found between the muscle fibers, which they separate and dissolve. The connective tissue normally envelops the pansporoblasts in a capsule produced as a result of a normal muscular defensive reaction. The oval spores are found inside the pansporoblasts, measuring 4–6 microns × 3 microns. The spores are liberated on rupture of the pansporoblasts, and an amoeboid organism is released from them to enter the musculature and give rise to new pansporoblasts. By this means an auto-infection occurs in the fish, and the disease affects ever increasing zones of musculature. In a transverse section of the body, Thieme found up to two thousand pansporoblasts. Apart from this auto-infection, there is a further way whereby other fish may become infected. Spores from the skin and musculature fall into the water. Since the kidney is also attacked (according to Thieme), the spores may be voided with the urine. These spores enter the gastro-intestinal tract of healthy fish together with the food, and become firmly fixed to the intestinal wall, by means of their polar filament, and liberate amoeboid forms which penetrate through the wall of the intestine. They are carried in the blood stream to the muslces, in which they divide and form new pansporoblasts. Certain authors (Sterba) believe that there is a possible ovaric infestation which contaminates the embryos from birth, but others (Thieme) deny this assumption. The question must remain open to the light of future research on the problem. It appears that low temperatures favor outbreaks of this disease.

Wales and Wolf (1955) reported the occurrence of a species of *Plisto-phora* in wild and cultured rainbow trout, red salmon and sculpin (*Cottus* sp.). In their paper, they give a good description of the pathology and symptomatology of the disease, together with details of the Epizootology and size of the parasite.

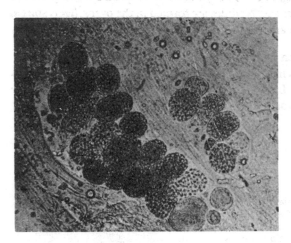

Figure 124. Spore-filled pansporoblasts of *Plistophora hyphessobryconis* in musculature. (Steffens)

HISTOLOGY AND HISTOCHEMISTRY: the pansporoblasts of *Plistophora hyphessobryconis* are situated one after another all along the muscle fibers, or grouped together in little piles (*Figure 124*). The infected muscle surrounds the pansporoblasts with a layer of connective tissue. The cysts which are situated in the periphery of the muscular fibers have a thicker covering of connective tissue. The muscle fibers separate and partially lyse, so that in severe cases only parasites are found in the place of muscle tissue. This is the cause of the pale zones in the musculature which are observed externally. The connective tissue may be parasitized, and cysts in this have a thicker capsule and are normally pigmented on the suface. THERAPY, PROPHYLAXIS AND HYGIENE: there is no cure for plistophorosis, and my own experiments with antibiotics were not successful. For this reason prophylactic measures are of such great importance, and among these are the sanitary controls to which all tropical fish breeders should be periodically subject. If the presence of plistophorosis is confirmed, the aquaria must be thoroughly disinfected. For this concentrated hydrochloric acid or chloramine are recommended. Filters and air diffusors should also be disinfected to prevent their passing on the disease by means of spores. The best procedure is to keep all these utensils in a concentrated solution of potassium permanganate, and to wash them under the tap immediately prior to use. Efficient hygiene is the keyword to successful fish breeding, and my own personal visits to fish hatcheries have brought home to me how little this rule is practiced as well as how much more hygiene is still required.

Glugea pseudotumefaciens

The disease, described by Pflugfelder (1952), is caused by *Glugea pseudotumefaciens* Pflugfelder. The parasite lives predominantly in the cells of the connective tissue. Nodules are formed in the ovary, liver, spleen, kidney, nervous tissue and eyes. It appears to be a rare disease.

Glugea anomala Moniez (Figure 125)

This microsporidian most frequently attacks the three-spined stickleback (*Gasterosteus aculeatus* L.). It forms white colored pea-sized swellings (up to 4 mm. in diameter) on the lateral sides of the body. It frequently gives rise to fatal epizootics.

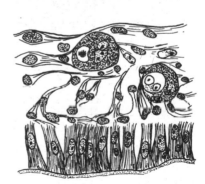

Figure 125. *Glugea anomala* within intestinal wall of a stickleback, showing two giant cells in which parasites may be seen; above the section are two cells, each possessing a mononuclear parasite. (Slightly modified after Weissenberg)

Species of *Glugea* also seem to be of importance in marine aquaria in which young flatfish are kept. A serious disease outbreak caused by *Glugea stephani* among young plaice was described by Bückmann (1952).

CILIATES (CILIOPHORA)

The ciliates are unicellular organisms usually having a fixed shape, although certain exceptions to this rule are known (*Ichthyophthirius*). They possess a tough striated cell wall, in the grooves of which are lines

197

of cilia whose function is locomotory. They are provided with a cytostome (cellular mouth) and a cytopharynx (cellular pharynx) which lead to the endoplasm. In some of them there is a cytopygium (cellular anus). Food vacuoles and a single contractile vacuole are to be seen within the cytoplasm. Each individual cilium is attached to the cytoplasm by means of a basal corpuscle. Both ciliary and body movements are controlled by neuronemes which transmit impulses to the myonemes. The ciliates possess a macronucleus (somatic) and a micronucleus (sexual). Reproduction may be asexual (by simple division) or sexual (conjugation).

Chilodonella

CLINICAL PICTURE AND SYMPTOMS: the skin of the infected fish shows a bluish-white opaqueness. In the neck region, above all, up to the beginning of the dorsal fin, the affected skin may show a stony relief which may be so pronounced as to resemble smallpox. Later on, if the attack is very severe, the skin may fall away in strips. The gills are also attacked. The fish scrape themselves against the bottom and the sides of the aquarium tank, and swim listlessly and with considerable fatigue. Some of them breathe with difficulty.

TECHNIQUE OF INVESTIGATION: only living fish are suitable for study, since *Chilodonella* rapidly leaves dead fish. Smears are made from the skin and gills. Indian ink may be added to the preparation if required. Preserved material serves no useful purpose whatsoever for diagnosis.

ETIOLOGY; MORPHOLOGY AND TAXONOMY OF THE CAUSATIVE AGENT; COURSE OF THE DISEASE: *Chilodonella cyprini* Moroff measures 60 microns in length and 45 microns in width. It is oval in shape, and has a small indentation in the posterior part of the body. This latter feature has given rise to their being called heart-shaped skin parasites, owing to a certain faint resemblance to a heart. I would like to add at this stage that too much attention should not be given to this characteristic, since in living parasites the indentation is rarely seen. What does attract attention however is the coarsely granular cytoplasm due to the presence of numerous small vacuoles, and this feature, together with the shape of the body, are useful criteria for their identification (see *Plate*). The macronucleus is oval and its size is about a third that of the body. The micronucleus is round and its position varied. In Indian ink preparations, from 5–15 lines of cilia may be counted on the ventral surface. There are some large cilia situated immediately anterior to the cytostome. At this point 14–26 of the so-called pharyngeal pillars terminate. Reproduction is asexual. *Chilodonella* parasitizes the skin and gills in a manner which makes it an obligate ectoparasite.

The form in which it feeds is not known, but it is assumed that *Chilodonella* feeds upon the destroyed cells of the epidermis and branchial epithelium. *Chilodonella* is an obligate parasite, but it multiplies in debilitated fish and thus comes to attack healthy ones. Contagion is direct from one fish to another, as shown in *Figure 126*. Its numbers increase by continual division, and it exercises a destructive effect on the skin and gills. *Chilodonella* is insensitive to temperature fluctuations, and is found as much in aquaria as in open waters.

In serious infestations the course of the disease is fatal because it reduces the respiratory surface of the gills, and destroys the skin, whose function is also vital.

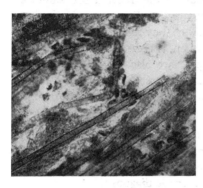

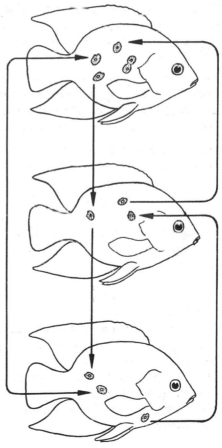

Figure 127. Squash preparation of the gill of *Pterophyllum scalare* (invasion by *Chilodonella*), showing the gill epithelium destroyed down to the cartilaginous areas of the gill laminae and with the parasites revealed as dark oblong formations. (Original)

Figure 126. Diagram showing growth of *Chilodonella cyprini* and spread of infestation among fishes. (Amlacher)

HISTOPATHOLOGY AND HISTOCHEMISTRY: apart from causing loss of the epidermis, it may completely destroy the gill epithelium, as I observed in *Pterophyllum scalare* (*Figure 127*). Frequently there remains nothing more than the cartilaginous rays of the gill laminae.

THERAPY, PROPHYLAXIS AND HYGIENE: for those fish which are destined for consumption, a 1% sodium chloride bath for 10 minutes is used. Malachite green (0.15 mgm./liter) safely destroys all the parasites. In the case of aquarium fish, the best results are obtained by using a trypaflavine bath coupled with a raise of temperature to 28° C. Under such conditions, *Chilodonella* dies within 10 hours. Aquarol may also be used, adding it to the aquarium on three occasions, at three day intervals over a period of nine days (for dosage see *Table 2*). Aquarol is useful as a preventive measure for dealing with aquarium fish. In home aquaria, the following rule applies: do not put too many fish together (allow 5 liters of water per fish). Guarantee the optimum conditions, adequate oxygen, pH and water hardness for each species; suitable water temperature; moderate feeding; periodical change of water. Put all new fish into quarantine. These same rules apply *mutatis mutandi* to fish farms and hatcheries.

Ichthyophthirius

CLINICAL PICTURE AND SYMPTOMS: in the aquarium trade ichthyophthiriasis is better known as "Ich" or white spot disease. The diseased fish (*Figure 128*) appear to be covered with small white spots, and as the disease progresses the spots may join together and form areas of a dirty white color which later fall away as strips of skin. The fins are held close to the body and the fish swim violently in an attempt to rid themselves of this annoying skin irritation. The progress of the disease is quite rapid, especially should the water temperature be high. The gills are also affected. Ichthyophthiriasis appears when the fish are in very close contact with each other, as is the case with aquaria and certain types of breeding tanks.

TECHNIQUE OF INVESTIGATION: living fish are to be preferred for examination, even though the parasite may be encountered in dead fish if these are in water and not too much time has elapsed since they died. Wet smears of the skin and gills are examined. Preserved material is not always of use for study.

ETIOLOGY; MORPHOLOGY AND TAXONOMY OF THE CAUSATIVE AGENT; COURSE OF THE DISEASE: *Ichthyophthirius multifillis* Fouquet is related to *Chilodonella*, and is also a holotrichous ciliate. According to the stage at which it is found, it may be pyriform or rounded. It is important to note that *Ichthyophthirius* may change its form when it invades the skin and gills in such a way as to not appear rounded, but frequently shows cytoplasmic outgrowths in the direction of movement. The protoplasm appears to be

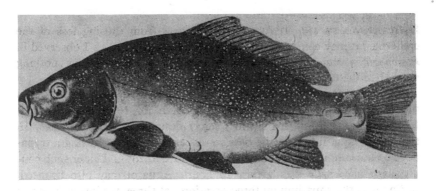

Figure 128. Carp attacked by *Ichthyophthirius multifiliis*. (Hofer)

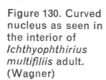

Figure 129. *Ichthyophthirius*: parasite appears dark-colored because of ingested food, and the nucleus is visible as a long clear zone. (Wagner)

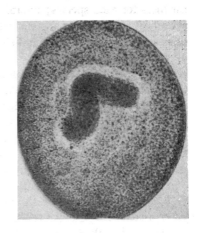

Figure 130. Curved nucleus as seen in the interior of *Ichthyophthirius multifiliis* adult. (Wagner)

grossly granular, and contains many small vacuoles. Generally speaking the macronucleus is bent in the living animal, and for this reason is quite easy to see. The nucleus is blackish and opaque, except when the animal is full of food particles (*Figure 129*). Alongside the macronucleus, a small and rounded micronucleus is to be found with a certain amount of difficulty (*Figure 130*). *Ichthyophthirius* measures between 0.2–1 mm. The parasite appears to be in constant movement due to the movements of the vibratile cilia. It is an obligate parasite. We may distinguish in its life cycle an epidermal, a benthonic, and an agglomerative phase respectively.

The benthonic phase is a cyst out of which proceed numerous pyriform elements measuring 30–50 microns. These bodies attack the fish (*Figures 131 and upper part of 132*), and rapidly perforate the epidermis (*Figure*

201

132a and b); they establish themselves between the epidermis and the dermis, and make a ball (*Figure 132c*).

Here the invaders keep growing and the skin shows a reactionary epithelialization, which is a cellular proliferation encompassing the parasite and visible externally as a little white spot measuring up to 1 mm. in diameter. *Ichthyophthirius* does not penetrate the dermis, but may move from the point of entry, and the joining together in one cavity of 3–6 different parasites has in fact been observed. The parasites grow and feed themselves on tissue fluids and the remains of epidermal cells. According

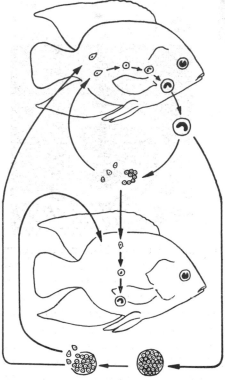

Figure 131. Life cycle of *Ichthyophthirius multifiliis* and its transmission among fishes: (above) infective elements which develop on the skin of a fish during the epidermal phase; (below) benthic phase in which infective elements are produced in a cyst and then disseminated (smaller circle) representative of an atypical development, without any benthic phase. (Amlacher)

to the water temperature (warm water accelerates growth) the parasite grows within 1–3 weeks until it reaches a definite size (*Figure 130*) and perforates the skin towards the exterior. It falls to the bottom, surrounds itself with a gelatinous capsule, and fixes itself onto any solid object. The benthonic phase lasts only for a short time (*Figure 133c*). Inside the cyst asexual reproduction takes place by means of successive divisions which may commence within about an hour. For this the whole cytoplasmic mass of the cyst divides, as was clearly demonstrated by Wagner (1960), (*Figures 133a, b*), with the formation of two cells, and later of four. Quite frequently

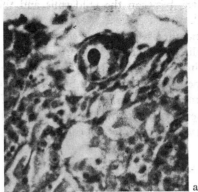
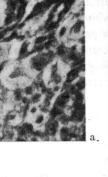
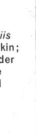

Figure 132. *Ichthyophthirius multifiliis*
(a) infective body penetrating the skin;
(b) taking on a spherical shape under
the epidermis; (c) grown under the
epidermis, wlth a long nucleus and
beginning of a covering
epithelization. (Wagner)

the first four cells divide in such a way that four blastomeres remain, separated from each other, but which all together resemble four cysts grouped in one (Wagner). Generally each one of these cysts produces its own orifice for escape. The division is completed within some 15–20 hours, and altogether produces from 20–1000 infective elements (*Figure 133*), rounded, and highly motile while they remain within the cysts, and pear-shaped when they leave them. These infective elements (or invasive phase) come to attack the same or another fish, where the cycle is repeated (*Figure 131*). Exceptions to this cycle occur in cases such as when the unattached adult parasites divide in the water without prior formation of cysts, due to lack of oxygen etc. (*Figure 131*). The vitality of these infective elements is limited to some 33 hours (Buschkiel, 1911) or 48 hours (Schä-perclaus, 1954). Within this period of time, the parasite must find a new host or it will die. *Ichthyophthirius* is extremely sensitive to a lack of oxygen.

Finally, a few words on the so-called latent infections. In this respect Wagner (1960) demonstrated that gudgeon infected experimentally failed to show the ordinary clinical picture, but rather that they behaved normally. However parasites were isolated from the skin and the gills of all

203

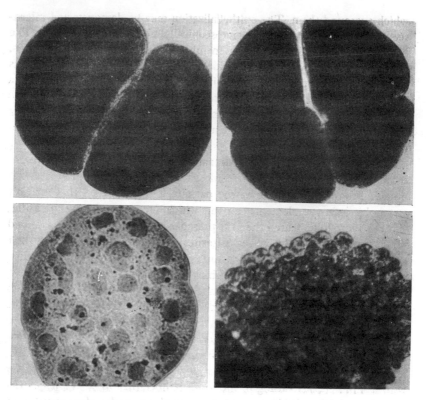

Figure 133. Formation of cysts and infective elements in *Ichthyophthirius multifiliis*: (a) bipartition; (b) tetrapartition, formation of quadrants; (c) multinucleate cysts; (d) intra-cystic infective elements, ready to leave the cyst. (Wagner)

of them. When these gudgeon were put together with other fish, the disease made its appearance in the latter but the gudgeon remained completely unaffected. These observations point to the dangers inherent in the tropical fish trade, because they serve to explain the occurrence of unexpected outbreaks, particularly among new arrivals. The parasites which are present on the gills may pass by undetected, even though careful sanitary inspections be carried out. When the water conditions become modified, or as a result of some special predisposition of the fish (for example, transport), the disease is liable to suddenly appear.

It has now been shown that rainbow trout have an immune response to *Ichthyophthirius* and produce a serum element which will kill the parasite on contact.

HISTOPATHOLOGY AND HISTOCHEMISTRY: the epithelial tissue engulfs the younger parasites by a precocious migration of isolated epithelial cells which surround them. The epithelialization may be demonstrated microscopically after six days, and macroscopically after from 10–14 days. The parasites penetrate up to the basal membrane, but fail to reach the dermis. In the dermis, according to Buschkiel (1936), and Sikama (1938), stasis is produced. In the area of epithelialization the nuclei are intermixed in a disorderly fashion, and flask cells are absent (Becker, 1941). According to Buschkiel *Ichthyophthirius* also penetrates into the dermis and lesions the blood vessels. Pflugfelder (1950) demonstrated an invasion of the conjunctiva and of the cephalic muscles.

THERAPY, PROPHYLAXIS AND HYGIENE: any attempt to fight against *Ichthyophthirius* will be doomed to failure unless the degree of infestation is determined. From the life cycle of the parasite it may be seen that a heavy attack by infective elements, among which are many young parasites, is much more to be feared than the presence of a few adults. This is based upon the fact that the young parasites grow and the degree of their destructive action in the skin is much greater than that of the adults, which soon become detached and which in any case die when the infective elements are formed. For this reason the treatment of heavily infected fish leads to rather doubtful results. According to our present experience, the parasites cannot be killed directly, as can *Chilodonella* for example, because they are localized under the epidermis. Control must therefore be based on the destruction of free-swimming infective bodies. In aquaria, this is best carried out by means of a long term trypaflavine bath together with a simultaneous raising of the water temperature to 30° C. Since the growth of *Ichthyophthirius* may last up to three weeks, the trypaflavine bath should be applied throughout this period, particularly when the skin of the fish cannot be examined regularly and microscopically. Should circumstances permit, treatment may be terminated before this period has ended, always on the condition that no new infestations are detected with the microscope. For aquaria, Stolk recommends a change of the temperature from 33° C. in the morning (6 hours) to 21° C. at night, repeating this procedure from three to five times in succession.

It is well worth the trouble to mention the technique of changing over aquaria. The fish are put into a new receptacle every 12 hours. The tanks used previously are freed from parasites every three days, since the parasites themselves die out during this time. To apply this method in practice, seven aquarium tanks are required altogether.

A similar technique may be used in fish farming practice, where a large number of empty tanks are available. Apart from this the removal of fish to larger tanks is always of value.

Recently, good results have been obtained with malachite green. According to Deufel (1960), 1 gm. of malachite green/10 sq. meters of tank

205

serves to cure trout and carp. My own experience (Amlacher, 1961) has shown that *Ichthyophthirius* is destroyed after 10 days in malachite oxalate (0.15 mgm./liter) at 4–10° C. A known quantity of malachite green stock solution is added gradually to the tank until it reaches the required concentration. The entry of water into the tank should be closed during the duration of the treatment. This method can only be used in carp farming, and in any case only young fish should be treated. It is not altogether clear whether malachite green has any direct action on *Ichthyophthirius*, but it seems likely that it produces a destruction of cytochrome c, together with a stimulus that obliges the parasite to emigrate rapidly from the skin of the fish. In larger fish rearing establishments, all recently arrived fish are placed into quarantine for a period of 4 weeks.

We shall give consideration to a method which has recently become quite popular in aquarist circles. It is claimed that *Ichthyophthirius* is unable to live in acid water, and that fish which prefer an acid pH remain free from the parasite. Without going into any great detail, my own experience has shown that the parasite remains quite alive on fish placed into water of pH 5. As mentioned by Wagner (1960), the cysts die at pH 5.5 and this prevents the formation of infective elements. This may perhaps explain why acid-loving fish remain free from ichthyophthiriasis. Therapeutically the observation is of little value, owing to the fact that fish which prefer a neutral or alkaline pH cannot be treated in an acid water. Trypaflavine, malachite green and formalin are at the moment the best methods available for the treatment of this particular disease.

Hatcheries and large aquarium establishments must take great care to ensure a frequent disinfection of all their utensils, keeping them for long periods in concentrated solutions of potassium permanganate, rivanol, or trypaflavine.

Trichodiniasis

Trichodina domerguei Wallengreen is a ciliate rarely giving rise to pathological manifestations of disease. It may be sporadically found in living fish, but it will only multiply in weakened ones. A macronucleus, micronucleus, and numerous food vacuoles are to be seen in the cytoplasm. The body is circular in shape when seen from below, and bell-shaped when seen from the side. The parasite possesses a ring of small hooks resembling a circular saw (see *Plate*), and its diameter is 48–50 microns. Schäperclaus has also found smaller forms of 25 microns grouped together in masses. *Trichodina* parasitizes the skin, gills, and urinary bladder of the fish, and is found both in freshwater and the sea.

A mass mortality from the White Lake (Berlin) due to this parasite is on record. Its control is as for *Costia* and *Chilodonella*.

Chapter 9

HELMINTHIASIS (WORM DISEASES)

In fishmongers' shops it is quite common to see diseases produced by parasitic worms, while in fish farms and aquaria such diseases are comparatively rare. This is due to the fact that helminths are highly specialized parasites and require a specific (or definitive) host. Furthermore, their development may require an intermediate host, and in the event of the fish itself being an intermediate host, then the final definitive host is not present in the aquarium, and conditions are thus not favorable for the parasite. This explains why aquarium fish from different climates and ecological conditions tend to lose their helminth parasites in the aquarium.

Some helminths and their larval forms are skin and gill parasites, whereas others live in the visceral cavity, the internal organs and the musculature. In the following taxonomic synopsis the ecto- and endoparasites (worms) of fish are briefly mentioned. See Hoffman (1967) for a complete synopsis of North American fish parasitic helminths.

Phylum: PLATHELMINTHES (flat worms)

    Class. Trematodes

        Order: Monogenea (monogenetic)

            fish pathogens: *Dactylogyrus vastator* Nybelin; *Dactylogyrus anchoratus* Dujardin; *Dactylogyrus minutus* Kulwiec; *Gyrodactylus elegans* Nordm.; *Monocoelium monenteron* Wag.; *Diplozoon paradoxum*, and other species from marine and freshwater fish;

        Order: Digenea (digenetic)

            fish pathogens: *Proalaria spathaceum* La Rue; *Sanguinicola inermis* Plehn; *Sanguinicola armata* Plehn; *Sanguinicola intermedia* Ejsmont; *Bucephalus polymorphus* Baer, and other species from marine and freshwater fish;

    Cestodes

    Class: Cestodaria

        fish pathogens: *Amphilina foliacea* and others;

    Class: Cestoda

Order: Proteocephalidea
fish pathogens: 37, particularly in sharks and rays. *Proteocephalus* in freshwater fish;
Order: Diphyllidea
fish pathogens: 4, in the intestines of sharks and rays only;
Order: Tetrarhynchidea
fish pathogens: very numerous, in the intestines of marine fish;
Order: Pseudophyllidea
fish pathogens: *Dibothriocephalus latus, Ligula intestinalis* L., *Triaenophorus nodulosus* (Pall.) Rud.; *Cyathocephalus truncatus* Pall.; *Schistocephalus gasterostei* Fabr.;
Phylum: NEMAHELMINTHES
Class: Nematoda
Order: Ascarididea
fish pathogens: very numerous. The sub-family Anisakinae, with the genera *Contracaecum, Porrocaecum, Raphidascaris, Anisakis, Paranisakis,* and the sub-family Acanthocheilinae are of importance, particularly in the case of marine fish;
Order: Spiruridea
fish pathogens: *Camallanus trunctatus,* in numerous freshwater fish; *Cucullanus cirratus, Cucullanus minutus,* in marine fish; *Dacnitis truttae* in freshwater fish;
Order: Filariidea
fish pathogens: *Filaria sanguinea* in the goldfish; *Philometra abdominalis* in the abdominal cavity of cyprinids attacked by *Ligula;*
Phylum: ACANTHOCEPHALA
Order: Neoechinorhynchidea
fish pathogens: *Neoechinorhynchus rutili* Müller;
Order: Echinorhynchidea
fish pathogens: *Rhadinorhynchus pristis* Rudolphi; *Pomphorhynchus laevis* Müller; *Acanthocephalus anguillae* Müller; *Acanthocephalus lucii* Müller; *Echinorhynchus salmonis* Müller; *Echinorhynchus truttae* Scharank; *Echinorhynchus gadi* Müller, and others in marine and freshwater fish;
Phylum: ANNELIDA
Order: Rhynchobdellida (leeches)
fish pathogens: *Branchellion torpedinus* Sav.; *Pontobdella muricata* L.; *Callobdella nodulifera* Malm.; *Callobdella lophi* Beneden and Hesse; *Piscicola geometra* L.; *Cystobranchus mammillatus* Malm.; *Cystobranchus respirans* Troschel; *Platybdella anarrhichae* Diesing; *Hemiclepsis marginata* Müller;

Class: Oligochaeta
species pathogenic to crayfish: *Branchiobdella parasita* Henle; *Branchiobdella pentodonta* Whitman; *Branchiobdella hexodonta* Gruber.

TREMATODES

Within this Class, there are numerous families which are parasitic for fish. The ingestion of food is made comparatively easy for them. Those which parasitize the skin and gills have characteristic hooks at the caudal end of the body, by means of which they fix themselves onto their host. Other trematodes, and more especially their larvae, are found in the skin, eyes, gills, blood and internal organs of fish.

MONOGENETIC TREMATODES

These are ectoparasites of the skin and gills. In the posterior part of the body they possess one or more acetabuli and hooks for fixation. Their development occurs directly within the host, or conversely by passing through free-swimming larval forms which later seek out a suitable host.

Dactylogyrus and Monocoelium

CLINICAL PICTURE AND SYMPTOMS: external symptoms are not observed, except in cases where the infestation is severe when the edges of the gills become thickened and the opercula appear to be somewhat opened. The gill edges have a grayish coloration. The worms are localized chiefly on the gill filaments, but when they are present in large numbers they become distributed all over the body (*Figures 134 and 135*).

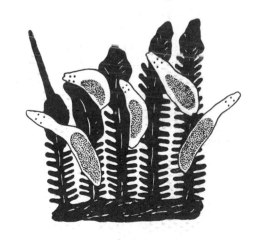

Figure 134. *Dactylogyrus* on gill filaments: to the left, a large prolongation of a filament as a tissue reaction against invasion by the parasite. (Amlacher)

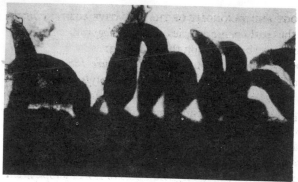

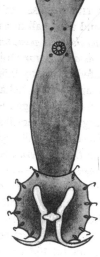

Figure 135. *Dactylogyrus* in the gill filament of a flame fish (probably referring to *Hyphessobrycon flammeus*. (Original)

Figure 136. *Dactylogyrus vastator*. (Amlacher)

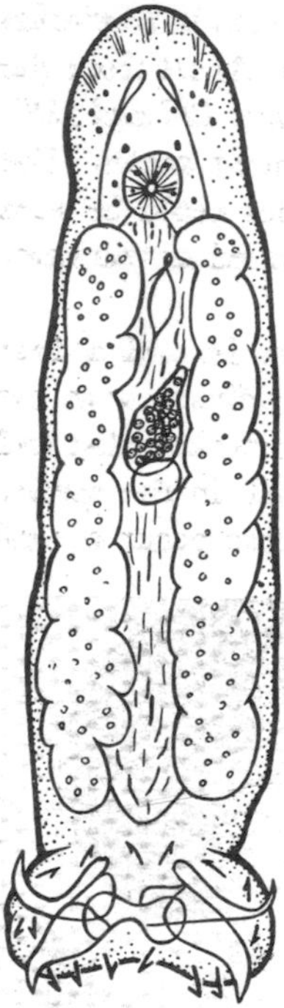

Figure 137. *Monocoelium monenteron*. (Reichenbach-Klinke)

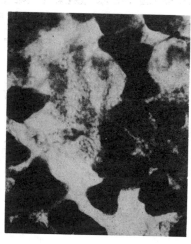

Figure 138. *Monocoelium* eggs on gill of *Tetraodon fluviatilis*. (Original)

TECHNIQUE OF INVESTIGATION: microscopical examination is carried out at a magnification of ×45–120. Several gill filaments are cut or a skin smear made, placed under a coverslip in a drop of water, and examined. The smears are made in a rapid fashion, without any need for staining (see the corresponding chapter).

Etiology; morphology and taxonomy of the causative agent; course of the disease: of the pathogenic species of *Dactylogyrus*, which are found above all in carp, we shall mention the following:

Dactylogyrus vastator Nybelin (up to 1 mm. long) (*Figure 136*), *Dactylogyrus anchorator* Dujardin (up to 0.6 mm. long), and *Dactylogyrus minutus* Kulwiec (up to 0.5 mm. long). *Dactylogyrus* is comparatively rare in aquarium fish. Schäperclaus (1954) found numerous small *Dactylogyrus* in fish of the genus *Lebistes*. *D. formosus* is known in aquaria, and is recognized scientifically. However in aquaria a related trematode called *Monocoelium* (*Ancryocephalus, Figure 137*) seems to be more common than *Dactylogyrus*. Schäperclaus found large numbers of it in *Pterophyllum scalare* and in *Ambassis*. I myself have observed *Monocoelium* in *Heniochus acuminatus* and *Tetraodon cutcutia* from marine aquaria. Apart from the parasite itself, numbers of its eggs were also found (*Figures 138 and 139*). The shape of these eggs was triangular and with rounded angles. The filiform prolongation which is to be found in trematodes could be seen (*Figure 139*). An isolated attack of oodiniosis also occurred at the same time.

The anterior point of *Dactylogyrus* has four points, in which four black eyes and a ventral sucker are clearly visible. It adheres with the help of a special fixation apparatus consisting of a characteristic disc and two typical central hooks. These are of value, above all, in the species determination of the parasite. On the border of the disc occur several

Figure 139. *Monocoelium monenteron* in gills of *Tetraodon fluviatilis*. (Original)

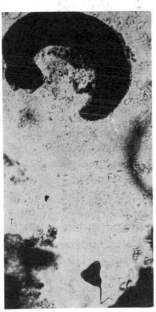

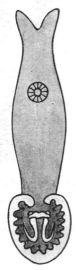

Figure 140. *Gyrodactylus elegans*. (Amlacher)

211

marginal hooks (*Figure* 136). All species of *Dàctylogyrus* and *Monocoelium* produce eggs, from which are born ciliated larvae which develop and are converted into adults, facilitating in this manner the invasion of other fish.

The genus *Monocoelium* is differentiated from *Dactylogyrus* chiefly because its fixation apparatus has four central hooks. It proved to be of little use to make any measurements on the worms which I examined, since they were from material preserved in formalin. As a small detail for reference, I will say that the fixed specimens measured 0.5 mm. in length, so that the living ones must be larger. The four black eyes and the four central hooks were perfectly visible.

Reproduction takes place by means of resistant eggs. After having laid these, the adults die. Larvae are seen in winter and in spring.

HISTOPATHOLOGY AND HISTOCHEMISTRY: in cases of severe invasion of the gills, apart from thickening of the gill edges already mentioned previously, destruction of the branchial epithelium and rupture of the blood vessels produce a respiratory hyperfunction and death of the fish due to asphyxia.

In carp it was observed that the gills reacted by the formation of fine prolongations 1.8 mm. in length. Wunder (1929) assumes that the purpose of these is to eliminate the parasites. I was myself able to demonstrate something similar to this in *Tetraodon* and *Heniochus* (*Figure 134*). Numerous eggs are also to be found on the gills (*Figure 138*).

THERAPY, PROPHYLAXIS AND HYGIENE: in fish hatchery operations the best method to combat, and at the same time to prevent these parasites is to make the fry resistant to their attacks as soon as is possible by administering a suitable diet prior to the growth of the fish. In aquaria, apart from the usual precautions of maintaining all new fish in quarantine, or at least submitting them to a sanitary control, the following therapeutic measures may be adopted:

(*a*) short bath in formalin (20–25 cc. 40% formalin in 100 liters of water for 30 minutes);

(*b*) short bath in salt water (see Table of drugs).

With reference to the salt-water bath, some doubts may be entertained as to whether this would be successful against salt-water trematodes, as for example in the case of *Monocoelium* sp. which I myself have had cause to observe.

Gyrodactylus

CLINICAL PICTURE AND SYMPTOMS: in contradistinction to species of *Dactylogyrus*, those of *Gyrodactylus* live on the fish skin. Seriously infected fish show an opacity of the skin, often with inflamed and reddened areas. Flashing will occur. Schäperclaus observed turbidity of the cornea followed by blindness in carp severely infested by this parasite.

TECHNIQUE OF INVESTIGATION: a microscopical investigation is performed by placing a thin scraping of skin or gill in a drop of water under a cover-slip, and examining it at ×45–120 magnifications. Dead fish are of less use for this observation, since *Gyrodactylus* rapidly abandons the body, even though it is true that observations have been reported (Reichenbach-Klinke) on the presence of abundant living *Gyrodactylus* in *Lebistes reticulatus* some 12 hours after death had taken place. Preserved material is inadequate for the investigation of this parasite. In living fish, when the invasion is considerable, the worm may be seen with the naked eye because of its movements on the skin.

ETIOLOGY; MORPHOLOGY AND TAXONOMY OF THE CAUSATIVE ORGANISM; COURSE OF THE DISEASE: of all the most frequently encountered species of *Gyrodactylus* in Europe, we shall mention *G. elegans* von Nordmann (*Figure 140*) and *G. medius* Kathariner. *G. elegans* measures 0.5–0.8 mm. in length, and *G. medius* 0.25–0.5 mm. The anterior end of the body has two points. *Gyrodactylus* has no eyes. The sucking disc has two central hooks, but these are smaller than those in *Dactylogyrus* (*Figure 140*). *Gyrodactylus* is not oviparous as in *Dactylogyrus*, but viviparous with the peculiarity that inside each worm lives a young animal, in whose interior is another one, and within this yet a further one (scatulation). *Gyrodactylus* infections are almost always the result of keeping the fish in bad conditions, for example in aquaria where metabolic by-products are allowed to accumulate. The parasite feeds on epidermal cells. *Gyrodactylus gracilis* Kathariner is a species measuring 0.18–0.32 mm. in length.

HISTOPATHOLOGY AND HISTOCHEMISTRY: generally speaking it only produces lesions on the superficial layers of the epidermis.

THERAPY, PROPHYLAXIS AND HYGIENE: short duration baths in formalin are excellent for combatting this disease (see *Dactylogyrus*). *Gyrodactylus* dies in such baths within 16 minutes, as was discovered by Schäperclaus from his experiments.

Diplozoon

Diplozoon is encountered with relative frequency in open waters, and has also been observed in aquarium fish. It lives on the gills, and when there are many parasites present, they impede respiration (proliferations and inflammations of the gills). It does not possess eyes. From the eggs of this parasite are born larvae which are free-swimming, and they reach other fish upon which they fix themselves. The larvae at birth are provided with what is known as a dorsal cone, which is a protruberance of the body important to the continuance of development: on drawing near to another one, each imprisons the dorsal protruberance of the other with its ventral acetabulum, and in this way they grow together and form the double animal.

213

The anterior portion of the body is flattened like a leaf and shows in the interior a ramified vitellum. These are two acetabuli at the anterior end.

Diplozoon paradoxum Nordmann, measuring 4–5 mm., is known from Central European fish. The two worms unite to form a cross. Reichenbach-Klinke observed *Diplozoon barbi* Reichenbach-Klinke in barbs (*Barbus* and *Puntius*). The length of this latter parasite is from 1–1.3 mm. Unlike *Diplozoon paradoxum*, this species does not unite in the form of a cross, but rather by the flattened face in the center of the body. *D. barbi* produces grayish pustules in the gills. This parasite probably originated in Asia Minor. *Diplozoon tetragonopterini* Sterba was found by that author in aquarium fish, and it seems that it only attacks salmonids.

It is difficult to detach the diplozoons, but they may be combatted by long duration baths in trypaflavine, or by a short bath in common salt (15 gm./liter).

DIGENETIC TREMATODES

These are endoparasites. Development is metagenetic, and implies a change of host. The fish may be either a definitive or an intermediate host.

Diseases produced by trematode larvae (cercariae and metacercariae)

Tropical aquarium fish become infected by cercariae in their native countries, just the same as the fish of our own waters are infected. This disease may also come to be produced in aquaria whenever diseased water snails are introduced from open natural waters. In wild fish the investigation is made by examining preparations obtained by the dissociation of material from the eyes; in tropical aquarium fish the material is taken chiefly from the musculature. In wild fish the disease is recognized in the majority of cases by the opaque appearance of the eye.

The life cycle is as follows: from the fertilized eggs of the trematode (in Germany for example, *Proalaria spathaceum*; in the tropics and Europe, the genus *Clinostomum*) is produced a free-swimming ciliated larva (miracidium). This, after some little time, penetrates the body walls of an aquatic snail (1st intermediate host) and migrates towards the liver. These snails are, in Europe *Limnaea stagnalis*; in South America *Helisoma nigricans*; in North and Central America *Helisoma trivolvis* and *H. tumidum*; in Asia *Planorbis*. In the first intermediate host the miracidium grows until it is converted into a sporocyst, inside which within two weeks are formed parthenogenetically the rediae and daughter rediae. Inside the redia are formed cercariae which leave the host and, swimming freely, search out a fish, fix themselves onto it, lose their characteristic forked tails, and perforate the skin. The fish (2nd intermediate host) forms a membrane (*Figure 141*) around the parasite, which as of this moment receives the name of metacercaria. This latter grows until it becomes a nodule visible externally, a process which takes place within three weeks, a fact which means that after a 3–4 week quarantine period it is possible to tell whether imported fish have metacercariae or not.

In nature the life cycle concludes when the fish is eaten by the definitive host, which is usually an aquatic bird, for example a gull. The membrane surrounding the metacercariae dissolves in the digestive tract of the definitive host, but they do not attack this latter. Within 4 days they are converted into adult trematodes which migrate to the pharynx and esophagus of the bird, and reach their sexual maturity. The fertilized eggs reach the water together with the excrement of the final host, and the life cycle commences once again.

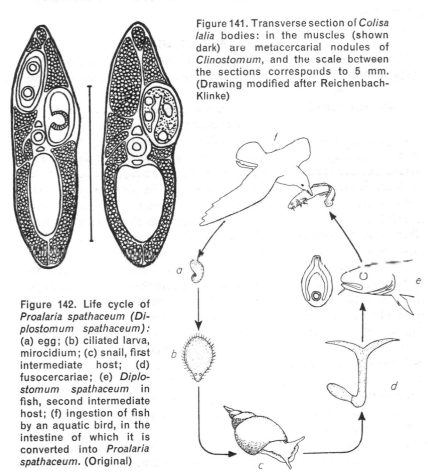

Figure 141. Transverse section of *Colisa lalia* bodies: in the muscles (shown dark) are metacercarial nodules of *Clinostomum*, and the scale between the sections corresponds to 5 mm. (Drawing modified after Reichenbach-Klinke)

Figure 142. Life cycle of *Proalaria spathaceum (Diplostomum spathaceum):* (a) egg; (b) ciliated larva, mirocidium; (c) snail, first intermediate host; (d) fusocercariae; (e) *Diplostomum spathaceum* in fish, second intermediate host; (f) ingestion of fish by an aquatic bird, in the intestine of which it is converted into *Proalaria spathaceum*. (Original)

Diplostomiasis of indigenous European freshwater fish is produced by the metacercariae *Diplostomum spathaceum* von Nordmann, of the trematode *Proalaria spathaceum* La Rue, Rudolphi (*Figure 142*). The eggs (0.1 × 0.06 mm.) reach the water with the feces of the host bird; from them comes the miracidium which swims freely and penetrates the liver of the following species of snails: *Limnaea stagnalis*, *Radix ovata*, *Radix auricularia* and *Galba palustris*. The sporocyst develops within the hepatic tissue, and gives rise to fork-tailed furcocercariae in 6 weeks (their body measures 0.26 × 0.08 mm. and their tail 0.24 × 0.04 mm.). These remain quiescent above 9° C. in a typical flexible position ready to fix themselves onto any fish swimming nearby. They do not live longer than 2 days. After passing through the skin or the gills of the fish, during which operation they lose their tail, the cercariae develop and grow into the metacercariae which are known as *Diplostomum spathaceum* in a period of 45 days (the juvenile larvae measure 0.4 mm.). The metacercariae, at the end of a few hours (or at the most after 7 days) emigrate towards the eye (*Figure 143*) where they may be encountered alive for more than 8 months. When an aquatic bird eats a diseased fish, the trematode *Proalaria spathaceum* develops in its intestine. The ocular invasion of *Diplostomum spathaceum* lesions the lens and vitreous body, swells the cornea through accumulation of liquid in the anterior chamber of the eye (aqueous humor) and produces a milky turbidity of the lens.

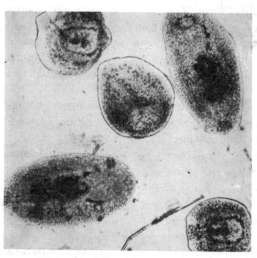

Figure 143. *Diplostomum spathaceum* in the eye of a fish. (Schäperclaus)

In the Gulf of Koenigsberg, a great mortality of fish due to cercarial infestation has been recorded. The fish went to the coast in order to spawn, and found abundant vegetation in which there were numerous infected *Limnaea stagnalis*, the metacercariae which invaded then.

Diplostomum spathaceum is not important to fish farming operations. In certain places almost 100% of the burbot may be attacked. *D. spathaceum* is occasionally found in trout hatcheries. The fight against the disease is carried out by killing aquatic birds and destroying all types of aquatic snails (leave the tanks to dry and then add quicklime).

Tropical aquarium fish may suffer damage in the event of a massive invasion, as was observed by Reichenbach-Klinke, because the metacercarial nodules grow inwards and may produce muscular atrophy through compression (*Figure 141*). An atrophy of this type, for example, in the caudal peduncle or in the muscular zones of the trunk, gives rise to loss of movement and metabolic disturbances.

Schäperclaus (1954) describes an infestation of *Diplostomum spathaceum* (metacercariae of *Proalaria spathaceum*) in *Pterophyllum scalare*. Reichenbach-Klinke (1956b) observed *Colisa lalia* attacked by metacercariae.

From the foregoing it may be seen that snails are undesirable in aquaria since they act as vectors for rediae which liberate cercariae. In aquaria, however, it is uncommon to see fish infested with metacercariae, and this is almost always confined to recently imported individuals.

Sanguinicola

CLINICAL PICTURE AND SYMPTOMS: among young carp losses may be produced over a long period of time. The fish show pale gills, partly decolorized and clear; they swim slowly and listlessly.

TECHNIQUE OF INVESTIGATION: the investigation is carried out in teased preparations of gills and kidney, at a magnification of × 120–600. Permanent mounts may be made by the usual methods where required (see Histological Techniques).

ETIOLOGY; MORPHOLOGY AND TAXONOMY OF THE CAUSATIVE AGENT; COURSE OF THE DISEASE: the causative agent is a trematode of the genus *Sanguinicola*. I shall mention the following species:

(a) *Sanguinicola inermis* Plehn; 1 mm. maximum length; carp parasite;

(b) *Sanguinicola armata* Plehn; 1.5 mm. maximum length; the edges of the body are provided with spines. It lives in tench;

(c) *Sanguinicola intermedia* Ejsmont; less than 1 mm. in length; the edges of the body are provided with spines except on the anterior and posterior ends. It is a parasite of goldfish.

The sexually mature worm lives in the circulatory system, especially in the bulbus arteriosus and in the gill vessels of the fish. Its movements are similar to those of a trypanosome, although they are much slower. The female genitalia always have no more than one egg. The eggs are formed from May to November, and after being released they enter the blood stream and grow to more than twice their original size. They become localized in the gills, cardiac muscle, liver and kidney, and may also be found in certain other internal organs. Their length is from 40–70 microns, and their width from 30–40 microns. Their hat-like shape is characteristic (*Figure 144a*); they appear like a triangle with two rounded angles and one acute angle. Inside them, as maturity takes place, is seen an embryo or larva with a characteristically rounded patch of black pigment. From the eggs localized in the gills is formed a ciliated larva or miracidium, which attacks an aquatic snail (generally *Limnaea stagnalis* and *Radix ovata*), in the liver of which the sporocyst develops, containing rediae and cercariae. The free-swimming cercariae have an undulating crest (*Cercaria cristata*), and move out through the gills and skin of the snail and infect another fish, losing their forked tails in the process (*Figure 144*). They develop within the new fish until they become sexually mature worms.

HISTOPATHOLOGY AND HISTOCHEMISTRY: the large numbers of eggs obstruct the branchial blood vessels and capillaries, giving rise to a fatal thrombosis. Large numbers of eggs may also be found in the kidney. The gills become necrotized. The eggs which pass to the kidney, and those which fail to mature in the gills, are encapsulated by the connective tissue

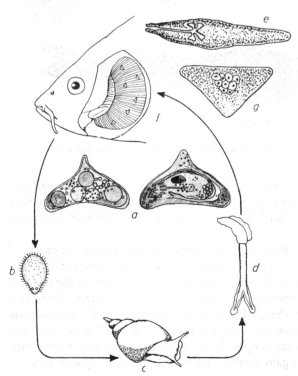

Figure 144. Life cycle of *Sanguinicola inermis*: (a) eggs; (b) ciliated larva; (c) snail, intermediate host; (d) *Circaris cristata*; (e) sexually mature *Sanguinicola*; (f) eggs in the gills; (g) degenerated and agglutinated eggs in the kidney. (Original)

and degenerate. They are frequently found in groups, surrounded by a multi-stratified capsule in the invading connective tissue (*Figure 145*). THERAPY, PROPHYLAXIS AND HYGIENE: the snails may be destroyed with quicklime on fish farms, and this constitutes an important preventive and hygienic measure.

"Black spot" (Neodiplostomum cuticola Ciurea)

The metacercariae of this worm is known as *Neascus cuticola* von Nordmann, and gives rise to small black-pigmented nodules on the skin, trunk musculature, and fins. It especially attacks perch and ruffe (*Figure 146*). The black patches on the dermis are caused by the concentration of melanophores which encapsulate the metacercariae (*Figure 147*). In the

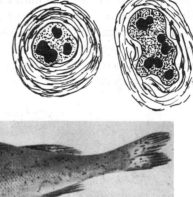

Figure 145. Degenerated eggs of *Sanguinicola*. (Original)

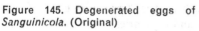

Figure 146. Perch attacked by *Neodiplostomum cuticola*. (Original)

oval nodules, about 0.8 mm. thick, is found the metacercarial larva (0.7–1.4 mm.) inside a transparent membrane. The worm reaches its sexual maturity in an aquatic bird. No damage in fish has so far been observed.

Nodules produced by metacercariae in the internal organs

Nodules produced by metacercariae are frequently encountered in the pericardium, peritoneum, lens, eye chamber, and in various of the internal organs. Gulls are frequently the definitive hosts. I found *Tetracotyle variegata* Creplin in the pericardium of the pike-perch. *Diplostomum clavatum* von Nordmann lives in the lens. In the internal organs we may find *Cotylurus variegatus* Creplin (also known as *Tetracotyle ovata*). The cysts in the internal organs measure 1 mm. and possess very thin walls.

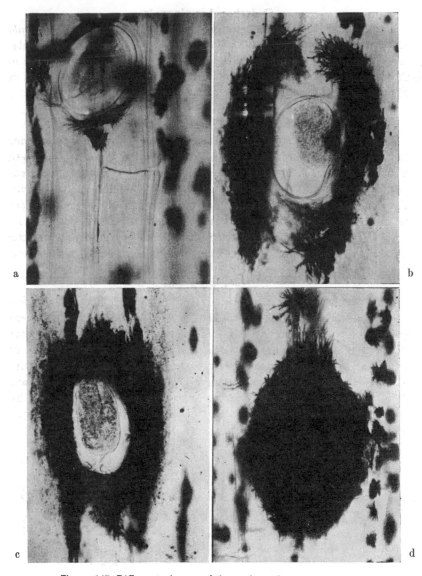

Figure 147. Different phases of the melanophore response to encapsulation of the metacercoriae of *Neodiplostomum cuticola*: (a) beginning of the closing in by isolated melanophores; (b) closing of the capsule, from both sides, around the cercaria (clearly visible in the interior); (c) complete encapsulation; (d) encapsulation of the metacercaria, which is seen externally as a black nodule in the skin. (Original)

Opisthorchis sinensis

The eggs of this trematode are ingested by the snail *Bithynia striatula japonica*. The cercariae which leave the snail attack the skin and musculature of cyprinids (e.g. *Carassius auratus*). The eating of raw fish leads to the development of the sexually mature worm in the pancreatic ducts of Man, cats, and dogs. The metacercariae are non-pathogenic to fish.

CESTODES

The body of the cestodes is flattened and ribbon-shaped. The anterior end bears the scolex or head, which is followed by the segments, the length of which may reach up to 10 meters. The strobila consists of different proglottids which basically contain only the male and female sexual organs. They have no intestine, and the nervous system and pronephridia are rudimentary. The eggs reach the water together with the proglottids. The larval stages of cestodes are: the oncosphere (hexacanth embryo within the egg), and the coracidium (ciliated larva) which swims freely in the water.

Caryophyllaeus

The sexually mature *Caryophyllaeus laticeps* Pall. lives in the fish intestine, and fish are therefore the final hosts of this parasite. This worm may reach up to 3 cm. in size. It is unsegmented, and thus one of the most primitive of all the typical cestodes. It would appear that this lack of segmentation is a phenomenon of neoteny, in the sense that sexual maturity takes place within the plerocercoid larval phase (*Figure 148*). Schäperclaus (1954) observed the death of large numbers of carp and bream caused by *Caryophyllaeus*. On autopsy the parasite is seen through the damaged intestinal wall of the diseased fish.

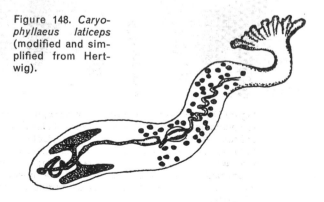

Figure 148. *Caryophyllaeus laticeps* (modified and simplified from Hertwig).

The oncosphere ingested by *tubifex* (or another tubificid) leaves the egg when in the intestine, crosses this organ, and migrates towards the anterior part of the visceral cavity, where up to ten 2 mm. larvae have been observed. When a fish ingests a tubificid worm, the parasite continues its growth and develops into a sexually mature worm. It lays its eggs in autumn, after which it leaves the fish.

When *Caryophyllaeus* makes its appearance in fish tanks, all tubificid worms should at once be destroyed, and the tanks themselves limed and left dry during winter.

Ligula

CLINICAL PICTURE AND SYMPTOMS: the diseased fish show retarded growth. Intensive attacks cause the belly to swell in the post-cephalic region. The fish may become thin. Autopsy shows peritonitis, atrophy of the internal organs, hemorrhages, necrotic white areas, and ascites.

TECHNIQUE OF INVESTIGATION: an autopsy is more than enough to obtain a good idea as to the extent of the disease and the percentage of fish which are attacked.

ETIOLOGY; MORPHOLOGY AND TAXONOMY OF THE CAUSATIVE AGENT; COURSE OF THE DISEASE: Ligulosis is caused by the larvae of the cestode *Ligula intestinalis*, which lives in the intestine of aquatic birds, and its larvae (*Ligula simplicissima* Creplin) in the visceral cavity of fish. *Ligula* has no proglottids, and its body shows a median furrow and a fine secondary segmentation, both dorsally and ventrally. The anterior end has two bothridia. The coracidium escapes from the egg when this falls into the water with the excrement of the host bird. This is eaten by a copepod *Diaptomus gracilis* (1st intermediate host), and in its abdominal cavity grows into a procercoid after having penetrated the intestinal wall. If this small crustacean is eaten by a fish, then the procercoid continues its growth in the abdominal cavity until it forms the plerocercoid, which is *Ligula simplicissima* and may weigh 10% of the fish's weight. The length of this is from 20–40 cm., and its width 0.5–1.5 cm. Its color ranges from white to ivory. After ingestion of the plerocercoid by an aquatic bird, the sexually mature adult worm develops within 2 days under the influence of the somewhat higher temperature in the bird's intestine (*Figure 149*). The worms die after having spent some time in the intestine of the bird.

Ligula chiefly attacks bream (*Abramis brama* L.). The smaller bream are principally infected since these show a preference for small crustaceans. From 4–80% of the whole population may be infected. In larger bream the number of diseased fish is lower. A secondary infection by *Ergasilus* and sporozoans may occur simultaneously. Perch, pike-perch, numerous cyprinids, darters, blackbass, trout, and suckers are also susceptible.

HISTOPATHOLOGY AND HISTOCHEMISTRY: histopathologically it is possible to demonstrate angiorrexia, compression atrophy (especially in the liver), local necrosis and hemosiderin deposits in the periphery of the liver. The hemosiderin gives a positive reaction with Prussian blue.

THERAPY, PROPHYLAXIS AND HYGIENE: in lakes the fish must be exhaustively fished and any sick individuals removed, particularly small bream. Preventive measures must be taken to prevent the free entry of fish-eating birds.

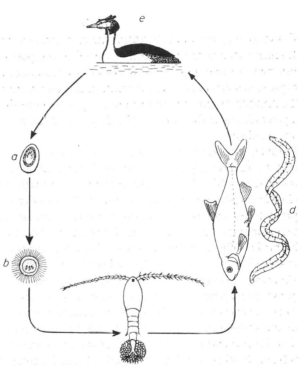

Figure 149. Life cycle of *Ligula intestinalis*: (a) egg with performed oncosphere; (b) ciliated larva, *coracidium*; (c) *Diaptomus gracilis*, first intermediate host; (d) fish, second intermediate host and in the visceral cavity of which the plerocercoid *Ligula simplicissima* develops; (e) aquatic bird, ultimate host in the intestine of which the sexually mature *Ligula intestinalis* develops. (Original)

Schistocephalus

Schistocephalus, like *Ligula*, reaches sexual maturity in the intestines of aquatic birds, where the temperature is a prerequisite. Such birds include ducks and sea gulls, and these are the definitive hosts in the life cycle of *Schistocephalus*. The eggs reach the water either loose or inside a whole worm, and within these the coracidium (miracidium) develops. The ciliated larva is eaten by water fleas (e.g. *Daphnia* and *Cyclops*) and here (the crustacean is the 1st intermediate host) the first larval stage, or procercoid,

223

of the worm takes place, as has been shown in the following species of
Cyclops: C. bicuspidatus, C. serrulatus, and *C. viridis.* If a stickleback
should eat one of these cyclops which was infested, it would be invaded by
Schistocephalus. Under the influence of the digestive juices, the procercoid
is freed into the gastro-intestinal tube, it perforates the intestinal wall and
is localized in the peritoneal cavity where it becomes the second larva, or
plerocercoid. In this fashion the stickleback plays the part of second
intermediate host in the life of the parasite. Inside the stickleback, the
plerocercoid reaches a size of 2–4 cm. × 6–9 mm. They show a fine
segmentation, visible to the naked eye, which imparts a finely ragged
appearance to the outer side of the plerocercoid. The color is snow white,
or in very few cases weakly ivory-colored. The definitive hosts (aquatic
birds) frequently acquire the second larva directly from the water, to
the bottom of which have fallen the worms from the visceral cavity of the
stickleback, or by eating the fish host directly. In this way the parasite life
cycle is completed. In severely parasitized sticklebacks the attention is
drawn to the angular appearance of the body profile. On opening the
abdominal cavity numerous plerocercoids are visible. So that these may be
better appreciated, they are shown beneath the host fish from which they
had been removed in *Figure 150.* Internally the organs are frequently
compressed; the liver and kidney show an obvious compression atrophy.

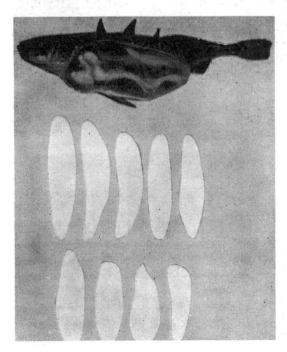

Figure 150. Three-
spined stickleback
with the visceral
cavity dissected;
below, nine plero-
cercoids of *Schisto-
phalus gasterostic*
taken from the vis-
ceral cavity. (Am-
lacher)

The general picture is completed by the presence of adhesions between the viscera and the peritoneum.

Dibothriocephalus latus (Diphyllobothrium latum)

The definitive host of *Dibothriocephalus latus* L. is man. The parasite is the largest of all the human cestodes. Its maximum length may be up to 10–12 meters (the beef tapeworm *Taenia saginata* is 4–10 meters, and the pork tapeworm *Taenia solium* is 2–8 meters). It is also parasitic in the small intestine of dogs and cats. The proglottids mature in the intestine, and into this they release their eggs. These eggs, together with old and degenerated proglottids, leave the body with the feces. Should they fall into the water, the oncosphere or hexacanth larva is released and converted into the miracidium. This latter swims freely by means of its ciliated epithelium and enters a copepod (*Cyclops, Diaptomus*), the 1st intermediate host, in whose abdominal cavity it develops into a procercoid of some 500 microns in length. The pike, perch, burbot, salmon, trout, grayling and eel (2nd intermediate hosts or vectors) eat the infected crustaceans. The larva, freed by the action of the host digestive juices, crosses the intestinal wall and enters either the musculature or the liver, in which it grows into a plerocercoid of 1–2 cm. in length. The plerocercoid, contrary to what occurs in the cysticercus, is not included in a bag full of liquid. It shows transverse furrows, an invaginated head, and great contractability (*Figure 151*). The ingestion of raw fish helps the plerocercoid to fix itself in the small intestine of man, dogs and cats. *Dibothriocephalus* causes acute anemia and many other typical symptoms of helminthiasis.

Triaenophorus

Triaenophorus nodulosus (Pall.) Rudolphi is one of the cestodes which has the fish either as an intermediate or as a definitive host. This parasite is most frequently found in pike, for which reason Schäperclaus has proposed that it be called "pike worm." The head possesses four chitinous hooks provided with three points, which serve to fix it to the intestine. In length it may reach 15 cm. Up to twenty of these parasites have been observed in the intestines of infected pike. However the most important lesions are not caused by the worm itself, but rather by its larvae. Development is as follows: eggs are laid from December to May; from these comes a miracidium which may live up to three days in the water, and following this it dies unless eaten by a copepod, the first intermediate host. The miracidium migrates to the abdominal cavity of the crustacean, and here becomes a procercoid of about 0.5 mm. long. This invasion may produce the death of the copepod. The cyclops are eaten by pike, burbot and other

225

fish, in whose intestine the procercoid is transformed into the plerocercoid within 2 days. This latter perforates the intestinal wall and invades the liver. If a pike eats one of the aforementioned fish, then the adult worm develops in its intestine. Typical symptoms of the disease are produced by the invasion of the liver by the plerocercoid. The invading larva is encapsulated by the connective tissue and may even be calcified. The number of cysts may be such that the whole of the liver tissue is lesioned and suffers a cirrhosis accompanied by a total loss of glycogen, after which the fish immediately dies. According to Scheuring (1929) the tunnels which the larvae produce in the liver give rise to hyperemia and ascites. The cysts

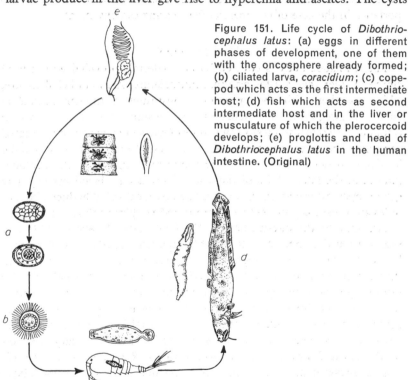

Figure 151. Life cycle of *Dibothriocephalus latus*: (a) eggs in different phases of development, one of them with the oncosphere already formed; (b) ciliated larva, *coracidium*; (c) copepod which acts as the first intermediate host; (d) fish which acts as second intermediate host and in the liver or musculature of which the plerocercoid develops; (e) proglottis and head of *Dibothriocephalus latus* in the human intestine. (Original)

formed round the parasite are composed of a layer of connective tissue with fusiform cells and a layer of polyhedral cells continually being attacked and destroyed by the larval enzymes, and the plerocercoid uses these for its nutrition (by osmosis). For this reason the second layer suffers a continual neoformation. As a result of all this there appears an intestinal inflammation (enteritis), which is also caused in part by the worms themselves. These adhere to the mucosa near to the stomach. The sub-mucosa may react and produce conical or racemose connective proliferations. The growth and resistance of the fish become diminished, and they are increasingly sensitive to hunger and lack of oxygen.

In the case of massive outbreaks, the only measure which can be taken is an intensive fishing and removal of the July–December pike, and destruction of the vectors of the plerocercoids. No pike should be present in the water used to supply any trout hatchery.

In aquarium practice, any water fleas used as food may act as carriers of the plerocercoids. For this reason it is important that such crustaceans be maintained in tanks free from fish. This precaution is of particular importance in the case of commercial fish rearing establishments.

NEMATODES

The nematode body is covered by an epidermis provided with a hard cuticle. Under this is a longitudinal musculature of an epithelial nature, which together with the epidermis constitutes a tubular muscular-cutaneous integument. The nematodes have a simple body cavity in which is found a cylindrical intestine which terminates in an anal orifice situated ventrally. The nervous system consists of an esophagal ring from which the longitudinal nerves are derived. The excretory organs are the protonephridia of the lateral lines of the skin. There are no blood vessels. The gonads open externally on the ventral side, by means of gonoducts. Nematodes are unisexual, and both oviparous and viviparous forms occur.

Fish may be the intermediate or the final hosts of the nematodes, or even both at the same time. If they are intermediate hosts, the nematode larvae are found in the integument, muscles, and internal organs, when they are encapsulated by the connective tissue and form small nodules measuring approximately 0.5–1 mm. The taxonomy of all of these nematodes has been little studied up to the moment. Schäperclaus (1954) observed a massive inflammation in eels resulting from a nematode invasion by the species *Spinitectus mermis* Zeder and a secondary infection by *Aeromonas liquefaciens*. In flatfish, larvae of *Raphidascaris* and *Cucullanellus* encysted in the intestine, liver and mesentery have been found. Röhr, Borkenhagen and Kudak (1959) described a case of invasion of the cod liver. In 27 cod products they found a massive infestation by larvae of *Anisakis*, and also saw some isolated adults (*Figure 152*). Marine fish are intermediate hosts of larval nematodes. The final hosts are seals, sharks and rays, among others. The larvae of *Anacanthocheilus rotundatus*, according to Kahl (1939, 1940), are the most widespread (hake, mackerel, *Gadus carbonarius*, *Molva byrkelange* Walb., *Ciclopterus lumpus* L., *Glyptocephalus cynoglossus* L.), being localized in the stomach, peritoneal cavity, internal organs and muscles. Adult *Ascaris* are frequently found in

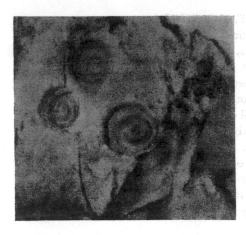

Figure 152. Larvae of
Anisakis in a cod liver
product. After Rohr, Borkenhagen & Knaak)

the intestines of fish. *Ancyracanthus cystidicola* Rud. is found in the swim bladder of freshwater fish, and massive infections result in an anemia. *Camallanus lacustris* Zoega lives in the intestine and pyloric appendages of both marine and freshwater fish. *Philometra abdominalis* Nyb. appears in the bream, together with *Ligula*. Female *Filaria sanguinea* Rudolphi live in the dorsal and caudal fins of the European golden carp. The intermediate host of this parasite is *Cyclops* sp.

The genus *Capillaria* Zeder is frequently found in the intestines of aquarium fish.

Heinze described *Capillaria pterophylli* from the dorsal fins. Schäperclaus found nematodes and larvae of nematodes in perch. *Capillaria piscicola* Travassos, Artigas and Pereira lives in the intestine of Brazilian characins, and Brazilian salmon are attacked by *Capillaria minima* Travassos, Artigas and Pereira. I myself have shown a *Capillaria* infection in the guppy (*Lebistes reticulatus*). Its intestine contained 32 nematodes of different sizes. The intestinal wall showed disseminated lesions chiefly in those parts in which the parasites seemed to be united together. Some of them were also found in the ovary. Furthermore, the much debilitated fish was also infected by *Trichodina*.

The length of those species of *Capillaria* found in aquarium fish is, according to their sex, from 10–20 mm. *Capillaria piscicola* measures from 4–6 mm. and *C. minima* from 1–2 mm. In freshly imported fish from Peru (*Hyphessobrycon innesi*) I was able to see nematodes encapsulated in the muscle tissue and liver.

According to Rankin, infected aquarium fish should be given dry food previously moistened in para-chloro-metaxylenol.

ACANTHOCEPHALA

The Acanthocephala are intestinal parasites which measure from a few millimeters to several centimeters, and possess a tip with hooks, by means of which they fix themselves to the intestinal wall. They have neither mouth nor anus, and do not possess any intestine. They absorb their food by osmosis over the entire body surface. The excretory organs are generally rudimentary; the gonads are well developed.

The intermediate hosts in which they live are isopods, *Gammarus*, aquatic insect larvae and fish. Acanthocephalans attain their sexual maturity in the fish as their final or definitive host. There may also be two intermediate hosts, in which case the first is followed by a fish as second intermediate host or vector, and this latter is afterwards eaten by a warm-blooded animal. The following species are of importance from the point of view of the fish hatcheryman:

(a) *Echinorhynchus truttae* Schrank.; length: male 8–11 mm., female 15–20 mm. In those infections which affect all of the trout intestine, symptoms of emaciation and exophthalmos appear. The larva lives in *Gammarus pulex*;

(b) *Neoechinorhynchus rutili* Müller; length: male 2–6 mm., female 5–10 mm.; this is chiefly known in rainbow trout kept in hatchery pools. The larvae probably live in *Sialis*;

(c) *Pomphorhynchus laevis* Müller; length: male 6 mm., female 13 mm.; found in barbel, in those parts of the river where this fish occurs. Infected barbel are very thin. The intestinal wall is perforated and reacts (Wurmbach, 1937) by encapsulating the parasite with connective tissue, when yellow nodules appear on the external parietal wall of the intestine. The life cycle of *Pomphorhynchus* is not altogether clear. In the sea it lives in gadids, flatfish and eels, among others;

(d) *Acanthocephalus anguillae* Müller; length: male 5–7 mm., female 12–20 mm.; this lives in the eel, perch, salmon and other fish. The intermediate host for the larva is probably *Asellus aquaticus* L. (an isopod crustacean);

(e) *Acanthocephalus lucii* Müller; length: male 4–8 mm., female 8–17 mm.; it lives in the pike, perch, ruffe, and tench;

(f) *Echinorhynchus gadi* Müller; length: male less than 20 mm., female up to 45 mm.; occurs in marine fish, particularly the cod; Prakash and Adams (1960) and Bullock (1963) have described the histopathology associated with infestations of these parasites.

Measures with which to combat these parasites can in reality consist of little more than removal of thin fish and those which appear to be ill; their viscera must be destroyed. In the fish hatchery both the parasites and their hosts may be destroyed by means of quicklime and drying out of the tanks.

FISH LEECHES

Leeches may be considered as modified annelids, flattened dorso-ventrally, and adapted to an ectoparasitic mode of life. Their external segmentation is secondary, and bears no relation to their internal segmentation. The body cavity is a coelom, or is reduced to open spaces. An anterior and a posterior sucker serve to enable the leech to move (to contract and expand itself). The anterior sucker contains the oral orifice, or the opening of the sheath of the mouth. Before reaching the pharynx there may be dentate mandibles or a protractile mouth. Both of these organs serve to inflict the wound on the host. Any blood which passes through it is rendered non-clottable by the action of hirudin, an enzyme produced in the anterior intestine. The stomach has numerous lateral blind sacs. The gonads are hermaphroditic.

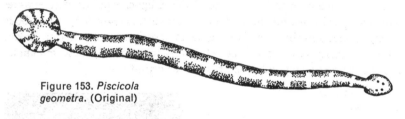

Figure 153. *Piscicola geometra*. (Original)

Of all the leeches of fish, which belong to the Order Rhincobdella, we shall only make mention of one, *Piscicola geometra* L. (*Figure 153*). Externally this may be recognized by characteristic transverse bands and by its prominent suctorial discs. Its length varies between 2–4 cm. This leech, as was shown by Dombrowski, is capable of filling itself with blood in 48 hours. After fixing its mouth in position, it removes 150 cc. of blood. In severe infections, the hemoglobin concentration and the red cell count are both decreased. The fish are restless and are more sensitive to *Trypanoplasma* and *Aeromonas liquefaciens*. When the leeches are full of blood, they leave the fish. In the water, they remain almost always near to the bottom, held fast by their posterior sucker. As soon as any fish swims past they immediately attach themselves to it by means of the anterior sucker. They lay eggs several times from spring to autumn, on plants or other fixed objects. *Piscicola geometra* lays its eggs one by one in oothecae of up to 4 mm. in length.

The fish which have been attacked (*Figure 154*) may be bathed in lysol or priasol (see Table of drugs and treatment). Tanks in which leeches have been seen should be emptied and powdered with quicklime.

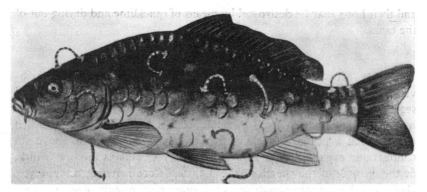

Figure 154. Carp infested
with *Piscicola geometra.*
(Hofer)

LEECHES OF CRUSTACEA

These annelids, members of the Order Oligochaeta, are ectoparasites
which attack the integument and gills of crayfish (*Figure 155*). Their body
is segmented, and the three last segments constitute the posterior sucker.
The oral cavity has two dentate chitinous mandibles. These mandibles
may be large and triangular, or small and pectiniform.

Figure 155. *Branchiobdella pentodonta*
on the ventral surface and the antennae
of *Astacus liptodolylus.* (Amlacher)

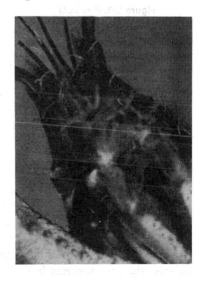

To the first group (triangular mandibles) belong:

(*a*) *Branchiobdella parasita* Henle (4–10 mm. long). The mandibles, all
of the same size, have a larger central tooth surrounded by three smaller
ones on each side in *B. parasita.* It lives on the carapace of crayfish.

231

(b) *Branchiobdella astaci* Odier measures up to 12 mm. in length; its superior mandible is bigger than the inferior one; the lateral teeth are retrograde and lie on a mandibular plate. It lives in the gills of crayfish.

To the second group (small pectiniform mandibles) belong:

(a) *Branchiobdella pentodontata* Whitman, from 3–4 mm. long, long mandibles of equal size, with a larger central tooth flanked by two or three small ones on each side. It lives on the ventral surface of the abdomen and the articular membranes of crayfish.

(b) *Branchiobdella hexodonta* Grüber measures 6 mm. in length, has equal sized mandibles, with two larger teeth and 3–4 smaller central ones. It lives in the gills of crayfish. I (Amlacher, 1954), and Schäperclaus before me, observed an extensive leech infestation in crayfish from Galicia co-existent with aphanomycosis. According to Sterba, crayfish leeches favor the development of aphanomycosis. Severely attacked crayfish should be removed and burned.

Chapter 10

CRUSTACEAN PARASITES OF FISH

The crustaceans are almost without exception aquatic animals which breathe by means of gills. Their appendages, with the exception of the first pair, are ramous legs. The first and often the second pair of appendages act as antennae. The excretory organs are specialized glands, and the eyes are frontal and tripartite (nauplii) or paired and compound. The gonads are unisexual, seldom hermaphroditic. Sexual dimorphism is common among parasitic crustaceans (dwarf male; female reduced to a tube filled with eggs). The greater part of the crustaceans undergo a metamorphosis which frequently includes a nauplius phase. The following taxonomic list indicates the distribution of parasitic crustaceans in the different Orders:

sub-Phylum: BRANCHIATA (Diantennata)
  Class: Crustacea
    sub-Class: Copepoda
      Order: Cyclopidea
        fish pathogens: *Ergasilus sieboldi* Nordmann; *Ergasilus minor* Halisch; *Ergasilus boettgeri* Reichenbach-Klinke; *Acanthochondria* Oakley; *Sphyrion lumpi* Kröyer;
      Order: Caligidea
        fish pathogens: *Caligus rapax* Milne-Edwards, *Caligus lacustris* Steenstrup and Lütken; *Lepeophtheirus* Nordmann; in freshwater and marine fish; *Lernaeocera branchialis* L.; *Lernaea cyprinacea* L.; *Lernaea esocina* L.; *Achtheres pseudobasanistes* Zandt; *Achtheres percarum* Nordmann; *Tracheliastes polycoppus* Nordmann; *Tracheliastes maculatus* Kollar; *Clavella* Oken; in freshwater and marine fish;
    sub-Class: Branchiura
      Family: Argulidae
        fish pathogens: *Argulus foliaceus* L.; *Argulus coregoni* Thorell; *Argulus pellucidus* Wagler;
    sub-Class: Cirripedia

Order: Rhizocephala
fish pathogens: *Sarcotaces arcticus*
sub-Class: Malacostraca
fish pathogens: among the isopods of the Order Cymothoidea should be mentioned as fish parasites *Anilocra physodes* L. and *Cymothoa punctata.*

Ergasilus

CLINICAL PICTURE AND SYMPTOMS: nothing exceptional is noted externally in the diseased fish, but in a heavy infestation (100–1000 parasites on the gills of a fish weighing 250 gm.) there is a marked emaciation (razor-back). If the opercula are lifted up, the crustaceans are seen as oval points on the gill filaments (*Figure 156*).

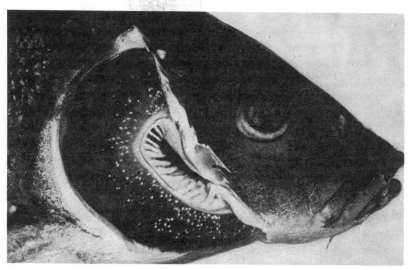

Figure 156. Tench with *Ergasilus* infestation. (Schäperclaus)

TECHNIQUE OF INVESTIGATION: the best way in which to discover if a fish has *Ergasilus sieboldii* is to have an assistant hold the fish and to lift the opercula, first on one side and then on the other. The investigator passes a pair of artery forceps or the handle of a spatula over the gills, raising them one by one. To carry out a taxonomic classification and identification, the cut gill filaments of an already dead fish are examined. Examination for *Ergasilus minor* can only be carried out under the microscope, using a wet mount, since in this way the gill filaments may be more easily separated. Preparations of individual crustaceans may be made using the rapid technique.

ETIOLOGY; MORPHOLOGY AND TAXONOMY OF THE CAUSATIVE AGENT; COURSE OF THE DISEASE: the most common ergasilids parasitizing the gills include the following:

(a) *Ergasilus sieboldii* Nordmann: length 1.3–1.7 mm., width 0.4–0.7 mm. More than 100 eggs per egg-sac. Length of the egg-sac 1.04 mm. It lives on the gills of many freshwater fish and on those of the herring (*Figure 157*). It is characterized by a bluish pigmentation.

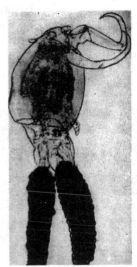

Figure 157. *Ergasilus sieboldii*. (Original)

(b) *Ergasilus briani* Markewitch: length 1 mm., width 0.22 mm. Lives on the gills of freshwater fish.

(c) *Ergasilus boettgeri* Reichenbach-Klinke: length 0.63–0.75 mm., width 0.3 mm. Number of eggs per sac approximately 100. Length of the egg-sac 0.45–0.5 mm. Lives on the gills of tropical fish(*Mollienesia petenensis*).

(d) *Ergasilus minor* Halisch: length 0.65 mm., width 0.18 mm. Number of eggs per sac approximately 36. Length of the egg-sac 0.32–0.34 mm. They are localized at the base of the gill filaments of tench. No blue pigment present (*Figure 158*).

(e) *Ergasilus gibbus* Nordmann: length 1.5–2.0 mm., length of the egg-sac 4.5–6.0 mm. It lives on the gills of eels and roach.

Morphologically the ergasilids resemble cyclops, with the difference that the antennae are transformed into large hooks which fix onto the gills. In the interior of the cephalothorax an accumulation of blue pigment is found. Development takes place after release into the water after having passed through a nauplius phase. The males do not live for longer than 14 days, and die after releasing the spermatophores. For this reason

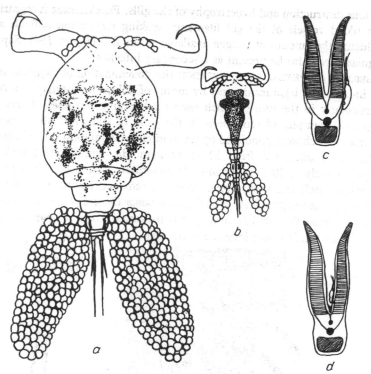

Figure 158. *Ergasilus sieboldii*; (b) *Ergasilus minor*; (c) *Ergasilus sieboldii* localized in a gill filament; (d) *Ergasilus minor* between gill filaments. (Holisch)

therefore, the individuals we find on the gills are always females. In summer two generations occur, the first in June and the second, five times greater in numbers, in September. *Ergasilus*, in the free-swimming stage, remains in the lower layers of the water and is positively geotropic (Gnadeburg, quoted by Schäperclaus, 1954), and therefore by swimming against the current attaches to the gills of the fish. By their slower manner of swimming, tench are the most frequently attacked fish, followed by the pike and the bream in that order. The carp is not infested as a result of its quicker movements. The pectoral fins may also become attacked, as I was able to observe in *Coregonus albula*. Infestation of fish in open waters and particularly those near the bottom, is more intensive than is the case when the fish remain among the vegetation. Bream are carriers of *Ergasilus*. *E. minor* Halisch only lives on tench measuring less than 20 cm. in length. HISTOPATHOLOGY AND HISTOCHEMISTRY: *Ergasilus* feeds on the gill epithelium by means of extra-intestinal digestion (Halisch, 1939). For this reason, as well as the fact that it can change its position, it gives rise to

236

serious destruction and hypertrophy of the gills. Furthermore it constricts the blood vessels of the gill filaments, making respiration difficult and reducing the amount of oxygen available to the fish (*Figure 159*). Saprolegniasis may also be present as a secondary infection.

THERAPY, PROPHYLAXIS AND HYGIENE: the dissemination of *Ergasilus* may be impeded by legal means and by means of obligatory sanitary controls, particularly in the case of tench used for breeding purposes. There are concrete examples of reductions in the yield of lakes and other masses of water which were populated by tench intensively infested with *Ergasilus*. The yields decreased from 32 to 14 kgm./Ha. which corresponds to approximately a 50% reduction. Therefore in waters of this type all diseased tench and small bream must be removed by intensive fishing.

To combat the propagation of *Ergasilus minor* the use of sexually mature tench of more than 20 cm. in length is suggested, since the parasite does not live on tench whose length exceeds this.

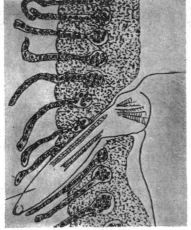

Clasping Hook

Figure 159. Section through a gill filament showing the antenna of *Ergasilus sieboldii*. (Neuhaus)

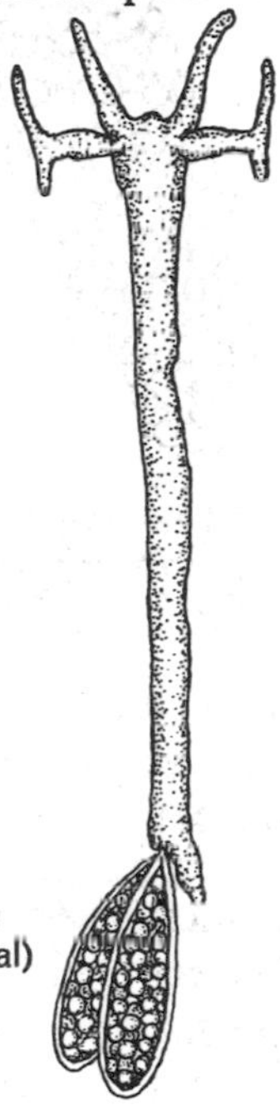

Figure 160. *Lernaea cyprinacea*. (Original)

Lernaea

A modification of the typical copepod type is found in *Lernaea cyprinacea* L., *L. lumpi*, *L. minuta* and *Lernaeocera branchialis*. *Lernaea cyprinacea* parasitizes fish in ponds, although it has also been observed in aquaria on *Nandus nandus*, *Carassius auratus gibelio* (veiltails) and *Cichlasoma* sp. The other species mentioned above occur in marine fish (gadids, pleuronectids, *Cyclopterus lumpus* and *Gobius minutus* among others).

Lernaea cyprinacea L. (*Figure 160*) measures from 9–22 mm. in length and lives in the muscles, although the greater part of its body is outside the body of the host. The cephalic region is characterized by four horns, known as cephalic horns, of which the anterior two are digitiform and the posterior two in the shape of a "T." These cephalic horns are situated around the mouth and enable the parasite to fix itself into the host musculature. During its growth it passes through a nauplius phase without changing hosts. The old adults die following the deposition of eggs.

Some other species of *Lernaea* are *L. esocina* Burmeister, with 4 lobuliform cephalic horns, and *L. phoxinacea* Kröger, with forked anterior cephalic horns.

Lernaeocera is of a dark red color and measures up to 4 cm. in length. Its head bears chitinous cephalic horns, by means of which it fixes itself to the base of the gill filaments. It also penetrates as far as the bulbus arteriosus. In young gadids infestations of up to 80% have been recorded. The life cycle is similar to that of *Lernaea*.

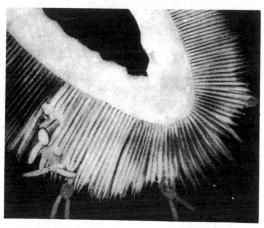

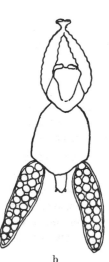

a

Figure 161. Gill of pike-perch attacked by *Achtheres*. (Schäperclaus)

Figure 162. *Achtheres percarus*: (a) from a perch; (b) from a pike-perch. (Jara)

b

238

Achtheres

In a manner resembling that of *Ergasilus sieboldii*, *Achtheres percarum* Nordmann lives on the gills and in the gill cavity, but it may also be localized in the buccal cavity, particularly in the case of the pike-perch (*Figure 161*). It also attacks perch and ruffe. Its reproduction takes place during the summer. The length of the female is from 2–2.5 mm. (*Figure 162*). Since the parasites are well covered by the mucus, they may be discovered by carefully washing the gills in water, particularly important when one wishes to demonstrate the presence of the young parasites. *Tracheliastes maculatus* Kollar (7–20 mm. in length) is very similar to *Achtheres*. This former species is found in freshwater and in bays; principally found to attack the bream.

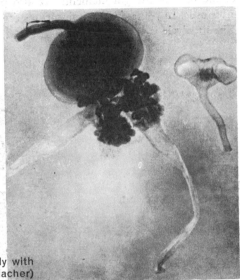

Figure 163. *Sphyrion lumpi*: body with ovary sacs and (right) head. (Amlacher)

Sphyrion

Another lower crustacean which parasitizes marine fish is *Sphyrion lumpi* Kröyer (*Figure 163*), and this is also a copepod. Its length is from 45–60 mm. The anterior part of the body is drawn out rather like a neck, the length of which may reach up to 35–45 mm. The trunk is cordiform or rounded and measures 12–16 mm. *Sphyrion* attaches itself strongly onto the skin by its anterior end, and the posterior end remains free. The caudal region of the body bears two 8–16 mm. long appendices. These parasites fix themselves to the lateral surfaces of the fish (redfish, *Sebastes marinus*), and also penetrate the oral and branchial cavities. Their pathogenicity is a subject of considerable controversy.

CLINICAL PICTURE AND SYMPTOMS: parasitized fish may show reddening of the skin. Spawning trout show an opacity at the base of the dorsal fin, and occasionally even an epithelial neoplasm. Secondary mycosis may be a complicating feature of the disease.

TECHNIQUE OF INVESTIGATION: carp lice may easily be recognized with the naked eye.

ETIOLOGY; MORPHOLOGY AND TAXONOMY OF THE CAUSATIVE AGENT; COURSE OF THE DISEASE: *Argulus foliaceus* L. is the most common carp louse known to us (in central Europe). Together with this species, *Argulus pellucidus* Wagler and *Argulus coregoni* Thorell are also widely distributed.

(*a*) *Argulus foliaceus* L.: maximum length 8.5 mm. Abdomen rounded and provided with spines. Attacks carp, trout and other fish (*Figure 164*);

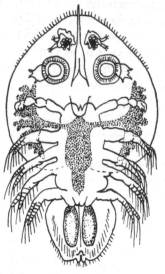

Figure 164. *Argulus foliaceus.* (Wagler, after Sterba)

(*b*) *Argulus pellucidus* Wagler: maximum length 8.5 mm. Abdomen more deeply divided than *A. foliaceus.* Legs covered by the carapace. Attacks carp;

(*c*) *Argulus coregoni* Thorell: maximum length 13 mm. Bicuspid abdomen, smooth edges. Attacks salmonids and percids.

Besides the three species mentioned above, more than 50 others are known. Carp lice have a flattened shield-like body. They adhere to the body by means of their suckers and their extremities. They perforate the skin with their jaws, the mandibles being formed like a sting. This organ is provided with a poison gland and surrounded by a mouth tube, which is introduced into the wound and enables blood and tissue fluids to be withdrawn. The toxin of the carp louse may be fatal to aquarium fish.

On the other hand the string of *Argulus* may lead to the transmission of the causative agent of bacterial hemorrhagic septicemia, or at the very least favor the invasion of this organism.

After leaving the fish the parasite lays from 20–250 eggs on plants and fixed objects. There are six larval stages following the egg, including a nauplius and copepodia phase, and after the seventh moult the adult animal is formed.

The external symptoms described are caused by the repeated biting and continuous rapid movements of the legs of the parasite during the time it is fixed to the host.

HISTOPATHOLOGY AND HISTOCHEMISTRY: the irritation caused by the parasite gives rise in the first place to a cloudiness of the skin according to Becker (1942). The epithelial cells undergo changes due to coagulation of the protoplasm. The secretion of mucus increases considerably, which same histologically gives rise to an increase in the number of claviform and calcifium cells, from 47 to 125/unit of the surface area. The parasite toxin causes a lymphocytic degeneration, the cells being eliminated from the skin. The inter-fibrilar spaces of the dermis disappear, owing to breakage of the fibers, which in turn produces a slight depression on the skin surface just beneath the parasites. The numbers of claviform and calciform cells increase, while that part of the epithelium lying immediately underneath the parasite suffers nuclear degeneration, atrophy of the mucilage cells, and lymphocytic infiltration.

THERAPY, PROPHYLAXIS AND HYGIENE: fish attacked by lice are bathed in lysol or priasol, or in potassium permanganate or an insecticide. Fish lice in pools may be killed by desiccation.

Cirripeds

From time to time fish are rejected by commercial aquarium establishments because they are parasitized by cirripeds. In *Molva byrkelange* Walb., some 3% of all specimens received show the presence of *Sarcotaces arcticus*. This organism is a cirriped, and was described for the first time by R. Collet (1874) and by H. Hjort (1896). According to these workers it affects the abdominal muscles. My own researches (Amlacher, 1958a) have shown an invasion of the lateral body muscles, with parasitic cysts localized at an equal distance between the skin and the vertebrae, near the costal apophyses. Contrary to what has been affirmed by other workers (Lübbert and Ehrenbaum, 1936), the presence of cysts alone could not be confirmed by touch.

The parasite feeds on blood; the cysts which are formed measure from 3–5 cm., according to the bibliography. Within the cyst is a fluid which resembles Indian ink, and this is formed by decomposed blood. The three cysts which I myself have observed measured 4×6 cm., 2×4 cm., and 3×7.5 cm. respectively. A parasite was removed from one fish and preserved. Its location on the host is shown in *Figure 165*. The body had one part in the form of a sac, full of this black-colored fluid. The saccate portion terminated in an articulated point (*Figure 165*). The total length was 4.5 cm., and the average diameter 2.0 cm. The cyst cavity holding the parasite had a length of 5 cm. and a diameter of 2.4 cm. These measurements would obviously be subject to considerable variations according to the stage of fullness at which the parasite occurred (for example, full or empty). The pointed part appeared to be composed of six segments of decreasing size. The saccate portion was divided into four parts by three external annular furrows. Two longitudinal opposed and deeper grooves gave the impression of bilaterality or dorso-ventrality. All of this part of the body was covered by numerous papillae measuring 1–1.5 mm. in diameter, irregularly situated. The numbers of these papillae decreased towards the base of the pointed part, but in the immediate vicinity of this they measured 2–2.5 mm. in diameter. The saccate part is separated from the muscles by a dense capsule of connective tissue. The interior of the body is adherent.

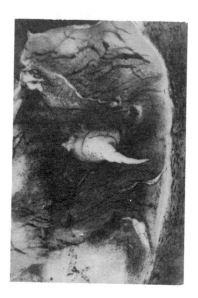

Figure 165. *Sarcotaces arcticus* in trunk muscle of *Molva byrkelange*. (Amlacher)

Several representatives of the Order Isopoda are important as parasites of marine fish. Many genera parasitizing freshwater fish from Argentina have been described by Szidot (1955), and thus it has been clearly established that freshwater isopods do occur as fish parasites.

It was not possible to classify with precision this parasite.* Apparently it occupies a position between the sub-Order Lepadida and the Rhizocephala. There is a similar parasite from the Lepadida, which occurs in rays, and this is a transition form leading to the Rhizocephala (*Anelasma squalicola*, Lov.).

* *Sarcotaces arcticus* is now recognized as a copepod and is not classified as a cirriped.

Chapter 11

ECOLOGICAL DISEASES PRODUCED BY CHEMICAL AND PHYSICAL FACTORS

Lack of oxygen (hypoxia and anoxia)

The requirements for dissolved oxygen are different for each and every species of fish. The carp normally requires 5 mgm./liter, and 3 mgm./liter constitutes the absolute minimum. The latter acts in a negative manner on the metabolism of the carp. Without doubt, the carp is capable of living with 3 mgm./liter, but a concentration of 0.5 mgm./liter has a definitely lethal effect.

In the case of trout, the normal oxygen requirements are 8 mgm./liter. In summer, the normal minimum is 5 mgm./liter; 4 mgm./liter produces dyspnoea; 3 mgm./liter slow death; and 2 mgm./liter rapid death.

The development of the spawn is also largely dependent on the amount of oxygen available, and growth is reduced when the latter is lacking. Lieder's (1955) research with artificially inseminated perch eggs incubated with little oxygen (the actual amount is not stated) at the optimum temperature (14° C.), showed that with very little oxygen development stops after 4–7 hours in the 2- or 4-cell blastomere stage. More developed eggs (32–64 blastomeres) also ceased their development in water deficient in oxygen. On progressively decreasing the oxygen concentration up to the time when the eyes appeared, embryonic malformations and anomalies were produced (fatty cell degeneration as a result of metabolic disturbances, with the usual abnormal mitosis, and simultaneous hydropericarditis and vitelline sac dropsy, together with acephaly, microcephaly, and anencephaly, and also microphthalmia, monophthalmia and anophthalmia). Even though the quantity of oxygen was increased to above normal levels, the young fish showed debility and mortalities.

In open waters and in reservoirs or other artificial masses of water, the oxygen is used up or its concentration decreases following the addition of rotting and decomposing organic substances (domestic residues, sugar and flour mill residues, distillery by-products, manure etc.). The consumption of oxygen is particularly great during winter, even more so when there is a layer of ice covered by snow.

Oxygen deficiency is also a frequent cause of mass mortalities in aquarium tanks. It usually occurs when the water is overpopulated, when there is a lack of aeration, or when decomposing remains of food use up oxygen at the bottom of the tanks. High temperatures, above 25° C., favor oxygen consumption by accelerating the oxidative processes in the aquarium. In old filters putrefaction may also take place, as a result of which oxygen is used up and the total volume is correspondingly decreased. The behavior of the fish in the event of a pronounced oxygen deficiency is typical: they reach the top of the water and gasp on account of the fact that they are asphyxiating. Contrary to what happens in a total lack of oxygen (anoxia), when there is an insufficient quantity which still permits respiration (hypoxia), the fish appear to be quite normal externally. It is just these threshhold concentrations near to the minimum limit which debilitate the natural reserves of the fish and make it more susceptible to different sorts of diseases. For this reason, the oxygen concentration in the water must be regulated. It can be measured in the following manner: an oxygen bottle of precisely 50 ccm. capacity (available commercially from laboratory apparatus suppliers) is completely filled with water and stoppered with a ground glass stopper, taking care that no air bubbles are trapped. The stopper is later removed and with a pipette 3 or 4 drops of sodium hydroxide solution containing a little potassium iodide are added. Following this, 3–5 drops of manganese chloride solution are added with a graduated pipette. A brown precipitate is formed, and the color intensity of this permits the oxygen concentration in mgm./liter to be determined by reference to a colorimetric scale.

The reagents for performing this test are available commercially. An oxygen concentration of 5–8 mgm./liter is sufficient for the majority of fish.

Such a color scale may be found in Plehn's "Praktikum der Fischkrankheiten." In practice, it is just as simple, and considerably more precise, to perform a normal Winkler's estimation of the amount of dissolved oxygen, the details of which may be found in any text on water analysis.

When oxygen is lacking, care should be immediately taken to restore it by forced aeration, partial renewal of the water, and adjustment of the temperature.

Gas bubble disease

Gas bubble disease is caused by a sudden decrease of the gas pressure in the water. The blood of fish which have been breathing in water with a high gas pressure is saturated with gas at the same pressure.

If this pressure is decreased through consumption of oxygen, decrease in temperature, or the addition of new water with a lower gas pressure then the gases in the blood are freed as bubbles, as a result of the higher pressure they still maintain. When there is supersaturation with oxygen and the nitrogen pressure remains constant, then gas bubble disease is also produced as and when the oxygen concentration becomes diminished too rapidly. This situation may be found in aquaria, when these have too many plants, or where there is an asphyxiating growth of algae. If the solar radiation is intense, the plants give off so much oxygen from their metabolic activities that they may come to produce a supersaturation in the water. When the solar radiation ceases, the gas pressure of the water falls rapidly the same as that of the blood, together with the oxygen formation by the plants.

The bubbles are made up principally of nitrogen. They accumulate under the skin, usually in the eye region, giving rise to the so-called gas bubble disease. The bubbles in the blood may cause death due to gaseous embolism.

Pauley and Nakatani (1967) have published a comprehensive description of the histopathology of gas bubble disease in salmonid fingerlings.

The best measure is to change the affected fish to normal water. Oxygen supersaturation in aquaria may be prevented by means of a strong aeration. Aquarium aeration is of decisive importance to achieve a normal equilibrium of the gas pressure.

Transportation carried out with excessive oxygenation may serve to endanger the fish should these be placed in ordinary water following a period in the saturated water. For this reason it is much better to aerate the water with compressed air. Aquaria containing much vegetation must be protected from intense solar radiation.

In hatcheries, gas bubble disease often results from physical conditions which allow air to be entrained in the water. (Harvey and Smith, 1961). The use of high nitrogen fertilizers on the watershed of a hatchery may also be a factor.

pH ACIDOSIS AND ALKALOSIS

In the same way as variations and oscillations in the oxygen concentration affect fish, so pH changes in the water are likewise of prime importance. It is also useful here to perform periodical readings as a control measure. Water chemistry has provided us with simple methods for the investigation of the pH, and these methods enable us to obtain rapid results. General indicators, and instructions for their use are obtainable commercially. Electrical pH meters are also available and are very accurate.

The pH limits are not the same for all species of fish. Some prefer acid water (species of *Rasbora*: 5.5); others require more alkaline water (the barbs: up to 8.5).

The greater majority of fish live between pH 6–8; others between 6–7, 7–8 or only 7–7.5. If the pH is lower than 7 (6.9), the water is said to have an acid reaction (pH 6 is weakly acid); if it is higher than 7 (7.1–14), its reaction is alkaline. Strongly acid water (pH below 5.5) produces the same results as strongly alkaline water (pH above 9), although the lethal limit is different for each species. In acid water, the number of respiratory movements is greatly increased, indicating that only a small part of the available oxygen is being utilized. For this reason, gasping at the surface may also suggest a rather acid water.

Acidosis

As its name suggests, acidosis is found in waters which are too acid, or in fish which normally require a neutral or alkaline pH. If such fish are introduced into acid water (pH below 5.5), or if the water becomes acid for any reason (this may occur as a result of a lack of calcium salts in the earth, from the entry of humic acids from the soil, or from acid mine water), they come to show very rapid swimming movements, gasping, and a tendency to jump out of the water. Death generally occurs rapidly, but it may also have a slower course. In the latter case, the fish die in a natural position, often hidden between the aquatic plants.

Dark grayish deposits, darkening of the edges of the external gills, and mucus secretion may be seen in the gills of carp (Schäperclaus, 1929). The skin has a milky turbidity and reddening of the ventral region. The fish swim indolently and die in a natural position towards the shore.

Mixed aquaria are frequently the scene of death due to acidosis, because species with very different pH and water hardness requirements are often kept together. According to Sterba the water of mixed community tanks must not be too soft, and its pH should lie between 6.5–7.5.

In the event of mortalities due to acidosis, the pH must be normalized. This emphasizes the need for frequent checks.

Tanks and ponds which run the risk of acidification should be limed with powdered calcium carbonate (*never* with quicklime), so as to keep the pH within normal limits. Iron bearing water, at pH 5, produces flocculation of colloidal iron which is deposited on the gills and impedes their normal respiratory function.

Alkalosis

According to the species of fish, this begins at pH 8–9. In the presence of soft water, profuse vegetation and abundant solar radiation, the assimilative activities of the plants add oxygen to the water so that insoluble calcium carbonate is formed from the calcium bicarbonate (biogenic decalcification). From the remains of the calcium carbonate still dissolved, calcium oxide is produced by elimination of carbon dioxide, and the oxide corrodes the branchial epithelium and fins, causing a typical fraying of the latter. A weak opacity of the skin may also be observed. Brandt (1936) determined the following lethal pH values:

trout	9.2
perch	9.2
bream	10.4
pike	10.7
carp	10.8
tench	10.8

To prevent alkalosis the water should be buffered by means of a suitable calcification. Excessive plant growth should be avoided. Aquaria containing many plants should be protected against solar radiation, particularly when the water is soft. The occurrence of ammonium compounds may give rise to the formation of lethal amounts of ammonia if the pH is alkaline (see ammonium intoxications).

Intoxications

Intoxications or toxicities are not always detected by chemical analyses. They generally proceed in the following way: the toxic substance being investigated (for example, rubber tubing) is put into clean water, fish are added to the container and their behavior is observed. The *Daphnia magna* test is also employed, where these animals are used instead of fish. Absorption of toxic substances usually takes place through the gills or the skin.

Among the toxic agents associated with aquaria and fish tanks are included the following:

(a) red, yellow, or black rubber tubing. In aquaria yellow tubing is highly toxic;

(b) aquarium putty;

(c) unsuitable dyes;

(d) cement: the cemented wall of an aquarium should be washed for 14–20 days, with frequent renewal of the water;

(e) impermeabilizing paints: unsuitable ones are toxic because they give off phenol;

(f) nitrogenous compounds: these occur in aquaria as a result of the disintegration of proteinaceous materials (decomposition of food remains, rotten plants, feces etc.); in fish farming operations they also arise from the decomposition of manures and fertilizers. Their concentration at determined levels has a very definite toxic action. The most important nitrogenous compounds are ammonia, nitrites, nitrates, and urea. The lowest limits of toxicity are: nitrates 100–300 mgm./liter; nitrites 10–20 mgm./liter; ammonia 0.2–0.5 mgm./liter. According to Mann, 150 mgm./liter of nitrites are noxious to guppies (*Lebistes reticulatus*). 0.6 mgm./liter of ammonia is the lower limit of toxicity for sardines, 1.2 mgm./liter for certain other varieties, and 0.4 mgm./liter for trout fingerlings.

The decomposition of nitrogenous compounds requires oxygen, and insomuch as its lack retards the formation of nitrites and nitrates, it favors the formation of the first of the by-products of protein decomposition, which is ammonia, the toxicity of which makes it the most dangerous of all the nitrogenous products previously mentioned. In this regard, the great importance attached to a regulation of the aquarium oxygen supply becomes self-evident. With reference to the toxic action of ammonia, the investigations of Wuhrmann and Woker (1949) have demonstrated that the non-dissociated molecules of ammonia (free ammonia) are much more toxic than the dissociated ions (NH_4).

$$NH_4^+ + OH^- \longleftrightarrow NH_3. H_2O$$

The amount and toxicity of these free ammonia molecules in solutions of ammonium salts depends fundamentally on the pH (*Figure 166*). Later Schäperclaus (1952) was able to demonstrate practically this dependence in fish hatchery operations. He observed dead carp in masses where the pH had risen to 9 and above, as a result of the metabolic activities of an intense planktonic growth. At the same time, the non-dissociated ammonia increased to above 2 mgm./liter (see the limits given above). Ammonia is a nerve toxin. Burrows (1964) reported gill hyperplasia in chinook salmon exposed to as little as 0.006 ppm. non-dissociated ammonia for 6 weeks.

Hydrocyanic acid (Prussic acid)

Contrary to what happens in the case of ammonia, the toxicity of hydrocyanic acid solutions decreases with a corresponding increase in pH. The cyanide reaches running water with residues from iron and steel works among others. The lethal dose for trout, the chief victims, is 0.2 mgm. KCN/liter. Cyanide is toxic to the blood, and acts even more violently when in association with ammonia (synergism).

Free chlorine

An increase in the usual concentration of chlorine from 0.2 mgm./liter to 0.4 mgm./liter or more (recognized by the smell of chlorine in tap water) kills aquarium fish when allowed to act over a long time. It attacks above all the gills (paleness); destroys the branchial epithelium (respiratory tissue), and its toxic action affects all the body. Chlorine is a toxic substance

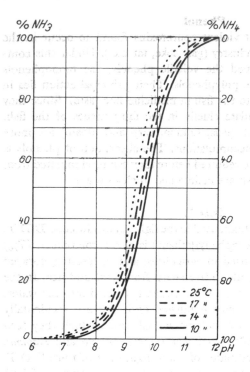

Figure 166. Percentage dissociation
of ammonium hydroxid in relation to
the pH and temperature: the curves
indicate the percentage of ammonia
dissociated and undissociated at
different temperatures and pH levels.
(Woker, after Bandt)

of slow action, which remains for a long time in cold water. 0.2 mgm./liter
of free chlorine at 4–5° C. can kill carp in 20 days. 4 mgm./liter is a fatal
concentration within only 8 hours. Strongly chlorinated water may be
neutralized with sodium thiosulfate (see *Table 2*).

Metals

In galvanized aquaria, the compounds of bivalent iron which frequently
occur in acid stream waters or slightly chalky waters may form a fine dark
precipitate of ferric hydroxide. This precipitate is deposited on the gills,
where it impedes breathing and destroys the branchial epithelium. The
fish die in a normal position. The discus fish is particularly sensitive to
ferric hydroxide. Bivalent manganese compounds behave in a similar
manner.

Phenol

Phenol is one of the most violent neurotoxins found to occur in the residual waters of the coal industry (gas, coke, tar etc.). Under this common denominator are grouped the volatile phenols, the monophenols (cresol, phenic acid), and the polyphenols. Their principal action lies in the taste which they impart to the fish (a medicine-like taste). Since they are liposoluble, they accumulate chiefly in the fatty tissues of the fish. For this reason the fatty fish (eels, salmon, carp and bream) are more subject than others to such accumulations. The absorption of phenols is extremely rapid, but weeks are required before they can be eliminated from the tissues, even when the fish are maintained in clean water.

D.D.T.

This is a liposoluble neurotoxin used in the fight against insects. D.D.T. (1,1,1-trichloro-2,2-bis[p-chlorophenyl]ethane) is also a component (5%) of Gesarol. This product is used in agriculture and in forestry, sprayed from the air, or as an insecticide to free sheep from ticks and lice. In the course of such operations as these, it is frequently carried into the water. By this means, stretches of water populated with fish are accidentally contaminated, and both the fish and the animals upon which they feed are killed. Schäperclaus (1950) stated that *Daphnia magna* and *Daphnia pulex* die in one day at a concentration of 0.001 mgm./liter of pure D.D.T. *Carinogammarus roeselii* perishes in two days at a concentration of 0.01 mgm./liter; *Rhodeus amarus* in 7 days at 0.2 mgm./liter. According to Roegner-Aust (1949) the toxic action of D.D.T. to carp starts at 0.005 mgm./liter. The capacity to recuperate after intoxication with D.D.T. is quite good (Cherrington, Paim and Page, 1969).

Temperature disturbances

Sudden temperature changes hasten death, especially in aquaria and among food fish. Small fish are in grave danger should they be suddenly placed in water which is too cold for them. A drop from 24° to 4° C. produces hemolysis *a frigore*, with vacuolar degeneration of the erythrocytes, which become rounded and allow the escape of hemoglobin which colors the blood stream. Death occurs at the end of about 3 days. In a general manner, it may be said that temperature fluctuations of up to $\pm 12°$ C. do not have serious consequences. On introducing fish into water which is too cold (4° C.) or too warm (25° C.) a thermal shock is produced. In aquaria, temperature fluctuations over a long period are unfavorable since they increase the oxygen consumption. A prolonged decrease in temperature is also prejudicial.

Metabolic disturbances

One of the greatest problems in the keeping and rearing of fish is that of providing them with a physiologically balanced and adequate food. Their vitality, growth and coloration, as well as the successful outcome of their breeding, are all dependent to a large scale on a suitable diet. For this reason the feeding of tropical fish should be rigorously adapted to that of their countries of origin.

By metabolism we generally understand the absorption of food, its decomposition and rebuilding within the body, and the elimination of certain determined end-products. In these processes energy is liberated, and this is converted into body movement. Three principal aspects of metabolism have to be considered:

(a) *energy metabolism:* this concerns the amount of food and the energy liberated after its assimilation. In this, three principal types of nutritive substances are involved—proteins, carbohydrates and fats—in different quantities and proportions, so as to maintain a positive energy balance.

(b) *anabolism:* this refers to the class or quality of the food. Its object is to repair and make up those parts of the body which have been used up (for example, cells), and important substances such as enzymes, hormones, plasma proteins, hemoglobin etc. Anabolism acts upon the three principal types of foodstuffs mentioned above, but also requires certain important complementary substances such as vitamins and inorganic salts. It plays an important role in growth and development.

Since fish are poikilotherms, whose temperature is controlled by that of the water, it is useful to know that all of their chemical (and by definition their anabolic) processes, increase with the temperature up to a limit, and develop best at a determined temperature which is different for each species of fish. This temperature is obviously the same as that of the ordinary aquarium tank, and every attempt should be made to keep it constant if our fish are to be maintained in a healthy condition. Fish may be divided into omnivorous, herbivorous, and carnivorous.

The omnivores form the great majority of fish species, and their name means nothing more than that they eat both animal and plant foods, and according to the type of food available they are quite capable of changing their dietary preferences.

Herbivorous fish are those which feed exclusively on plants, and as examples of these we may mention *Tilapia* and *Xiphophorus variatus.*

Finally most of the predatory fish such as pike, perch, pike-perch, *Aplocheilus lineatus* and *Pantodon* are carnivores.

The food of fish consists basically of the same constituents as we find in that of mankind: carbohydrates, fats, proteins, vitamins and minerals. All of these (with the exception of the vitamins) undergo breakdown in the body until they are reduced to their basic components, which the organism later builds up again in accordance with its own requirements. By means of metabolic processes the organism can, for example, make fat from a sugar, or sugar from a protein.

We shall briefly consider the decomposition and the transformation of foodstuffs. We may commence by making a balance, as in accountancy. The fish requires substances which it obtains in order to survive, these are the "profits." On the other hand it eliminates unwanted products, which constitute its "losses." If we put both of these together we end up with something resembling Fischbach's synopsis:

INPUT	OUTPUT
(a) carbohydrates	(a) carbon dioxide
(b) fats	(b) water
(c) proteins	(c) metabolic products in the waste
(d) inorganic salts and water	and water
(e) vitamins	
(f) oxygen	

(c) *intermediate metabolism*: the foods taken in, especially carbohydrates, fats and proteins, suffer breakdown in the intestinal tract under the influence of digestive enzymes. They reach the blood as metabolites absorbed through the cells of the intestinal mucosa, and are transported to the points of assimilation. Digestion and transformation of the principal nutrients retain many reversible relationships between each other, so that they take place in a harmonious manner. They fall under the general description of intermediate metabolism.

INTERMEDIATE CARBOHYDRATE METABOLISM: sugars and starch are included within the general concept of carbohydrates. Fish take up their carbohydrates from plant material, with the exception of the predatory species. The carbohydrates are digested until they are reduced to their simplest components, the monosaccharides, and as such they reach the blood stream. They enter the liver through the portal, and here they are assimilated in the form of glycogen, or animal starch. Glycogen as such is a reserve substance from which the liver may at any time liberate glucose, which is a most important energy source. The muscles also contain glycogen which is transformed into glucose during work, and this is finally converted into lactic or pyruvic acid. The synthesis of glucose occurs through the destruction of the liver glycogen. All of these processes are controlled by hormones, and performed by enzymes (*Table 9*).

TABLE 9

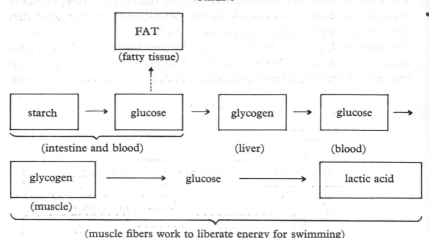

(muscle fibers work to liberate energy for swimming)

In pathological conditions such as fatty degeneration of the liver, or bacterial hemorrhagic septicemia, the liver glycogen disappears (Amlacher, 1956a).

INTERMEDIATE FAT METABOLISM: fats are composed of the trivalent alcohol glycerine and fatty acids. There are both saturated and unsaturated fatty acids. The fat of warm-blooded animals only contains saturated fatty acids, whereas that of fish is composed chiefly of unsaturated fatty acids. With the help of enzymes, the fat is broken down into glycerine and fatty acids in the gut, and these are absorbed by the intestinal wall. Within the intestinal cells they recombine to form fats, and in this way they are transported in the blood and lymph to the liver and adipose tissue. Whenever energy is required, the fat is oxidized by intermediate metabolism to form once again fatty acids and glycerine. Glycerine may be used to form hepatic glycogen, while the fatty acids are further broken down by means of special cellular organs (Krebs citric acid cycle, *Table 10*).

TABLE 10

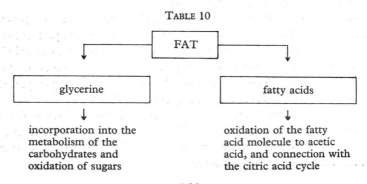

INTERMEDIATE PROTEIN METABOLISM: proteins, fundamental components of meat, are digested enzymatically in the gastro-intestinal tract until they form amino-acids. These amino-acids reach the bloodstream via the intestinal wall, pass to the liver, and continue their breakdown within specific protein cells. During the process of proteolysis in the liver, the well known final breakdown product of metabolism is formed, *id est*, urea.

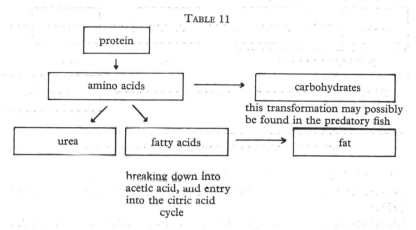

TABLE 11

Fatty acids and carbohydrates may also be formed from the breakdown of amino-acids. The transformation of proteins is a very important part of protein metabolism, as may be seen in the salmon. During the spawning period the trunk muscles come to form material which contributes to the sexual maturity of the gonads.

The transformation of proteins to carbohydrates is probably of great importance in predatory fish, as these ingest no plant material at all, and therefore their body sugar must have had its origin in proteins. For the synthesis of body proteins certain specific amino-acids must be present, and these are grouped together collectively under the name of essential amino-acids. For salmonids, these are the same ten required by man. The fish body also requires these for growth.

Vitamins have a favorable influence and actively direct the processes of metabolism. On the one hand, they form an important part of the enzymatic macromolecules which are of such importance in metabolism. Gastric pepsin for example, is an enzyme, and with the help of the gastric hydrochloric acid, digests the proteins found in meat. The part played by vitamins will be considered in greater detail further on.

Finally, the minerals are also important, and among these iodine may be particularly mentioned. Lack of iodine causes goitre in fish, and the therapeutic measures employed, which involve the administration of iodine, serve to cure this condition.

Let us now consider the pathological changes which may affect metabolism. We can distinguish the following varieties of metabolic disorders quite commonly encountered in fish pathology.

metabolic disorders due to feeding;

vitamin deficiencies;

enzymatic disorders;

glandular disorders affecting metabolism;

hereditary metabolic disorders which occur during growth; under this heading figure both hormonal manifestations of disease, as well as those caused by food;

metabolic disorders caused by pathogens.

The study of these problems does not correspond exclusively to the fish pathologist, but rather to the physiopathologist, whose conclusions are based on fundamental research in normal fish physiology, a field in which much information has still to be obtained. We shall now consider the following metabolic disorders and abnormalities:

(1) **metabolic disorders of alimentary origin:** Fatty infiltration of the organs. The keeping of fish in aquaria and tanks, even under the very best conditions, can never completely compare with life in the natural environment, and for this reason captivity tends to give rise to all types of metabolic disturbances. The most common of these is fatty infiltration of the internal organs, particularly of the intestine, ovary, liver and hepato-intestinal interstitial tissues, all of which contain numerous blood vessels. In squash preparations, the adipose tissue is seen as an accumulation of numerous little spheres all heaped together, which in the fish appear to shine when observed with reflected light. Older fish, particularly those which have spent considerable time in aquaria and fish tanks, almost always show some degree of fatty infiltration. In the tropics, many fish spawn when there is abundant food, which in this case signifies the rainy season, when ciliates multiply enormously. The excess of food ingested serves to aid the growth of the gonads. The usually superabundant food and lack of movement in an aquarium almost certainly leads to a pathological fatty infiltration (*Figures 167, 168*). This holds true for trout and carp in fish hatcheries, although in this instance the whole object of their being fed certain types of food is to obtain a variable degree of fatty infiltration. Those organs which play a key part in the metabolic process, such as the liver, may degenerate as a result of adiposis (fatty dystrophy of the liver), and so provoke the death of the animal. This observation may be made with particular emphasis in the case of trout fed with meat in bad condition and with too much fat; a toxic accumulation of non-saturated fatty acids takes place in the liver, followed by nephritis and hepatic degeneration. My own basic research on the physiology of hepatic metabolism

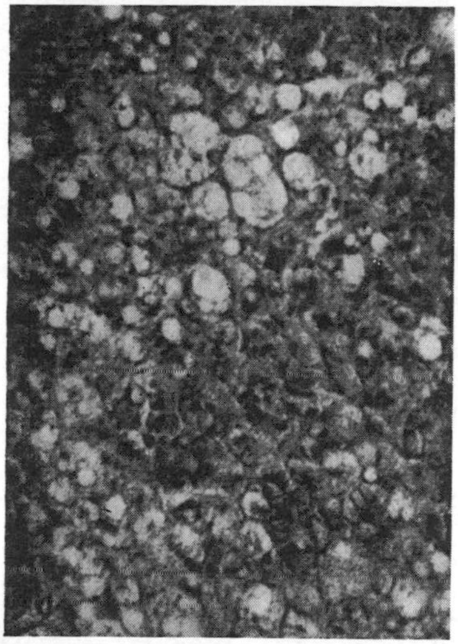

Figure 167. Fatty infiltration in the liver of a tropical fish: the fat appears microscopically in the form of clear globules. (Amlacher)

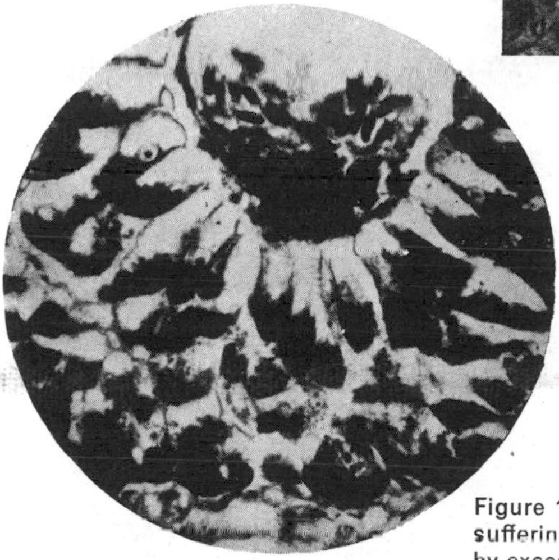

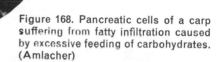

Figure 168. Pancreatic cells of a carp suffering from fatty infiltration caused by excessive feeding of carbohydrates. (Amlacher)

(Amlacher, 1958c) has shown the definite repercussions to be encountered in the liver as a result of any metabolic disturbance (see bacterial hemorrhagic septicemia). Livers having a pathological fatty degeneration show a brownish-yellow color, a piece of information which suffices to indicate necrosis of the hepatic cells. Fish suffering from fatty degeneration are more sensitive than are healthy ones to infectious diseases. Apart from this, experience has shown that fat fish are useless as breeding stock because the functional activity of the gonads is inhibited by the lipoid degeneration. Although the danger of fatty infiltration is of small consequence in young fish, in the case of the adults a more balanced feeding should be provided, since food is not used any longer for body building, but rather is accumulated as fat.

In carp maintained in the fish pools of the Dresden Zoo (*Figure 169*), which besides their normal food had an abundant extra supply of carbohydrates in the form of cakes and buns thrown to them by the tourists, I was able to show that the effects of the assorted buns and cakes was to give them eleven times more fat than in the case of similar carp fed with wheat in a hatchery. The abdominal fat of the Dresden Zoo carp weighed 90 gm., as against 2–8 gm. in the control fish (*Figure 170*). Furthermore the muscles of these carp had four times more fat than in the controls (25.4% against 6.25%, in the control carp) and showed fatty infiltration (*Figure 171*). The amount of fat in the internal organs, with the solitary exception of the heart (*Figure 172*) was practically the same. This was different to what occurred in golden orfe (*Idus melanotus*) from the same tanks as the carp. In this case the continual feeding with white bread causes a complete fatty infiltration, particularly of the liver, as I was able to observe in a pool from the botanical gardens of the University of Jena.

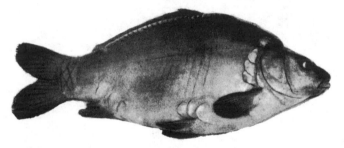

Figure 169. Carp fed with abundant carbohydrates. (Amlacher)

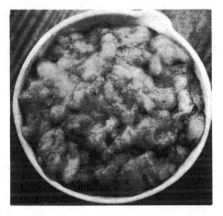

Figure 170. Fat extracted from abdominal cavity of a carp fed with abundant carbohydrates. (Amlacher)

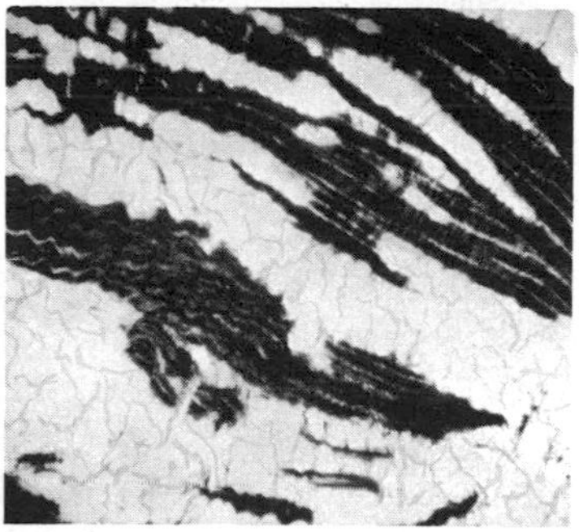

Figure 171. Fatty degeneration of trunk muscle of a carp excessively fed with carbohydrates. (Amlacher)

Epicardial Fatty Tissue

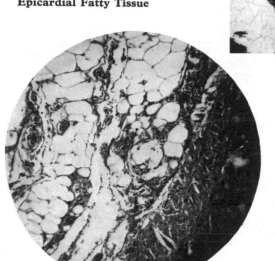

Figure 172. Heart of carp over-fed with carbohydrates, the epicardium showing a heavy increase in the quantity of deposited fat. (Amlacher)

Heart Musculature

(2) **Vitamin deficiencies:** there are specific vitamin deficiencies caused by lack of vitamins A, D, and B in the food. Theoretically vitamin D production during the darkest months of the year (winter) may be paralyzed due to insufficient sunlight. For the same reason, a lack of living plankton in the form of crustaceans gives rise to a decrease in available carotenes (vitamin A precursors) which are normally present in water fleas (*Daphnia*) and *Cyclops*. A lack of algae in an aquarium produces a partial lack or deficiency of carotene and of vitamin B. The following summary on vitamins in fish may be useful:

Vitamin A: the carotenes, precursors of vitamin A, are found chiefly in green plants. The transformation of carotenes into vitamin A probably takes place in the intestinal mucosa and the liver, for which reason this latter organ is especially rich in this vitamin. It is not fully known up to the present to what point fish obtain vitamin A from their food (algae and small crustaceans), or even up to what point they can synthetize it from

259

the corresponding provitamins. Together with vitamin A_1, which is well known to all of us, we find vitamin A_2 in the liver of freshwater fish. This latter is also biologically active.

Morton and Creed (1939), working with perch and whitefish (*Alburnus alburnus*), found that an absorption of carotene led to an increase in the amounts of vitamins A_1 and A_2 in the liver.

Vitamin A is also found in the eyes of fish, but the marine varieties probably have nothing more than vitamin A_1. Freshwater fish have A_2, and migratory species (eels, salmon) possess both vitamins together.

In accordance with the results of modern research, the carotene is transformed into vitamin A in the intestinal mucosa of the fish. It is taken in either directly with plant foods, or indirectly with copepods and *Daphnia*, whose chief source of food is made up of algae. In spite of all this, it appears as though in certain fish plant carotene is preferred to animal carotene (copepods). If a lack of carotene occurs, a fatty degeneration of the liver and necrosis of the hepatic cells (disturbances in protein metabolism) occur.

Trout, at least, can suffer from too much vitamin A (hypervitaminosis)—lowered hematocrit and fin necrosis.

Provitamin A, also formed in certain algae and diatoms, reaches the intestines of phytophagous fish together with such plants, and is converted into vitamin A_1 or A_2. This transformation is not possible in many carnivorous fish.

Finally the component of visual violet in freshwater fish eyes, retinett$_2$, is also a vitamin A derivative, and according to Wald, is chemically different to that found in the human retina.

Vitamin D: vitamin D is naturally found in very small quantities, contrary to the provitamins which are very widely distributed. According to Windaus, provitamin D is found in the earthworm and in certain freshwater oligochaetes (*Tubifex, Nais, Limnodrilus*). It is also found in certain snails, for example, in the red snail (*Buccinium ondulatum*). Vitamin D is found in small amounts in algae and zooplankton. We do not know how the fish obtain their hepatic reserves of vitamin D. Many marine species live at poorly illuminated depths, so that the theory of vitamin D formation from its provitamin as a result of solar radiation is not always applicable. Perhaps the fish synthetize it for themselves, or obtain it directly from their food. For the greater majority of freshwater and aquarium fish the well known scheme of vitamin D synthesis holds good.

Vitamin E: the presence of vitamin E (tocopherol or the anti-sterility vitamin) has been recorded in fish. As it also occurs in green plants, it is probable that certain phytophagous fish obtain it from green algae, among others. Deficiency causes reduced hematocrit. It is essential for salmonids.

Vitamins B_1 and B_2: these are found in green plants (algae) and in the active muscles of vertebrates (even in higher amounts in the heart). Lack of these cause gastric, intestinal and nervous disturbances, a slowing down in growth, and a general decrease in the overall capacity of resistance. Vitamin B_1 is indispensable for carbohydrate metabolism. The requirements of vitamin B_1 increase on the addition of carbohydrates to the diet. Vitamin B_1 as such is not active, but as an ester of pyrophosphoric acid it has the function of a cocarboxylase in the decarboxylation (oxidative decarboxylation) in the Krebs cycle. Fresh fish contains the enzyme thiaminase which destroys B_1 resulting in a deficient diet. Vitamin B_2 is of great importance for the growth of fish, as has been shown for trout. Under its influence the utilization of food for the formation of tissues (growth) is favored, principally by means of the synthesis of fats and proteins. For this reason trout foods are fortified with vitamin B_2 by the addition of yeast.

The occurrence of pantothenic acid and of the anti-anemic factor (folic acid) has been demonstrated in salmon, *Melanogrammus aeglefinus* L., *Trisopterus luscus* L., and in herring (the anti-anemic factor is found in fish liver). Pantothenic acid is an important component of coenzyme A, which occupies a key position in the citric acid cycle (intermediate metabolism). Its lack results in "nutritional gill disease" and possibly "blue slime."

Vitamin B_{12} (cyanocobalamin), is the so-called Castle's extrinsic factor, which together with the intrinsic factor (homogenase) is indispensable for red cell maturation, by means of the formation of folic acid, the anti-anemic vitamin (see VHS). Folic acid deficiency causes a macrocytic anemia in juvenile salmonids (Smith and Halver, 1969).

Vitamin C: vitamin C, according to research carried out up to the present time, is important for older fish. It was found in large amounts in the eggs of roach (*Leuciscus rutilis* L.), pike-perch (*Lucioperca sandra* Cuv. and Val.), carp and perch, in carp flesh, and in the glands of internal secretion (with the exception of the pancreas and thyroids). The same distribution would hold good for most of our aquarium fish. Green plants also contain vitamin C. Deficiency symptoms resemble scurvy of higher animals.

Vitamin K: is essential in blood clotting. A lowered hematocrit results from a deficiency.

Vitamin B_6 (pyridoxine): is associated with protein metabolism. Deficiency results in mass mortality.

Biotin: is associated with "blue slime" disease of salmonids.

Inositol: is essential to salmonids and is considered to be one of the anti-anemia factors.

Niacin (nicotinic acid; vitamin P): is associated with "sunburn" of salmonids.

In the feeding of aquarium fish, algae, plankton, tubificid worms and chironomids should be combined together in an adequate manner. A unilateral feeding, for example with *Enchytraeus* (white worms) alone causes serious metabolic disturbances and intense fatty degeneration of the internal organs. Fish should not be fed all at one go, but always be left a little hungry between meals. Frequent feeding in small portions is the method most resembling the ingestion of food under natural conditions. The precise amount of food to be given depends on observation and experience.

(3) **Bone degeneration:** bone degeneration is a metabolic disturbance caused by abnormalities in enzymatic activity. The bones become brittle and softened owing to a loss of calcium (Mann, 1940). Bone fragility is observed in necrosis of the mandible and operculum, and softness in cases of deformities of the vertebral column. Causes of the condition include hormonal disturbances, hereditary deficiencies, and bacterial infections. Such infections are particularly frequent in tuberculosis and bacterial hemorrhagic septicemia. Metabolic changes may also act as the chief cause of osteomas.

(4) **Gastritis and enteritis:** gastritis and enteritis are particularly common in tropical fish owing to a monotonous diet of nutritious and easily digested foods (*tubifex*, for example), or of dried foods. Vitamin deficiencies and lack of one of the three known basic foodstuffs (carbohydrates, proteins, fats) give rise to inflammation of the gastric and intestinal tracts. The enteritis which occurs in trout fed with diets excessively rich in fats, with spoiled food, or with foods such as fish meal containing more than 3% sodium chloride, is well known. A particularly dangerous disease is produced following the feeding of chironomid larvae or *tubifex* taken from the mud of waters contaminated by industrial pollution, and which contain toxic substances which severely damage or even kill the fish. The diseased fish show considerable swelling and a reddish inflammation, not only of the gastro-intestinal tract, but also of the liver. This swelling of the liver and other internal organs produced on one occasion symptoms of scale protrusion even though there was no accumulation of fluid within the abdominal cavity (*Figure 173*). It is, therefore, advisable to thoroughly wash chironomid larvae and other live foods before giving them to the fish. When the food is insufficient to satisfy the nutritional requirements of the fish, these latter often show symptoms which include a swollen belly and diarrhea (evacuation of coiled and stringy feces). In gastro-intestinal

disorders of fish, the administration of food is suspended for a period of ten days, and then small amounts of live food are cautiously given. In similar cases occurring in hatchery trout, the feeding schedule is likewise suspended. A proper feeding is quite obviously the safest way of avoiding this type of gastric and intestinal disorder.

(5) **Thyroid disturbances:** a disease which is not at all too infrequent in tropical fish is goiter or cancer of the thyroid gland. Although goiter (usually caused by a hormonal disturbance) is included together with the benign tumors, cancer of the thyroid is a rare, malignant and incurable disease. This condition was once epizootic in salmonid hatcheries but is rarely seen now. As with human goiter, adequate iodine in the diet has nearly eliminated the disease.

Thyroid tumors usually appear as reddish inflammations and growths, about the size of a pin-head, in the ventral part of the mouth (*Figure 173*). Thyroid tumors in *Copeina arnoldi* decrease in size over the course of two weeks when an iodine-potassium iodide solution is applied as a bath (Amlacher, 1957a). The following formula was used: 0.1 gm. iodine and 10.0 gm. of potassium iodide in 100 cc. of distilled water. From this stock solution 0.5 cc. is added for each liter of water. Apart from benign thyroid tumors caused by hormonal deficiencies, incurable malignant neoplasms are also found, and these will be described in greater detail in the section dealing with tumors.

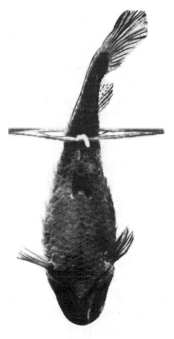

Figure 173. *Mollienesia velifera*: enteritis and hepatitis (after feeding with red chironomid larvae from waste waters) inflammation of the liver and raising of scales. (Amlacher)

Chapter 12

HEREDITARY DISEASES

We shall not concern ourselves at this point with the theoretical aspects of the origin of hereditary diseases. These diseases occur infrequently and are a result of domestication. In tropical fish, they are often the result of crosses, with the aim of obtaining certain anomalies such as color (black mollies) or of shape (veiltails). Certain tumors are also the result of such crossing.

(1) **Tumors of hereditary origin:** Breider (1938) has scientifically described malignant tumors due to hereditary factors in cyprinodonts. The melanophores, which are cells containing melanin granules, begin to multiply rapidly giving rise to melanosarcomas; connective tissue with melanophores of considerable size (macromelanophores). These pigment cell tumors frequently occur in the skin, muscles, bones and nerves of the tail region. Apart from malignant pigment cell tumors, others of a benign nature are sometimes observed.

(2) **Constitutional dropsy of the vitelline sac (hydrocoele):** this occurs in fish which have recently left the egg; their vitelline sac is greatly dilated with an aqueous fluid (*Figure 174*). The young fish dies from this cause. This type of vitelline dropsy must be differentiated from infectious vitelline dropsy caused by the bacterium *Diplobacillus liquefaciens piscium* Betegh. The latter bacterial infection has never been seen in aquaria. It has been suggested that fluorescent pseudomonads and viruses may be partly responsible for this condition.

(3) **Deformities:** lack of fins, swim bladder debility, and certain skeletal deformities occur as hereditary conditions, the origin of which seems to be due to an inherited disorder of vitamin D metabolism. Disturbances in segmentation of the egg give rise to "Siamese twins." Usually one of the twins is perfect, while the other appears as nothing more than an appendix to its other twin (*Figure 175*). The cause of these deformities is unknown, and they have been reported from trout, mollies (*Molliensia latipinna* Lesueur) and in guppies (*Lebistes reticulatus* Peters).

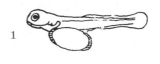

1

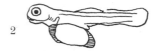

2

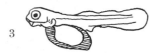

3

Figure 174. Stages in development of
dropsy in embryos; of the five phases
shown, 4 and 5 are usually fatal.
(Dietrich)

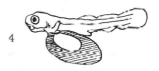

4

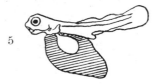

5

Figure 175. Formation of Siamese twins in *Lebistes reticulatus* resulting from faulty
segmentation. (Original)

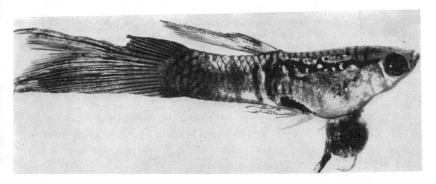

Chapter 13

TUMORS

The papillomas, characterized by cauliflower disease, constitute the most common fish tumors. Tumors are generally divided into benign and malignant (sarcomas, carcinomas). Benign tumors have a slow development, do not destroy the surrounding tissues, and do not spread by metastasis to other parts of the body. They are composed of mature homologous tissue and show an ordered cellular growth similar to that of the original tissue. At this stage it is convenient to give a classification of benign tumors according to strict scientific criteria:

(*a*) cutaneous tumors (epitheliomas);

(*b*) pigment cell tumors (melanomas);

(*c*) connective tissue tumors (fibromas);

(*d*) muscular tumors (myomas);

(*e*) glandular tumors (adenomas);

(*f*) bone tumors (osteomas);

(*g*) cartilaginous tissue tumors (chondromas);

(*h*) nervous tissue tumors (neuromas).

Between the principal types mentioned above are the transition forms, such as for example fibro-epitheliomas (tumors of the epithelium and connective tissues) or myofibromas (muscular and connective tissue tumors). Malignant tumors, on the other hand, grow by infiltration, which means to say that they destroy the surrounding tissue. Furthermore they produce metastasis, which results in the diffusion of the tumorous tissue throughout the entire body. Malignant tumors show a more or less disorganized cellular growth (heterologous tissue). In the strict sense of the word, carcinomas are malignant epithelial growths while sarcomas are malignant connective tissue tumors.

Benign tumors

(1) **Epitheliomas and fibro-epitheliomas:** epitheliomas are benign epidermal tumors, for example as in carp pox. These tumors have their origin in the action of well determined stimuli, and are reduced in size on the removal of such stimuli; they are for this reason pseudotumors,

for which motive they are designated under the general title of hyperplasia. I would like to make mention, among the fibro-epitheliomas, of the growths about the size of a plum or a pigeon egg which formed in carp after tagging them with perlon string (*Figure 176*). In the structure of these neoplastic formations, the epidermis, dermis and hypodermis were involved (*Figure 177*), with the formation of knots of epidermal masses which had proliferated towards the interior, and whose appearance in sections was quite striking due to their appearance as epithelial islands (*Figure 178*). The dermis is of interest because of the intense vascularization of the hyperplastic connective tissue, and the vessels themselves are filled with blood, for which reason the tumors have a definite red coloration.

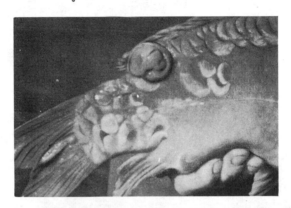

Figure 176. Fibro-epithelioma in a carp during the spawning period, when marked with perlon string. (Schäperclaus)

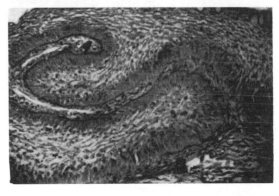

Figure 177. Structure of the fibro-epithelioma shown in Figure 176: the epidermis and the dermis take part in the formation of the neoplasm. (Amlacher)

The fibro-epithelial neoplasms in *Aspius rapax* showed a different histopathological aspect, even though their external appearance was the same (*Figure 179*). Histopathologically a papulous structure was demonstrated (see papillomas). The connective stroma presented vascular formations and hyperemia (*Figures 180* and *181*).

Figure 178. Con-
striction of an
epithelial island in
the periphery of the
fibro-epithelioma
formed by the ac-
tion of perlon string:
(a) epidermal fold;
(b) constriction of
the folded epider-
mal part. (Am-
lacher)

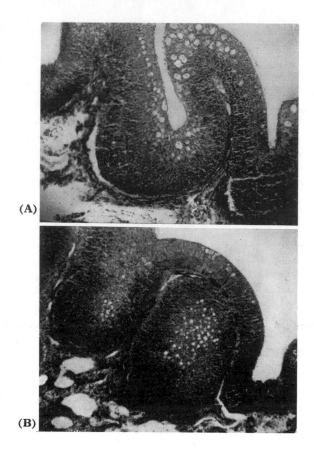

(A)

(B)

Figure 179. Papilloma of *Aspius rapax*,
of unknown origin. (Original)

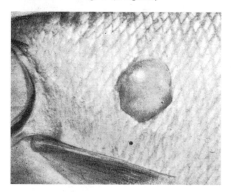

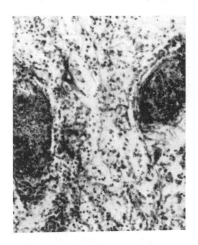

Figure 180. Infiltration of round cells, vascular neoplasm and hyperemia in the tumor shown in figure 179. (Original)

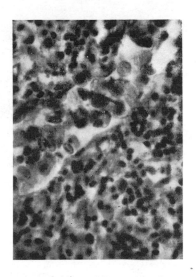

Figure 181. Portion of figure 180 showing within the tissue invaded by round cells, a capillary full of erythrocytes. (Original)

(2) **Epithelioma papulosum (carp pox):** an epithelioma which is frequently observed is that of the epidermal growths known as carp pox (also seen in tench and certain other fish). Carp pox is perhaps the oldest known fish disease, and was fairly widely distributed in Europe during the Middle Ages. The first description of it as a disease was that of Gessner, published in the mid-Sixteenth Century. They have a gelatinous milky appearance and at times cover the whole body of the fish (*Figure 182*).

Normally this condition begins with the fins. In general the behavior of the fish is not affected, but in spite of this carp affected by pox disease tend to become worse. When it is grave it produces emaciation and osteomalacia (softening of the bones). The fish can be bent in any position. Should the disease stop, the skeleton hardens again but even then deformities of the vertebral column are likely to remain.

In an excellent paper Schubert (1964) demonstrated, using electron microscopical techniques, that the infective agent of the carp pox is a virus (*Figures 183, 184 and 185*). Virus like particles found in the epidermis of carp are described. In the nuclei of the host cells round to ovoid particles, surrounded by a single layered membrane with a diameter of approximately 110mu are observed. In the cytoplasm the virus like particles have a double layered membrane and a diameter of about 140mu. The virus is placed in the Herpes group.

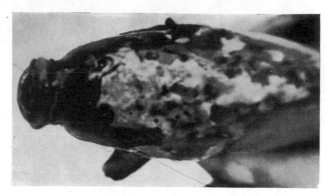

Figure 182. Carp affected by
pox disease. (Original)

Figure 183. Pox papillomas of carp. Virus particle transgressing
from the nucleus (N) to the cytoplasma (C). AK: outer nuclear
membrane, IK: inner nuclear membrane, NP: nuclear pore,
Vn: virus particles in the nucleus, VC: virus particle in the
cytoplasm. (After Schubert)

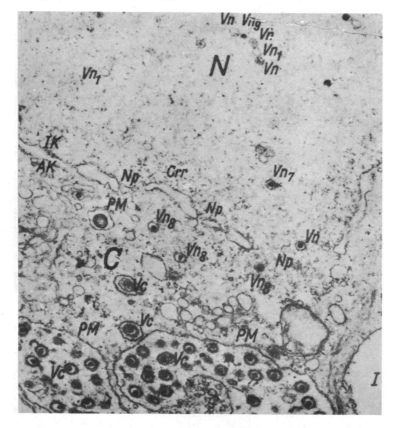

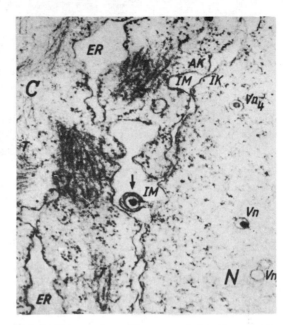

Figure 184. Pox papillomas of carp. Emergence of a virus particle from the nucleus (arrow). IM: space between the inner and outer nuclear membranes, N: nucleus, C: cytoplasma, Vn: virus particle in the nucleus, Vc: virus particle in the cytoplasma. (After Schubert)

Figure 185. Emergence of a virus particle from the nucleus, greatly enlarged. N, C, IK, AK, as in figures 184 and 185.

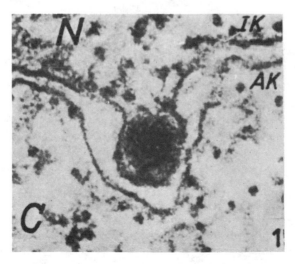

Histologically a thickening of the epidermis is observed. This hyperplasia is composed of homologous tissue. Calciform cells are present only in very reduced numbers in the tumor tissue of the carp, and the dermis is reduced to about a quarter of its normal thickness.

The diseased fish may be treated with drugs (see Table of drugs), but this is of no practical importance. Removal of the fish to another tank or to clean water may help to cure pox disease. Breeding carp whose offspring show a propensity to carp pox should be replaced by others.

(3) **Papillomas:** papillomas are a peculiar form of skin tumor. They look like cauliflowers, and in their interior they show a connective tissue stroma. Virus particles have been seen associated with several of the fish papillomas but, as yet, have not been proved to be the actual cause. These neoplastic formations or growths are frequently observed in eels, and of late their number has reached startling proportions. Schäperclaus (1934b) termed this condition "cauliflower disease" (see the description of the disease under the viral infections of fish). In 1957b, I described a similar tumor in bleak (*Alburnus alburnus*), the histological structure of which bore a great resemblance to the papillomatosis of eels. In the eel, the tumors are preferentially localized in the upper and lower jaws, although they may also be present on the body. The bleak which I studied had a growth between the pelvic and anal fins, which had developed on both sides in an upwards direction until it almost bent the fish in two. Its size was almost that of a hen's egg (*Figure 186*).

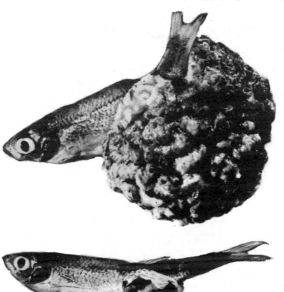

Figure 186. *Alburnus Alburnus* with a cauliflower-like papilloma in the ventro-caudal region: (a) localization of the tumor in the body of the bleak; (b) the fish after removal of the tumor. (Amlacher)

Wellings *et al* (1965) reported a high incidence of papillomas in *Hippoglossoides elassodon*. The papillomas originated as angioepithelial nodules. Virus like particles were observed but their relationship to the papillomas was not established.

Lucké and Schlumberger (1941) described a papilloma of brown bullheads found in Pennsylvania. This neoplasm resembles the cauliflower disease of eels in being a lesion of the lips. This lesion is still commonly found in several areas of Pennsylvania and has been reported to affect as high as 50% of some populations.

Papillomas are known from Atlantic salmon in the U.S.A. and Europe.

(4) **Adenomas:** as an example of adenoma in aquarium fish I should like to mention tumors of the thyroid gland, which according to my own research may be thought of as goiter, and have a benign course (Amlacher, 1957a). In *Copeina arnoldi*, I observed red pin-head sized bodies in the center of the region corresponding to the floor of the mouth (*Figure 187*).

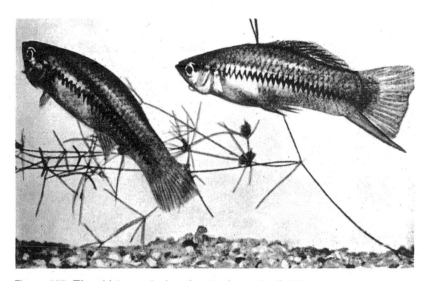

Figure 187. Thyroid tumor in basal part of mouth of *Xiphophorus montezumae.* (Gorbmann and Gordon)

This was due to an anomalous growth of the thyroid, which under normal circumstances is spread throughout the surrounding tissues, and of microscopical dimensions, (*Figure 188*). The tumors observed in *Copeina* were some 800 times larger than the normal thyroid of *Hyphessobrycon innesi* when this latter was taken as a comparison. They were composed of a glandular tissue proliferation which formed acuni and tubules. In the interior of the thyroid follicle there was abundant colloid, with numerous

273

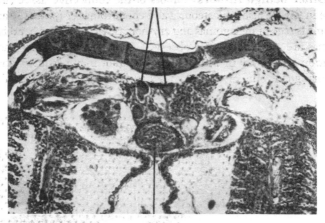

Aorta ventralis

Figure 188. Transverse section of gill region of a neon tetra, showing three thyroid follicles. (Amlacher)

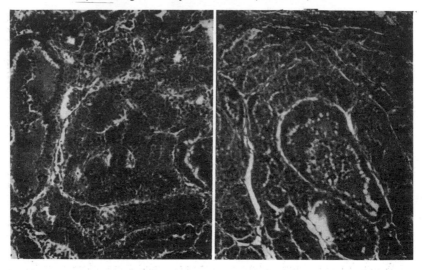

Figure 189. Sections through different areas of benign thyroid tumor in *Copeina arnoldi*: within the hyperplastic granular epithelium are follicles in which blood vessel may be seen, and in the proximity of the follicles there are numerous acini and neoplastic thyroid tissue, together with hyperemic inter-follicular vessels. (Amlacher)

erythrocytes and leucocytes (*Figure 189*), due to internal hemorrhage. A long bath in a 1:20000 solution of Lugol's iodine results in an apparent involution of the tumors at the end of a 10 day period.

(5) **Other benign tumors:** tumors of the connective tissue (fibromas) are rare in fish, as also are osteomas and chondromas (*Figures 190* and *191*). The same is true of melanomas and erythomas. On the other hand however, neuromas are more frequently observed. Thyroid tumors serve as a good illustration of the way in which a benign tumor may become transformed into a malignant one, or at least of a simultaneous appearance of the two

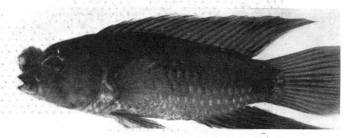

Figure 190. Chondrom in the nasal region. (Original)

Figure 191. Section through the tumor shown in figure 190. (Original)

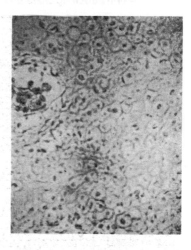

types in fish. They may be present as an adenoma (goiter) or as a carcinoma.

Wood, Yasutake and Lehman (1955) described a granulomatous lesion in brook trout which they considered to be produced by a fungus. The condition is common in some hatcheries rearing brook trout and results in the death of many because the fish cannot withstand stress.

The lesions are first seen on the anterior portion of the stomach as small nodules on the surface of the serosa. The nodules are composed of granulomatous connective tissue and continue to enlarge and spread throughout the visceral mass. Granulomas commonly form in the kidney but other organs acquire the lesions through invasion from the stomach.

Visceral granuloma, as it is now called, is not caused by a fungus but is related to the diet. The exact etiology is unknown but work is being done on the problem.

Malignant tumors

As has been mentioned above, malignant tumors such as epithelial tumors with connective stroma, are called carcinomas or cancers. Tumors of the connective tissues are called sarcomas. Among these may be differentiated fibrosarcomas, myosarcomas, adenosarcomas etc., according to the tissues which take part in their formation.

(1) **Carcinomas:** by virtue of its relationship to goiter, we shall consider the carcinoma of the thyroid gland.

At times small thyroid nodules which invade the surrounding tissues may break away; these enter the blood stream and reach other regions of the body where they begin to proliferate. In this way nodular carcinomas are formed, above all in the gills and floor of the mouth, which displace or compress the branchial blood vessels, producing stasis and respiratory difficulty. These tumors develop by infiltration and destroy the host tissue (Gorbmann and Gordon, 1951). In hatchery practice, Schereschewsky (1933) has observed an enzootic of thyroid cancer in 6–8 week old trout. Gaylord and Marsh (1914) had previously made similar observations to these, even though those authors were able to effect a cure by administering iodine-rich foodstuffs to the fish. Thyroid tumors have also been observed in cyprinodonts and in marine fish. In the cancerous tissue of trout, Schereschewsky found a considerable lack of nuclear chromatin and a glycogenic degeneration of the tumor cells and of the thryoid gland (accumulation of glycogen granules within the cell itself).

Wessing and von Bargen (1959) described a mesenchymal tumor in the guppy (*Lebistes reticulatus*). The infectious particles could be separated by centrifugation of the tumor extract at a speed of 40,000–50,000 revolutions/minute. Of nine species of fish studied, 4 were susceptible to the infection, and the remaining 5 were resistant. These tumors are frequently formed in the kidney, from where they invade the visceral cavity and destroy the muscles, heart, and intestine. The liver, spleen, ovaries and brain are exempt from attack. They are considered to be metastases resulting from the penetration of tumor cells into the blood stream.

Histologically the tumor tissue is composed of non-differentiated mesenchymal tissue, and it is likely that this may originate in different organs (*Figures 192, 193, 194, 195* and *196*).

(2) **Hepatoma:** In the early 1960's, hepatoma was found in epizootic proportions in rainbow trout in the U.S.A. (Wood and Larson, 1961). Pesticides or other added chemicals were suggested as possible causes.

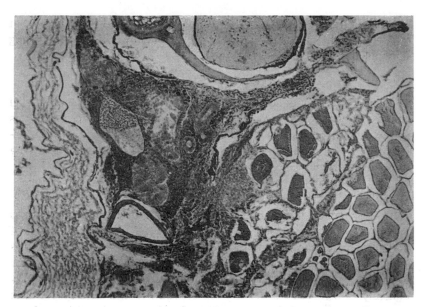

Figure 192. *Lebistes reticulatus*. Primary medullar tumor, with infiltration of the muscles and kidney. (Section and photograph: Dr. Wessing)

Figure 193. *Lebistes reticulatus*. Kidney tumor which grows and penetrates into the dorsal muscles, infiltrating and destroying them. (Section and photograph: Dr. Wessing)

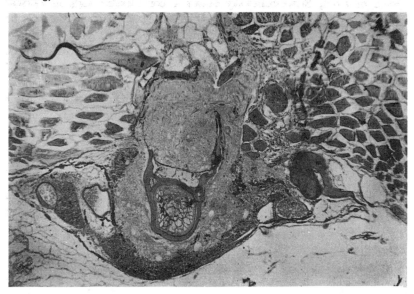

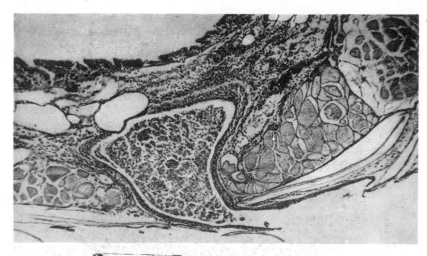

Figure 194. *Pristella riddlei.* Infiltrating growth of a tumor in the visceral cavity, with invasion of the abdominal musculature; the necrotic material is evacuated externally. (Wessing)

Figure 195. *Lebistes reticulatus* with large esophagal tumor, showing two zones of incipient necrosis. (Wessing)

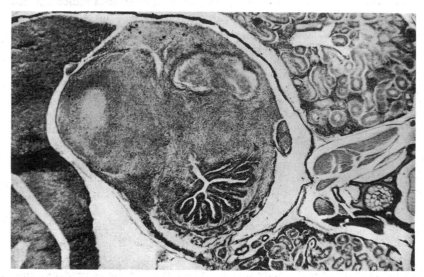

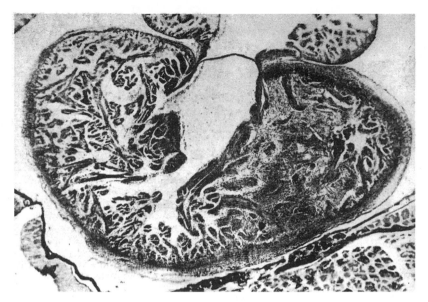

Figure 196. *Lebistes reticulatus* with necrosis of the venticle. (Section and photograph: Dr. Wessing)

However, Wales and Sinnhuber (1966) have reported data indicating that hepatoma outbreaks occurred in California in 1936. This would rule out most agricultural chemicals as possible causes.

Experiments at the Western Fish Nutrition Laboratory and other laboratories indicate that the primary cause of hepatoma in rainbow trout is the presence of aflatoxin in the diet. This toxin is produced by *Aspergillus flavus*, a common fungus (Ashley and Halver, 1967; Halver and Mitchell 1967).

This disease is rapidly becoming rare in the U.S.A. as feed manufacturers improve their feeds and hatchcrymen store their feed under better conditions.

(3) **Melanosarcomas:** in melanosarcomas the melanophores of the skin are subject to an abnormal growth (macromelanophores). These latter appear in extraordinarily large numbers in the connective tissue affected by the tumor. Breider (1938), Breider and Schmidt (1951), and Gordon (1950) have obtained great fame from their investigations and descriptions of melanosarcomas. These tumors appear chiefly at the base of the tail and over the body surface. There is a hereditary predisposition towards them, and they appear principally in hybrids. Their autonomous growth is self-destructive and leads to loss of the fins, rupture of the abdominal cavity, loss of the eyes, and lesions of the brain.

Chapter 14

BIOLOGICAL FACTORS WHICH ADVERSELY AFFECT AQUARIA, AND THEIR CONTROL

The fish in an aquarium is in close contact with the possibility not only of unfavorable factors such as temperature, pH and hardness, but also with what are known as biological factors, which vary according to the ecological conditions (live foods, aquatic plants, growth of undesirable organisms etc.). Even the very structure of the fish population may be the cause of adverse growth. The worst sin is to populate the aquarium too densely, on the one hand the danger of contagion is increased, while on the other certain fish such as male cichlids require their own minimum space for normal growth and development. These considerations make it immediately clear that the installation of mixed community tanks is quite a problem. Unfortunately it is all too common to commit two mistakes at the same time; first to populate too densely, and second to mix together fish with very different pH or water hardness requirements. As a result of this, one section of the fish tends to become diseased and in their turn transmit the disease to the healthy stock, so that in the long run all of them may be lost. For reasons such as these, special emphasis is placed on the need for keeping aquarium fish in conditions as closely resembling those of their natural environment as possible, at least as far as temperature and feeding are required. Throughout the whole of this book I have always insisted upon this, even though it may be true that in certain aquaria factors may come into play which are not directly related to the responsibilities of the aquarist. A few of these are briefly mentioned below:

(1) **Hydras:** *Hydra* is a freshwater cnidarian which paralyzes its prey by means of nematocysts situated in the tentacles. Hydras are not usually dangerous to fish, but in aquaria they grow well and may cause problems. Certain fish such as paradise fish and gouramis feed on hydras according to Flinsk. Ammonium nitrate (1 gm./10 liters of water) is used to prevent them. Two days later a second dose is added, and the hydras die within a few days. There is no need to remove the fish from the aquarium tank. Ammonium nitrate is useful as a fertilizer for the plants. Slawinski recommends a concentration of 0.5 gm. ammonium nitrate/10 liters of aquarium water, which is renewed after two days.

(2) **Turbellarians:** turbellarians also multiply actively in tropical aquaria, being brought in with the food. They are predatory in that on multiplying they feed on fish ova, and also compete with the fish for water fleas. Turbellarians are flat worms, similar to tapeworms, somewhat flattened or leaf-shaped, and of a brownish, yellowish or milky white color. Reichenbach-Klinke described an important growth of *Stenostomum leucops* in the Braunschweig Aquarium. He found it on dead and young living fish. *Stenostomum* occurs particularly where there is an increased consumption of oxygen as a result of an accumulation of organic debris.

The only way to combat turbellarians is to use a bait. A small bag filled with raw meat is hung in the aquarium overnight, near to the bottom of the tank. The well developed olfactory sense of the animals makes them concentrate on the bag, which is removed after a few hours and placed in boiling water. Hungry paradise fish and Siamese fighting fish may be introduced into the tank as a means of biological control.

(3) **Blue-green algae (Cyanophyceae):** the blue-green algae come to form a sticky, bluish-green, velvety layer on the bottom of the tank and on the surface of the plants, as a result of a strong solar radiation on water rich in calcium. Pieces of the algal mat may be removed by aspiration. According to Sterba (1954), when the algal growth becomes excessive, the aquarium may be treated with iron filings, which are spread evenly over the water.

(4) **Green algae (Chlorophyceae):** these algae usually form a layer on the glass sides of the aquarium, and this may be quite thick at times. The algal layer is formed by green algae of the Order Protococcales. Planktonic representatives of this Order may produce a deep green coloration in the water ("algal soup"). Filamentous varieties are the worst, since they form a thick network which eventually embraces almost everything in the tank. Fish enjoy removing green algae from the sides of the aquarium, since they contain provitamin A (carotene). Cleansing of the walls of the tank is achieved by means of a cotton wool swab. Snails should also be removed and well cleaned. The filamentous algae, to which members of the Conjugales belong, are removed by twisting a stick on its own axis in the center of the mat, which can by this means be wound up and removed.

Cases of histozoic algae in fish, including bluegills, have been described.

(5) **Diatoms:** diatoms are found in insufficiently illuminated vessels, forming a fixed layer on the bottom, on the plants, and on the walls. They may be scraped away from the walls and removed by siphoning the bottom. The illumination of the tank should be increased.

Chapter 15

SPECIAL SUGGESTIONS FOR VETERINARIANS, WITH REFERENCE TO DECISIONS ON FISH DISEASES

The veterinarian is frequently confronted with the necessity of making a decision on a fish mortality and its possible repercussions. Experience has amply shown that the great majority of veterinarians know nothing whatsoever about fish pathology, and as a result of this they almost always attempt to resolve the case in question according to the regulations and methods of their own particular speciality. This may give rise to differences of opinion, and even to legal proceedings, and an erroneous decision may frequently cause a considerable economic loss either on a local or a national scale.

The suggestions given below are intended to assist the veterinarian who may be called upon in a case of fish mortality, and to enable him to adopt adequate and precise measures to deal with the case, and also to prevent unnecessary loss of time and differences of opinion to the parties involved.

(1) When fish die without showing any definite macro- or microscopical symptoms of disease, a sample of the water should be taken and analyzed chemically.

(2) Where it is suspected that the water course has been polluted by waste waters, the facts should be presented to the local Fisheries Department. The assistance of Governmental laboratories may be requested in order to resolve this problem.

(3) If the presence of an epizootic is suspected, the veterinarian should carry out his investigation in accordance with the techniques set out in the corresponding chapter in the present book. Fixed material and cultures may be forwarded to the nearest Fish Pathology Laboratory for a concrete diagnosis.

(4) In accordance with what is known at the present time, none of the diseases of fish are transmissable to man, with the exception of the Cestode *Dibothriocephalus latus* and the Trematode *Opisthorchis sinensis*. Viral and bacterial fish diseases are not known to be transmitted to man.

(5) When an epizootic gives rise to a mass fish mortality, every attempt must be made to collect and destroy (burial or incineration) the dead fish.

(6) *The lack of transmission of fish diseases to man requires a special disposition with reference to the hygiene of foodstuffs. Thus carp which are infected with abdominal dropsy, but which die without any macroscopical symptoms, may be smoked and sold to the consumer. Any foul fish should be condemned for human consumption, but they may nevertheless be used fresh in the feeding of pigs, and it is not therefore obligatory to have them destroyed in the abattoir. No fish may be used for feeding pigs if it has been removed from polluted waters, as for example in the case of phenol, since the phenols as a group have an unpleasant taste and are carcinogens. In the case of any doubt as to what decision should be taken with regard to a fish disease, the competent authorities of the nearest Fish Pathology Laboratory should be consulted for a definite ruling on the question. The address of the appropriate Laboratory may usually be obtained from the Department of Fisheries.

* In the United States, the Federal Food and Drug Administration (FDA) prohibits the use of any animal for human consumption which died other than at slaughter. State regulations may vary.

BIBLIOGRAPHY

Alexandrowicz, J. S.: "Lymphocystis tumours in the red mullet (*Mullus surmuletus* L.)", J. Mar. Biol. Ass. U.K., *30*, 1951

Amend, D. F., W. T. Yasutake, and R. W. Mead: "A Hematopoietic Virus of Rainbow and Sockeye Salmon", Trans. Amer. Fish. Soc. 98(4): 796–804

Amlacher, E.: "Ein Fall von Aphanomycespest (Krebspest) im Kreis Güstrow/Mecklenburg", Dtsche. Fisch. Ztg., No. *1* and *12*, 1954

Amlacher, E.: "Das Serum und Gallenbilirubin normaler und künstlich mit *Pseudomonas punctata forma ascitae* (Zimmermann) Schäperclaus infizierter Karpfen (K_2)", Arch. Fisch., *7*, 1956a

Amlacher, E.: "Krankheitsablauf, natürliche Abwehr und Perspektiven der Heilung bei Befall von Zierfischen mit Ichthyophonus", Aquarien und Terrarien, *3*, 1956b

Amlacher, E.: "Die Jodtherapie von Schilddrüsengeschwülsten bei tropischen Zierfischen", Z. Fisch., *6* N. F., 1957a

Amlacher, E.: "Mikroscopisch-anatomische und histologische Studien an einer Blumenkohlgeschwulst beim Ukelei (*Alburnus lucidus* Heck.)", Abh. Ber. Naturk. u. Vorgesch., *10*, 1957b

Amlacher, E.: "Stoffwechsel und Fütterung bei Zierfischen", Aquarien und Terrarien, *4*, 1957c

Amlacher, E.: "Der Blutzucker normaler und an Infektiöser Bauchwassersucht erkrankter Karpfen (K_2)", Arch. Fisch., *8*, 1957d

Amlacher, E.: "Zierfischkrankheiten," Aquarien und Terrarien, *6*, 1958; *7*, 1959; *8*, 1959

Amlacher, E.: "Ein seltener und ein häufigerer parasitischer Krebs an Meeresfischen", Dtsche. Fisch-Ztg., *5*, 1958a

Amlacher, E.: "Die Blumenkohlkrankheit und was wir darüber wissen", Dtsche. Angelsport, *5*, 1958b

Amlacher, E.: "Pathologische Histologie und Histochemie der Leber normaler und an Infektiöser Bauchwassersucht erkrankter Karpfen (K_2)", Arch. Fisch., *9*, 1958c

Amlacher, E.: "Zusammenhang und Wechelwirkung der Bauchwassersuchtformen und ihre Symptomkomplexe beim Karpfen", Dtsche. Fisch. Ztg., *6*, 1959a

Amlacher, E.: "Das Verhalten der inneren Organe und der Muskulatur dreisömmeriger Karpfen aus dem Teich des Dresdner Zwingers bei extremer Kohlehydratfütterung. 1. Teil: Histologische Untersuchungen an Herz, Leber, Bauchspeicheldrüse, Milz, Niere und Darm", Z. Fisch., *8*, N. F., 1959b

Amlacher, E., & E. Mix: "Versuche mit Prowona-Nährhrefe als Zusatz im Futter von Regenbogenforellen", Dtsche. Fisch.-Ztg., *7*, 1960

Amlacher, E.: "Die Wirkung des Malachitgrüns auf Fische, Fischparasiten (*Ichthyophthirius, Trichodina*), Kleinkrebse und Wasserpflanzen", Dtsche. Fisch-Ztg., *8*, 1961a

Amlacher, E.: "Das Verhalten der inneren Organe und der Muskulatur dreisömmeriger Karpfen aus dem Teich des Dresdner Zwingers bei extremer Kohlehydratfüttereung. 2. Teil", Z. Fisch., *9*, N. F., 1961b

Amlacher, E.: "Pathologische und histochemische Befunde bei Ichthyosporidiumbefall der Regenbogenforelle (*Salmo gairdneri*) und am aquarienfisch *Ichthyophonus*", Zt. Fisch., *13*, 1965

Ammon, R., & W. Dirscherl: "Fermente, Hormone, Vitamine", Leipzig, 1948

Anderson, J. I. W. and D. A. Conroy: "The significance of disease in preliminary attempts to raise flatfish and salmonids in sea water", Bull. Off. int. Epiz., *69*, 1129–1137, 1968

Aronson, J. D.: "Spontaneous tuberculosis in salt water fish", J. inf. Dis., *39*, 1926

Ashley, L. M. and J. E. Halver: "Trout hepatomagenesis", Final Progress Report to National Cancer Institute, 1967

Auerbach, M.: "Bemerkungen über Myxosporidien heimischer süsswasserfische", Zool. Anz., *32*, 1907

Auerbach, M.: "Untersuchungen über *Henneguya psorospermica* Thel.", Verh. nat. Ver. Karlsruhe, *24*, 1911

Baker, J. A., and W. A. Hagan: "Tuberculosis in the Mexican platyfish (*Platypoecilus maculatus*)", J. inf. Dis., *70*, 1942

Bandlow, E.: "Das Vorkommen säurefester Stäbchen in den inneren Organen bei tropischen Zierfischen", Staats. Päd. Hochschule Potsdam, 1959

Bandt, H. J.: "Der für Fische 'tödliche pH-Wert' im alkalinischen Bereich", Z. Fisch., *34*, 1936

Bandt, H. J.: "Die tödliche Menge an gelöstem Eisen in Fischgewässern", Fisch.-Ztg., *41*, 1938

Bandt, H. J.: "Fischereischäden als Indikator für Flussverunreinigungen", Wasserwirtschaft-Wassertechnik, *3*, 1953

Bank, O.: "Winterschädigung und ansteckende Bauchwassersueht des Karpfens", Österr. Fisch., *13*, 1960

Bataillon, Dubard & Terre: "Un nouveau type de tuberculose", C. R. Soc. Biol., *49*, 1897

Bauer, H.: "Mikrosckopish-chemischer Nachweis von Glykogen und einigen anderen Polysacchariden", Z. mikr. anat. Forsch., *33*, 1933

Becher, J.: "Die Abwehreinrichtungen von Haut und Kieme beim Karpfen gegenüber mechanischen, chemischen und parasitären Reizen", Int. Rev. Hydrobiol., *41*, 1941

Becker, J.: "Die Abwehrreinrichtungen von Haut und Kiemen beim Karpfen gegenüber mechanischen, chemischen und parasitären Reizen", Intern. rev. d. ges. Hydrobiol. u. Hydrogr., *41*, 1942

Bell, G. R.: "Two epidemics of apparent kidney disease in cultured pink salmon (*Oncorhynchus gorbuscha*)", J. Fish. Res. Bd. Canada, *18*, 1961

Bell, G. R.: "A Guide to the Properties, Characteristics, and Uses of Some General Anaesthetics for Fish", Fish. Res. Bd. Canada Bull. No. 148, 1967

Bellet, R.: "Du syndrôme éntero-hepato-renal chez la truite 'arc-en-ciel' de pisciculture", Bull. franç. Piscicult., *198*, 1958

Bellet, R.: "L'ichthyophoniase des truites d'elevage", Coll. Trav. Path. comp. 1959a

Bellet, R.: "L'octomitiase des truites arc-en-ciel et fario", Bull. franç. piscicult., *31*, 1959b

Benisch, J.: "Über das Auftreten der Lymphocystis-Krankheit bei einigen Korallenfischen", "W", *34*, 1927

Benisch, J.: "Untersuchungen über *Costia necatrix* Leclerq.", Z. Fisch., *34*, 1936

Bergen, v.: "Eine kritische Bemerkung zur sulfitentfärbung des Tuberkelbazillus", Z. Bakt., *88*, 1922

Bergey: "Manual of determinative bacteriology", Baltimore 1957

Bergmann, A. M.: "Die rote Beulenkrankheit des Aals", Ber. a. d. Kgl. Mayer. Biolog. Vers. Stat. München, *2*, 1909

Bertarelli, E. and J. Bocchia: "Neue Untersuchungen über die Tuberkulose der Kaltblütter", Z. Bakt., *54*, 1910

Betegh, L. v.: "Weitere Beiträge zur experimentellen Tuberkulose der Meeresfische nebst Studien über die Transmutationsfrage der Warmblüterbazillen", Z. Bakt., *53*, 1910 and *54*, 1910

Besse, P.: "Epizootie à bacilles acido-résistants chez des poissons exotiques", Bull. Acad. Vet. France, *3*, 1949

Besse, P.: "La tuberculose des poissons", Bull. Fr. Piscid. 164, 1952

Besse, P.: "Recherche sur l'étiologie de l'anémie infectieuse de la truite", Bull. Acad. Vet. France, *28*, 1955

Blake, J. and E. J. M. Anderson: "The Identification of *Bacillus salmonicida* by the Complement-fixation Test—a further Contribution to the Study of Furunculosis of the Salmonidae", Fish. Bd. Scotland Salmon Fisheries No. 1, 1930

Breider, H.: "Die genetischen, histologischen und zytologischen Grundlagen der Geschwulstbildung nach Kreuzung verschiedener Rasen und Arten lebengebärender Zahnkarpfen", Z. f. Zellforschung u. mikr. Anat., *28*, 1939

Brown, E. M: "Note on a new species of dinoflagellate from the gills and epidermis of marine fishes", Proc. Zool. Soc. London, *1*, 1931

Brunner, G.: "Zur Bekämpfung der Karpfenlaus (*Argulus foliaceus* L.)", Fisch. Ztg., *46*, 1943

Bruun, A. F. and B. Heiberg: "Red disease of the eel in Danish waters", Medd. Komm. Danm. Fisk-og Nav-undersog. Ser. Fisk., *9*, 1932

Bruun, A. F. and B. Heiberg: "Weitere Untersuchungen über die Rotseuche des Aales in den dänischen Gewässern", Z. für Fisch., *33*, 1935

Bullock, G. L.: "A schematic outline for the presumptive identification of bacterial diseases of fish", Prog. Fish-Cult., *23*, 1961

Bullock, W. L.: "Intestinal Histology of some Salmonid Fishes with Particular Reference to the Histopathology of Acanthocephalan Infections", Jour. Morph. 112, 1963

Burrows, R. E.: "Effects of Accumulated Excretory Products on Hatchery-Reared Salmonids", Bur. Sport Fish. and Wild. Res. Report No. 66, 1964

Buschkiel, A. L.: "Beiträge zur Kenntnis des *Ichthyophthirius multifiliis* Fouquet", Arch. Protist., *21*, 1911

Canestrini, G.: "La malattia dominante delle Anguille", Atti Ist. Veneto Sci., Serie Settima, Tomo Quarto, Dispenoz Sesta, p. 809–814, 1893

Chaullery, M. and F. Mesnil: "Recherches sur les haplosporidies", Arch. Zool. Exp., 4, 1905

Cherrington, A. D., U. Paim, and O. T. Page: "In vitro degradation of DDT by intestinal contents of Atlantic salmon (Salmo salar)", J. Fish. Res. Bd. Can., 26, 47–54, 1969

Christiansen, M. and A. J. C. Jenson: "On a recent and frequently occurring tumour disease in eels", Report of the Danish Biological Station, 28, 1947

Cisar, J. O. and J. L. Fryer: "An epizootic of vibriosis in chinook salmon", Bull. Wildl. Dis. Assoc., 5, 73–76, 1969

Conroy, D. A.: "Studies on the Application of Kanamycin to the Control and Treatment of Some Bacterial Diseases of Fish", Jour. Appl. Bact. 26: 182–192, 1963

Conroy, D. A.: "Nocardiosis as a disease of tropical fish", Vet. Record 76 (25): 676, 1964

Conroy, D. A.: "A report on the problem of Bacterial Fish Diseases in the Argentine Republic", Second World Symp. of the Perm. Comm. of the O.I.E. on Diseases of Fish, Munich, 1965

Conroy, D. A.: "Observaciones sobre casos espontaneos de tuberculosis ictica", Microbiol. Espan. 19: 93, 1966

Conroy, D. A.: "Tuberculosis of poikilotherms", Fish Pathology (Japan) 2(1), 1967

Conroy, D. A. and J. L. Rodriguez: "Haematological Study of the Hake (Merluccius merluccius) from the Southwest Atlantic", Jour. Fish. Res. Bd. Cana. 22(3): 869–871, 1965

Conroy, D. A. and I. E. Valdez: "Un caso de Tuberculosis en peces tropicales", Rev. Latinoam. Microbiol. 5(1), 1962

Cornelius, W. O.: "Kaulbarschsterben durch Larven von Cotylurus variegatus (Tetracotyle ovata)", Z. Fisch., 33, 1935

Cotton, W. H.: "Ichthyophonus disease in fishes", Water Life and Aquaria World, 7, 1957

Daniel, G. E.: "Studies on Ichthyosporidium hoferi, a parasitic fungus of the herring (Clupea harengus). I. The parasite as it is found in the herring. II. The gross and microscopic lesions produced by the parasite." Amer. Jour. Hygiene 17, 1933

Davis, H. S.: "A new bacterial disease of freshwater fishes", Bull. U.S. Bureau Fish., 38, 1922

Davis, H. S.: "Cytophaga columnaris as a cause of fish epidemics", Trans. Amer. Fish. Soc., 77, 1949

Davis, H. S.: "Culture and diseases of game fishes", Univ. California Press, 1961

Dempster, R. P.: "The use of copper sulfate as a cure for fish diseases caused by parasitic dinoflagellates of the genus Oodinium", Zoologica, 21, 1955

Deufel, J.: "Neue Untersuchungsergebnisse über Darmentzündung, lipoide Leberdegeneration sowie über die Infektiöse Nierenschwellung und Leberdegeneration bei Regenbogenforellen", Fischwirt, 8, 1958a

Deufel, J.: "Untersuchungen über den Erreger der Infektiösen Nierenschwellung und Leberdegeneration der Forellen", Arch. Fisch., 9, 1958b

Deufel, J.: "Versuche mit T-Vitamin-Goetsch bei der Infektiösen Neieren-schwellung und Leberdegeneration", Fischwirt, 8, 1958c

Deufel, J.: "Untersuchungen, über die Wirkung von T-Vitamin-Goetsch auf Regenbogenforellen", Allg. Fisch.-Ztg., 83, 1958d

Deufel, J.: "Über das Virus der Infektiösen Nierenschwellung und Leber-degeneration und einige Bekämpfunsversuche", Fischwirt, 9, 1959

Deufel, J.: "Malachitgrün zur Bekämpfung von Ichthyophthirius bei Forel-len", Fischwirt, 1, 1960

Deufel, J. and K. U. Naumann: "Der Einfluss von Vitamin T auf Regen-bogenforellenbrut", Fischwirt, 8, 1958

Doflein, F. and E. Reichenow: "Lehrbuch der Protozoenkunde", Jena, 1951–1953

Dorier, A.: "Infection de. truites arc-en-ciel d'élevage par des échino-rhynques", Trav. lab. d'hydrobiol. piscic. Univ. Grenoble, 23, 1932

Dorier, A. and C. Degrange: "L'evolution de l'Ichthyosporidium (Ichthyo-phonous) hoferi (Plehn et Mulsow) chez les Salmonides d'elevage (Truite arc-en-ciel et Saumon de fontaine)". Trav. Lab. Hydrobiol. Piscicult. Univ. Grenoble 51, 52, 1960, 1961

de Drouin de Bouville, R.: "Maladie des abces du barbeau, myxoboliasis tuberosa", Bull. Soc. Sci. Nancy, 1908

Earp, B. J., C. M. Ellis and E. S. Ordal: "Kidney disease in young salmon", Spec. Report, Series No. 1, State of Washington Dept. Fisheries, 1953

Ebeling, G.: "Fischereischädigung durch Thuja occidentalis (Thuja oder Lebensbaum)", Z. Fisch., 28, 1930

Ebeling, G.: "Über Fischereischädigungen durch Zuckerfabrikabwässer", Z. Fisch., 29, 1931

Ebeling, G.: "Versuche über die Wirkung phenolhaltiger Abwässer im Zusammenhang mit Rheinuntersuchungen auf der Strecke Mainz bis Emmerich in den Jahren 1935–1937", Von Wasser, 7, 1933

Ebeling, G. and T. Schräder: "Uber freies Chlor im Wasser und seine Wirkung auf Fische und andere Wasserorganismen I, II, III", Z. Fisch., 17, 1929

Edlbacher-Leuthard: "Physiologische Chemie", Berlin 1954

Eichler, W.: "Malariabekämpfung und Fischerei", Allg. Fisch.-Ztg., 72, 1947a

Eichler, W.: "Die Karpfenlaus, Entwicklungsgang, Parasitismus und Bekämpfung", Allg. Fisch.-Ztg., 72, 1947b

Ejsmont, L.: "Morphologische, systematische und entwicklungsgeschitliche Untersuchungen an Arten des Genus Sanguinicola Plehn", Bull. Acad. Pol. Sci. Lett, B. Sci. Nat., 1925

Emmerich and Weibel: "Über eine durch Bakterien erzeugte Seuche unter den Forellen", Arch. f. Hygiene, 21, 1894

Engelhorn, O. R.: "Die Gasblasenkrankheit bei Fischen", Z. Fisch., 41, 1943

Fijan, N. N.: "Propagation experimentale de l'hydropsie infectieuse de la carpe", Second Symp. Comm. Perm. O.I.E. pour l'etude des maladies des poissons, Munich, 1965

Fish, F. F.: "A fungus disease in fishes of the Gulf of Maine", Parasitology 26, 1934a

Fish, F. F.: "Ulcer disease of trout", Trans. Amer. Fish. Soc., 64, 1934b

Fish, F. F. and R. R. Rucker: "Columnaris as a disease of coldwater fishes", Trans. Amer. Fish. Soc., *73*, 1945

Flemming, H.: "Untersuchungen über die Bluteiweisskörper gesunder und bauchwassersuchtkranker Karpfen", Z. Fisch. N. F., *8*, 1958

Flemming, H.: "Über das Blutbild bauchwassersuchtkranker Bleie (Braschen, *Abramis brama* L.)", Z. Fisch., *3*, N. F., 1954

Ghittino, P. and R. Penna: "Recherches microbiologiques Sur la nocardiose de la truite arc-en-ciel", Bull. Off. int. Epiz.. *69*, 1045–1056, 1968

Goncharov, G. D.: "Serologische Diagnostik als neuer Beweis der Virusnatur der 'Rotseuche' des Karpfens", Ryb. chozjajstwo, *4*, 1949

Goncharov, G. D.: "Rubella, a viral fish disease", Viral Diseases of Poikilothermic Vertebrates, N. Y. Acad. Sci. 126 (art. 1): 598–600, 1965

Griffin, P.: "The nature of bacteria pathogenic to fish", Trans. Amer. Fish. Soc. 83, 1954

Gröben, G.: "Beobachtungen über die Entwicklung verschiedener Arten von Fischmarotzern aus der Gattung *Dactylogyrus*", Z. Paras., *11*, 1940

Gröben, G.: "Neue Beobachtungen über Eiablage und Entwicklung von *Dactylogyrus vastator*", Fisch.-Ztg., *43*, 1940

Guseva, N. V.: "Fleckrötein bei Nutzfischen im Asowschen Meer", Priroda, *37*, 1949

Habs, H.: "Bakteriologisches Taschenbuch", Leipzig, 1954

Haempel, O.: "Vitamin- und Hormonwirkungen bei Fischen", Int. Rev. d. ges. Hydrobiol., *35*, 1937

Halisch, W.: "*Ergasilus minor*, ein neuer Parasit auf der Kieme der Schleie", Zool. Anz., *106*, 1934

Halisch, W.: "Ein Vergleich zwischen *Ergasilus briani* Markewitsch und *Ergasilus minor* Halisch", Zoll. Anz., *109*, 1935,

Halisch, W.: "Anatomie und Biologie von *Ergasilus minor*", Z. f. Parasitenk., *11*, 1939

Halisch, W.: "Neues über den Ergasilus", Fisch.-Ztg., *43*, 1940

Halisch, W.: "Der Grosse und der kleine Ergasilus der Schleie (*Ergasilus sieboldii* und *Ergasilus minor*)", Fisch.-Ztg., *38*, 1955

Hallmann, L.: "Klinische Chemie und Mikroskopie", Leipzig, 1954

Halver, J. E. and I. A. Mitchell: "Trout hepatoma research conference papers", Bur. Sport Fish. Wild. Res. Report 70, 1967

Harms, J. W.: "Zoobiologie", Jena, 1954

Harvey, H. H. and S. B. Smith: "Supersaturation of the water supply and occurrence of gas-bubble disease at Cultus Lake trout hatchery", Can. Fish Cult. No. 30, 1961

Hass, G.: "Myxoboliden als Gewensparasiten der Zanders", Z. Fisch., *38*, 1940

Herman, R. L.: "Effects of Gossypol on Rainbow Trout (*Salmo gairdneri*)", Fish Biology, in press

Herman, R. L.: "Fish Furunculosis 1952–1966", Trans. Amer. Fish. Soc. 97(3), 1968

Herzog, H.: "Zur Tuberkulose im Kaltbluterorganismus", Zentralbl. Bact. Orig. 31, 1902

Herzog, P.: "Die ansteckende Bauchwassersucht in Jugoslavien und ihre Bekämpfung", Die Binnenfischerei, *3*, 1950a

Herzog, P.: "Neueste russische, tschechische und jugoslawische Forschungen über die ansteckende Bauchwassersucht", Die Binnenfisch., *3*, 1950b

Heuschmann, O.: "Kiemenfäule bei Biebeln", Z. Fisch., *33*, 1935

Heuschmann, O.: "Die Drehkrankheit der Salmoniden", Allg. Fisch.-Ztg., *47*, 1949

Heuschmann-Brunner, G.: "Nocardiose bei Fischen des Susswassers und des Meeres", Tierarztliche Wocehnschrift 78(5), 1965

Hirschmann, H. and K. Parstch: "Der 'Colisaparasit'—ein Dinoflagellat aus der Oodiniumgruppe", Die Aqu. Terr. Z., *6*, 1953

Hofer, B.: "Eine Salmonidenerkrankung", Allg. Fisch.-Ztg., *18*, 1893

Hofer, B.: "Handbuch der Fischkrankheiten", München, 1904

Hoffman, G. L.: "Parasites of North American Freshwater Fishes", Univ. Calif. Press, 1967

Hoffman, G. L., C. E. Dunbar and A. Bradford: "Whirling disease of trouts caused by *Myxosoma cerebralis* in the United States", Bur. Sport Fish. Wild., Spec. Sci. Report No. 427, 1962

Hoffman, G. L., G. W. Prescott and C. R. Thompson: "*Chlorella* parasitic in bluegills", Prog. Fish-Cult. 27(3), 1965

Jahnel, J.: "Spontaninfektionen mit säurefesten Stäbcnen", Wein. Tierärztl. Monatschr., *13*, 1940

Japanische Autoren: "Untersuchungen über eine epidemische Krankheit bei Regenbogenforellen, die Leberdegeneration und Anämie erzeugt", 1958

Jara, Z.: "*Achtheres percarum* Nordm. als Parasit des Barsches (*Perca fluviatilis* L.) und des Zanders (*Lucioperca lucioperca* Cuv.)", Wiss. Ztschr. Ernst-Moritz-Arndt-Univ. Greifswald., *8*, 1958/59a

Jara, Z.: "Das Blutgerinnungssystem des Karpfens (*Cyprinus carpio* L.)", Wiss. Ztschr. Ernst-Moritz-Arndt-Universität Greifswald, *8*, 1958–9b

Jirovec, O.: "Parasitologie für Arzte", Jena, 1960

Johnson, H. E. and R. F. Brice: "Observations on columnaris in salmon and trout", Prog. Fish-Cult., *14*, 1952

Johnson, H. E. and R. F. Brice: "Further observations on columnaris in salmon and trout", Prog. Fish-Cult., *15*, 1953

Kaestner, A.: "Lehrbuch der speziellen Zoologie", Jena, 1954/55

Kahl, W.: "Nematoden in Seefischen", Z. Parasit., *10*, 1939, *11*, 1940

Kempter, H.: "Veränderungen im Blutbild bei Fischen infolge von Temperaturabfall", Z. Fisch., *31*, 1933

Keysselitz, G.: "Über durch Sporozoen hervorgerufene pathologische Veränderungen", Verh. Ges. dtsch. Vet. Artze, *79*, 1908

Klemm, E. and I. Freund: "Einige pathologische Beobachtungen an Fischen", Prager Arch. f. Tiermedizin und vergl. Pathol., *10*, 1930

Klingler, K.: "Die 'neue' Forellenkrankheit", Schweiz. Fisch-Ztg., *65*, 1957

Klontz, G. W., W. T. Yasutake, and A. J. Ross: "Bacterial diseases of the salmonidae in the Western United States: Pathogenesis of furunculosis in rainbow trout", Amer. Jour. Vet. Res. 27 (120), 1966

Kopp, K.: "Untersuchungen über den Einfluss längerer Hungerperioden auf den Karpfendarm und die in ihm auftretenden histopathologischen Veränderungen bei Erkrankung an Infektiöser Bauchwassersucht", Diss. Tierärztl. Fak., Univ. München, 1951

Krause, R.: "Mikroskopische Anatomie der Wirbeltiere in Einzeldarstellungen 4. Teleostier, Plagiostomen, Zyklostomen, Leptokardier", Berlin und Leipzig, 1923

Krauss, O.: "Über die Wirkung verschiedener gelöster Düngemittel und von K-, Na- und Ca-Salzen auf Haut und Kiemen von Fischen", Z. Fisch., *34*, 1936

Krockert, G.: "Herstellung und Prüfung eines Trockenfutters unter Berücksichtigung von Vitaminen, Mineralstoffen und Hormonen zur Aufzucht und Mast von Forellen", Z. Fisch., *36*, 1938

Kuster, E.: "Kaltblutertuberkulose", Handb. d. path. Mikroog. 5(2), 1928

Lajmann, E. M. and A. S. Spoljanskaja: "Einige neue Tatsachen zur Klinik und Epizootologie der Rotseuche der Karpfen", Ryb. chozjajstwo, *4*, 1949

Larsen, H. N.: "Comparison of various methods of hemoglobin determination on catfish blood", Prog. Fish Cult. 26(1), 1964

Larsen, H. N. and S. F. Snieszko: "Comparison of various methods of determination of hemoglobin in trout blood", Prog. Fish Cult. 23(1), 1961

Lauridsen, O.: "Untersuchungen über die sogenannte Viruskrankheit bei der Regenbogenforelle", Nord. Veterinärmed., *9*, 1958

Laveran, A. and A. Pettit: "Sur une épizootie des truites", C. R. Acad. Sci. Paris, *151*, 1910

Leaman, A. C.: "Control of furunculosis in impounded adult salmon", Nature 208(5017), 1965

Lederer, G.: "Fischtuberkulose", Zool. Garten (N.F.) 15, 1943

Léger, L.: "Sur la sanguinicolose maladie parasitaire de la carpe d'élevage", Trav. lab. hydrobiol. piscic., Univ. Grenoble, *21*, 1930

Liebmann, H.: "Ernährungsstörung und Degeneration als primäre Ursache der Bauchwassersucht bei Fischen", Münch. Berl. Tierärztl. Wochenschr., *69*, 1959

Lieder, U.: "Über Schädigungen von Fischeiern durch Sauerstoffmangel", Dtsche. Fisch.-Ztg., *2*, 1955

Lübbert and Ehrenbaum: "Handbuch der Seefischerei Nordeuropas", 2, Stuttgart, 1936

Lucké, B. and H. G. Schlumberger: "Neoplasia in cold blooded vertebrates", Physiol. Rev. 29(2), 1949

Lühmann, M. and H. Mann: "Beobachtungen über die Blumenkohlkrankheit der Aale", Arch. Fisch., 7, 1956

Lüling, K. H.: "Schmarotzende Ruderfusskrebse", Leipzig, 1953

Lühling, K. H. and H. Mann: "Schädliche Krebsparasiten beim Kabeljau", Fischereiwelt., *4*, 1952

Maie, S.: "Experimentelle Versuche bei Goldfischen (*Carassius auratus*) mit säurefesten Bazillen", Z. Bakt., I, *88*, 1922

Mann, H.: "Die Einwirkung von Chlor auf Fische und Fischnährtiere", Dtsche. Aqua. u. Terr. Ztg., *3*, 1950

Mann, H.: "Eine einfaches und billiges Mittel zur Entchlorung von gechlortem Leitungswasser", Fischwirt, *1*, 1951

Mann, H.: "Zur Frage der lipoiden Leberdegeneration bei Forellen", Fischereiwelt., *4*, 1952

Mann, H.: "*Lernaeocera branchialis* (*Copepoda parasitica*) und seine Schadwirkung bei einigen Gadiden", Arch. f. Fisch., *4*, 1952/3

Mannsfeld, W.: "Die Krepspest im Generalbezirk Lettland in den Jahren 1924–1938", Z. Fisch., *40*, 1942

Markewitch, A. P.: "Parasitische Copepoden und Branchiuren des Aralsees, nebst systematischen Bemerkungen über die Gattung *Ergasilus* Nordmann", Zool. Anz., *96*, 1931

Mattheis, T.: "Die Infektiöse Nierenschwellung und Leberdegeneration der Forellen (INuL)", Dtsche. Fisch.-Ztg., 7, 1960

McCraw, B. M.: "Furunculosis of fish", Fish and Wild. Ser. Spec. Sci. Report: Fisheries No. 84

Meierjürgen, A. G.: "Absterben von Aquarienfische als Folge ungeigneter Fütterung", "W", *32*, 1935

Miegel: "Entzündung der Afters und Darms bei Regenbogen- und Bachforellen infolge von Fütterung mit Abwasserzuckmückenlarven", Z. Fisch., *31*, 1933

Moroff and Fiebiger: "Über *Eimeria subepithelialis*", Arch. f. Protistenk., 6, 1905

Mrsic, W.: "Die Gasblasenkrankheit der Fische. Ursachen, Begleiterscheinungen und Abhilfe", Z. Fisch., *31*, 1933

Neresheimer, E. and C. Clodi: "*Ichthyophonus hoferi* Plehn & Mulsow, der Erreger der Taumenlkrankheit der Salmoniden", Arch. Protistenk., *34*, 1914

Neuhaus, E.: "Untersuchungen über die Lebensweise von *Ergasilus sieboldii* Nordmann", Z. Fisch., *27*, 1929

Neuhaus, E.: "Die Wasserhibbel, eine eigentümliche Hauterkrankung der Karpfen-züchter im Aischgrund", Allg. Fisch.-Ztg., *75*, 1950

Nietzke, G.: "Über die Giftwirkung der organisch-synthetischen Insektbekämpfungsmittel auf Zierfische", "W", *44*, 1950

Nigrelli, R. F.: "Causes of diseases and death of fishes in captivity", Zoologica, *28*, 1943

Nigrelli, R. F.: "Two diseases of the Neon Tetra", Aqu. Jour. 24, 1953

Nigrelli, R. F. and G. D. Ruggieri: "Studies on virus diseases of fishes. Spontaneous and experimentally induced cellular hypertrophy (Lymphocystis disease) in fishes of the New York Aquarium, with a report of new cases and an annotated bibliography (1874–1965)", Zoologica 50(2), 1965

Nigrelli, R. F. and H. Vogel: "Spontaneous tuberculosis in fishes and in other coldblooded vertebrates with special reference to *Mycobacterium fortunitum* Cruz from fish and human lesions", Zoologica, *48*, 1963

Nolte, W.: "Gefährdung der Bleiwirtschaft durch Bandwurmbefall (Ligulosis) in der Havel bei Spandau", Mitt. d. Fischereivereine, *25*, 1933

Nybelin, O.: "Untersuchungen über den bei Fischen krankheiterregenden Spaltpilz *Vibrio anguillarum*", Mitt. d. Anstalt f. Binnenfisch. b. Drottningholm, Stockholm, *8*, 1935a

Nybelin, O.: "Über die Ursache der Krebspest in Schweden", Fisch.-Ztg., *38*, 1935b

Offhaus, K., G. Brunner and S. Riedmüller: "Gedanken über die Entstehung der Bauchwassersucht des Karpfens auf Grund bakteriologischer Ergebnisse und elektrophoretischer Blutuntersuchungen", Arch. Fisch., 6, 1955

Opitz, H.: "Mikrosporidienkrankheit *Plistophora* auch bei *Hemigrammus ocellifer* und *Brachydanio rerio*", "W", *39*, 1942

Ordal, E. J. and B. J. Earp: "Cultivation and transmission of etiological agent of kidney disease in salmonid fishes", Proc. Soc. exp. Biol. & Med., *92*, 1956

Ordal, E. J. and R. R. Rucker: "Pathogenic myxobacteria", Proc. Soc. exp. Biol. & Med., *56*, 1944

Parisot, T.: "Tuberculosis of fish. A review of the literature with a description of the diseases in salmonid fish", Bact. Rev. 22, 1958

Parisot, T. and A. H. Decker: "A comparative study of the causative agent of a mycobacterial disease of salmonid fishes. I. A comparison of the staining characteristics of the fish disease with human tuberculosis in sections stained by the Fite-Faraco and Ziehl-Neelsen methods", Amer. Rev. Respir. Dis. 81(1), 1960

Pauley, G. B. and R. E. Nakatani: "Histopathology of 'gasbubble' disease in salmon fingerlings", Jour. Fish. Res. Bd. Cana. 24(4), 1967

Pescheck, E.: "Eine Konstitutionskrankheit küntlich erbrüteter Salmoniden", Wasser yu. Abwasser, 1958

Peskov, M. A.: "Krasnuha karpov kak samostojateljnoe virusnoe zabolevanie ryb.", Trudy Inst. Morfol. Zhivotn 5, 1951

Pettit, A : "Observations sur l'Ichthyosporidium et sur la maladie qu'il provoque chez la truite", Ann. Inst. Past. 27, 1913

Pettit, A.: "A propos du microorganisme producteur de la Taumelkrankheit. Ichthyosporium ou Ichthyophonus", C. R. Soc., Biol., *70*, 1911

Pfitzner, I.: "Beitrag zur Aetiolgie der 'Haemorrhagischen Virussepti-kaemie der Regenbogenforellen' ", Zentbl. Bakt., Par., Infek. und Hygiene 201, 1966

Pflugfelder, O.: "Ein neuer Fischparasit aus der Gruppe der Mikrosporidien", Die Aquar. und Terrarien., *5*, 1952

Pflugfelder, O.: "Zooparasiten", Jena, 1950

Plehn, M.: "Eine neue Karpfenkrankheit und ihr Erreger *Branchiomyces sanguinis*", Z. Bakt., *62*, 1912

Plehn, M.: "Die Gaskrankheit der Fische", Allg. Fisch.-Ztg., *46*, 1921

Plehn, M.: Praktikum der Fischkrankheiten", Handb. Binnenfisch. Mitteleuropas, *1*, 1924

Plehn, M.: "Pankreas-Fettnekrose bei karpfenartigen Fischen (Cypriniden)", Virchows Arch. Path., Anat., Physiol., *302*, 1938

Plehn, M. and K. Mulsow: "Die Erreger der Taumelkrankheit der Salmoniden", Z. Bakt. *59*, 1911

Prakash, A. and J. R. Adams: "A histopathological study of the intestinal lesions induced by Echinorhynchus lageniformis (Acanthocephala-Echinorhynchidae) in the starry flounder", Can. Jour. Zool. 38, 1960

Putz, R. E. and G. L. Hoffman: "Earliest susceptible age of rainbow trout to whirling disease", Prog. Fish Cult. 28(2), 1966

Rabb, L., J. W. Cornick and L. A. McDermott: "A macroscopic slide agglutination test for the presumptive diagnosis of furunculosis in fish", Prog. Fish Cult. 26(3), 1964

Rankin, J. M.: "New cure for fin rot", Water Life, 1953

Rasmussen, C. J.: "Nogle forelobige undersogelser over regnbuerredens virussygdom (Egtvedsygen)", Meddelelse nr. 10 fra forsogsdambruget, 1959

Reichenbach-Klinke, H. H.: "Massenauftreten weisser Strudelwürmer in Aquarien", Wschr. Aquar. Tech., *44*, 1950

Reichenbach-Klinke, H. H.: "Untersuchungen über die bei Fischen durch Parasiten hervorgerufenen Zysten und deren Wirkung auf den Wirtskorper 1, Teil", Z. Fisch., N. F., *3*, 1954

Reichenbach-Klinke, H. H.: "Die Dinoflagellat *Oodinium pillularis* Schäperclaus als Bindegewebsparasit von Süsswasserfischen", Giorn. Microbiol., *1*, 1956a

Reichenbach-Klinke, H. H.: "Muskelcercarien aus einem Zwergfadenfisch (*Colisa lalia*)", Mikrokosmos, *45*, 1956b

Reichenbach-Klinke, H. H.: "Krankheiten der Aquarienfische", Stuttgart, 1957

Reichenbach-Klinke, H. H.: "Ein neuer Ergasilide in europäischen Susswasseraquarien", Z. Paras., *18*, 1958

Reichenbach-Klinke, H. H.: "Schadigungen und Krankheiten der Fische", Gustav Fischer Verlag, Jena, 1966

Reichenbach-Klinke, H. H. and G. Elkan: "Diseases of the lower vertebrates", Academic Press, London, 1963

Robertson, M.: "Notes on a Haplosporidian belonging to the genus *Ichthyosporidium*", Proc. Royal Soc. Edinburgh, *17*, 1908

Robertson, M.: "Notes on an *Ichthyosporidium* causing a fatal disease in seatrout", Proc. Zool. Soc. Lond., 1909

Roegner-Aust, S.: "Die Wirkung von Gesarol auf Fische", Allg. Fisch.-Ztg., *74*, 1949a

Roegner-Aust, S.: "Einige Beobachtungen über die Wirkung von DDT unf Hexapräparaten auf Fische", Z. angewandte Entomol., *31*, 1949b

Roegner-Aust, S.: "Über die Wirkung der neuen Kontaktinsektizide auf Fische", Verh. d. Deutschen Gesselschaft. f. angewandte Entomol., 1949, 1951

Röhr, W., M. Borkenhagen and J. Knaak: "Nematodenlarven in Dorschleberkonserven", Arch. f. Lebensmittelhygiene, *10*, 1959

Romeis, B.: "Mikroskopische Technik", München, 1948

Ross, A. J.: "*Mycobacterium salmoniphilum* sp. nov. from salmonid fishes", Amer. Rev. Resp. Dis. 81(2), 1960

Ross, A. J. and F. P. Brancato: "*Mycobacterium fortuitum* Cruz from the tropical fish *Hyphessobrycon innesi*", Jour. Bact. 18(3), 1959

Ross, A. J., B. J. Earp and J. W. Wood: "Mycobacterial infections in adult salmon and steelhead trout returning to the Columbia River Basin and other areas in 1957", Bur. Sport Fish. Wild., Spec. Sci. Report—Fisheries No. 332, 1959

Rucker, R. R.: "Vibrio infections among marine and fresh-water fish", Prog. Fish Cult. 21(1), 1959

Schäperclaus, W.: "Karpfenerkrankungen durch saures Wasser in Heide- und Moorgegenden", Z. Fisch., *24*, 1926a

Schäperclaus, W.: "Fischsterben durch Cyclochaeten in einem See", Fisch.-Ztg., *29*, 1926b

Schäperclaus, W.: "Krebssterben und Krebskrankheiten in der Mark.", Mitteilg. der Fischereivereine f. die Provinz Brandenburg uws., *19*, 1927a

Schäperclaus, W.: "Lymphocystiskrankungen bei Flundern und Schollen und ihre Bekämpfung", Mitt. d. Dtsche. Seefisch., *43*, 1927b

Schäperclaus, W.: "Die Rotseuche des Aales im Bezirk von Rügen und Stralsund", Z. Fisch., *25*, 1927c

Schäperclaus, W.: "Die Hechtpest in Brandenburg und Rügen", Z. Fisch., 26, 1928a

Schäperclaus, W.: "Wieder ein pestartiges Krebssterben in der Mark.", Mitteilg. der Fischereivereine f. die Provinz Brandenburg usw., 20, 1928b

Schäperclaus, W.: "Beiträge zur Kenntnis der Kiemenfäule des Karpfens", Z. Fisch., 27, 1929

Schäperclaus, W.: "*Pseudomonas punctata* als Krankheitserreger bei Fischen, Untersuchungen über Süsswasseraalrotseuche, Leibeshöhlenwassersucht der Cypriniden, insbesondere des Karpfens und Fleckenseuche der Weissfische", Z. Fisch., 28, 1930

Schäperclaus, W.: "Das Lysolbad, ein neues Mittel zur Bekämpfung der Karpfenlaus in der Teichwirtschaft", Z. Fisch., 29, 1931a

Schäperclaus, W.: "Die Drehkrankheit in der Forellenzucht und ihre Bekämpfung", Z. Fisch., 29, 1931b

Schäperclaus, W.: "Die Furunkulose der Forellen und ihre Bekämpfung," Fisch.-Ztg., 37, 1934a

Schäperclaus, W.: "Untersuchungen über die Aalseuchen in deutschen Binnen- und Küstengewässern 1930 0 1933", Z. Fisch., 32, 1934b

Schäperclaus, W.: "Die Ursache der pestartigen Krebssterben", Z. Fisch., 33, 1935a

Schäperclaus, W.: "*Chilodon cyprini* (Moroff) als Krankheitserreger bei Forellenbrut und seine fischpathologische Bedeutung im allgemeinen", Z. f. Paras., 7, 1935b

Schäperclaus, W.: "Eine neue Mikrosporidienkrankheit beim Neonfisch und seinen Verwandten", "W", 38, 1941

Schäperclaus, W.: "Die Darmcoccidiosen, insbesondere die Knötchencoccidiose des Karpfens", Z. Fisch., 41, 1943

Schäperclaus, W.: "Fischfuttervergiftung durch DDT und Benzolhexachlorid", "W", 43, 1949

Schäperclaus, W.: "Über einen Fall von Flossenfäule beim Schwarzen Molly", "W", 44, 1950a

Schäperclaus, W.: "Auswirkungen der Insektenbekämpfung mit DDT und Benzolhexachlorid auf Fischgewässer", Abhand. a. d. Fisch. Liefg., 111, 1950b

Schäperclaus, W.: "Der Colisa-Parasit—ein neuer Krankheitserreger bei Aquarienfischen", Die Aqu. Terr. Z., 4, 1951

Schäperclaus, W.: "Fischerkrankungen und Fischsterben durch Massentwicklung von Phytoplankton bei Anwesenheit von Ammoniumverbindungen", Abhand. a. d. Fisch. Liefg., V, 1952

Schäperclaus, W.: "Die Blumenkohlkrankheit der Aale und anderer Fische der Ostsee", Z. Fisch., 2, N. F., 1953a

Schäperclaus, W.: "Fortpflanzung und Systematik von *Ichthyophonus*", Die Aqu. Terr. Z., 6, 1953b

Schäperclaus, W.: "Infektionsblauf und natürlich Infektionsabwehr bei der ansteckenden Bauchwassersucht des Karpfens", Z. Fisch., 1, N. F., 1953c

Schäperclaus, W.: "Die Bedeutung der Bakteriophagen von *Pseudomonas punctata ascitae* (Zimmermann) Schäperclaus für die Entstehung und Bekämpfung der Infektiösen Bauchwassersucht des Karpfens", Z. Fisch., 3, N. F., 1954a

Schäperclaus, W.: "Fischkrankheiten", Berlin, 1954b

Schäperclaus, W.: "Aufsehenerregende Heilungs- und Bekämpfungserfolge bei der Infektiösen Bauchwassersucht der Karpfen durch antibiotische Mittel", Dtsche. Fisch.-Ztg., *11*, 1955

Schäperclaus, W.: "Die Bauchwassersucht des Karpfens, eine bakterielle Infekstionskrankheit, und neue Methoden zu ihrer erfolgreichen Heilung und Bekämpfung durch antibiotische Mittel", Arch. Fisch., *7*, 1956a

Schäperclaus, W.: "Bekämpfung der Infektiösen Bauchwassersucht des Karpfens durch Antibiotika", Z. Fisch., *5*, 1956b

Schäperclaus, W.: "Ergebnisse der Versuche zur Bekämpfung der Infektiösen Bauchwassersucht in Karpfenteichen mit Chloronitrin im Jahre 1956", Dtsche. Fisch.-Ztg., *4*, 1957

Schäperclaus, W. and H. Mann: "Untersuchungen über die ansteckende Bauchwassersucht des Karpfens und ihre Bekämpfung", Z. Fisch., *37*, 1939

Scheuring, L.: "Beobachtungen zur Biologie des Genus *Triaenophorus* und Betrachtungen über das jahreszeitliche Auftreten von Bandwürmern", Z. Paras., *2*, 1929

Schikora, F.: "Zur Krebspest in der Neumark", Fisch.-Ztg., *8*, 1905

Schikora, F.: "Die Krebspest", Fisch.-Ztg., *9*, 1906

Schikora, F.: "50 Jahre Krebspest", Fisch.-Ztg., *29*, 1926

Schilling, V.: "Praktische Blutlehre", Jena, 1952

Schmidt, W.: "Untersuchungen über *Octomitus intestinalis truttae*", Arch. f. Protist., *40*, 1920

Schmorl, G.: "Die pathologisch-histologischen Untersuchungsmethoden", Berlin, 1934

Schreitmüller, W. and G. Lederer: "Krankheitserscheinungen an Fischen, Reptilien und Lurchen", Berlin 1930

Schubert, G.: "Elektronenmikroskopische Untersuchungen zur Pockenkrankheit des Karpfens", Z. Naturforschg. 19b, 1964

Shanor, L. and H. B. Saslow: "Aphanomyces as a fish parasite", Mycologia 36, 1944

Sikama, Y.: "Über die Weisspünktchenkrankheit bei Seefischen", J. Shanghai Sc. Inst. Sect., *4*, 1938

Sindermann, C. J.: "Diseases of fishes of the western North Atlantic. I.", Dept. of Sea and Shore Fish., Maine, Res. Bull., *18*, 1954a

Sindermann, C. J.: "Diseases of fishes of the western North Atlantic. II", Dept. of Sea and Shore Fish., Maine, Res. Bull., *19*, 1954b

Sindermann, C. J.: "Diseases of fishes of the western North Atlantic. III", Dept. Sea and Shore Fish., Maine, Res. Bull., *25*, 1956

Smith, C. E. and J. E. Halver: "Folic acid anemia in coho salmon", J. Fish. Res. Bd. Can., *26*, 111–114, 1969

Smith, I. W.: "The occurrence and pathology of Dee disease", Dept. Agric. Fish. Scotland, Freshwater & Salmon Fish., No. 34, 1964

Snieszko, S. F.: "Ulcer disease in brook trout (*Salvelinus fontinalis*): its economic importance, diagnosis, treatment and prevention", Prog. Fish-Cult., *24*, 1952

Snieszko, S. F. and P. J. Griffin: "Kidney disease in brook trout and its treatment", Prog. Fish-Cult., *17*, 1955

Snieszko, S. F., P. J. Griffin and S. B. Friddle: "A new bacterium (*Hemophilus piscium* n. sp.) from ulcer disease of trout", J. Bact., *59*, 1950

Snieszko, S. F., P. J. Griffin and S. B. Friddle: "Antibiotic treatment of ulcer disease and furunculosis in trout", Trans. N. Amer. Wildlife Conf., *17*, 1952

Snieszko, S. F.: "Microhematocrit as a tool in fishery research and management", Bur. Sport Fish. Wild., Spec. Sci. Report No. 341, 1960

Snieszko, S. F., G. L. Bullock, C. E. Dunbar and L. L. Pettijohn: "Nocardial infection in hatchery reared fingerling rainbow trout (*Salmo gairdneri*)", Jour. Bact. 88(6), 1964

Snieszko, S. F. and G. L. Hoffman: "Control of fish diseases", Lab. Animal Care 13(3), 1963

Sproston, N. G.: "*Ichthyosporidium hoferi* (Plehn et Mulsow), an internal fungoid parasite of the mackerel", J. Mar. Biol. Assoc., U.K., *26*, 1947

Stammer, I.: "Beiträge fur Morphologie, Biologie und Bekämpfung der Karpfenläuse", Z. f. Parasitenkunde, *19*, 1959

Stankowitch, S.: "Systématique et répartition des coccidies des poissons d'eau douce", Trav. labor. piscicult. Univ. Grenoble, *14*, 1924

Steffens, W.: "Weitere Beiträge zur Kenntnis der *Plistophora*-Krankheit", Die Aquar. und Terrarien Z., *6*, 1956

Steinsträsser, W.: "Acanthocephalen als Forellenparasiten", Z. Fisch., *34*, 1936

Stempel: "Zoologie im Grundriss", Berlin, 1935

Sterba, G.: "Aquarienkunde", 1954

Sterba, G.: "Aquarienkunde", Vol. 2, Leipzig/Jena, 1956

Szidat, L.: "Über ein Fischsterben im Kurischen Haff und seine Ursachen", Z. Fisch., *25*, 1927

Tack, E.: "Bekämpfung der Drehkrankheit mit Kalkstickstoff", Fischwirt, *1*, 1951

Tack, E.: "Ist die neu aufgetretene Forellenkrankheit ansteckend?", Allg. Fisch.-Ztg., *82*, 1957a

Tack, E.: "Beiträge zur Erforschung der Forellenseuche", Fischwirt, 7, 1957b

Tack, E.: "Über die Ergebnisse neuerer Albaumer Versuche zur Bekämpfung der ansteckenden Forellenseuche", Fischwirt, *9*, 1959

Thieme, H.: "Erkennung und Wesen der Neonkrankheit", Aquarien und Terrarien, *6*, 1956

Tomasec, I.: "Neueres auf dem Gebiet der Bw des Karpfens", Rib. Jugosl. 4, 1949

Tomasec, I.: "Untersuchungen über die Atiologie der Bauchwassersucht des Karpfens (*Cyprinus carpio* L.)", Veter. Arch. Knjuga, *21*, 1951a

Tomasec, I.: "Istrazivanja o etiologiji zarazne vodene bolesti sarana (*Cyprinus carpio* L.)", Vet. Arch. 21 (3–4), 1951b

Tomasec, I.: "Considerations generales sur le probleme de l'etiologie de l'hydropisie infectieuse de la carpe", 2. Symp. Comm. Perm. O.I.E. pour l'etude des maladies des poissons, Munich, 1965

Touraine, F.: "Kystes provoqués par la sanguinicolose dans le foie et le rein de la carpe", Trav. lab. d'hydrobiol. piscic. Univ. Grenoble, *23*, 1932

Vogel, H.: "Mycobacteria from cold-blooded animals", Amer. Rev. T.B. 77(2), 1958

Vogt, K.: "Experimentelle Untersuchungen über die Gründe von Masseninfektionen mit Plerocercoiden des Fischbandwurmes *Triaeonophorus nodulosus* Pallas", Z. Fisch., *36*, 1938

Wagler, E.: "Die deutschen Karpfenläuse", Zool. Anz., *110*, 1935

Wagner, G.: "Der Entwicklungszyklus von *Ichthyophthirius multifiliis* Fouquet und der Einfluss physikalischer und chemischer Aussenfaktoren", Z. Fisch., N. F., *9*, 1960

Wales, J. H. and R. O. Sinnhuber: "An early hepatoma epizootic in rainbow trout, *Salmo gairdnerii*", Calif. Fish and Game 52(2), 1966

Wales, J. H. and H. Wolf: "Three protozoan diseases of trout in California", Calif. Fish and Game 41(2), 1955

Walker, R.: "Fine structure of lymphocystis virus of fish", Virology 18(3), 1962

Walker, R.: "Viral DNA and cytoplasmic RNA in lymphocystis cells of fish", Ann. N. Y. Acad. Sci. 126, 1965

Walker, R. and R. Weissenberg: "Conformity of light and electron microscopic studies on virus particle distribution in lymphocystis tumor cells of fish", Ann. N. Y. Acad. Sci. 126, 1965

Warren, J. W.: "Kidney disease of salmonid fishes and the analysis of hatchery waters", Prog. Fish-Cult., *25*, 1963

Wasserburger, H. J.: "*Daphnia magna* als Testtier zum Nachweis von Kontaktinsektizid-Spuren", Die Pharmazie, *1*, 1952

Weissenberg, R.: "Lymphocystiskrankheit der Fische", in "Handbuch der pathogenen Protozoen von Prowazek-Nöller", *3*, 1921

Weissenberg, R.: "Positive result of a filtration experiment supporting the view that the agent of the lymphocystis disease of fish is a true virus", Anat. Rec. 111(3), 1951

Weissenberg, R. and R. F. Nigrelli: "Lymphocystis in the hogfish *Lachnolaimus maximus*", Zoologica, *22*, 1937

Wellings, S. R., R. G. Chuinard and M. Bens: "A comparative study of skin neoplasms in four species of pleuronectid fishes", Ann. N. Y. Acad. Sci. 126 (art. 1), 1965

Wessing, A. and von G. Bargen: "Untersuchungen über einen virusbedingten Tumor bei Fischen", Arch. f. d. ges. Virusforschung, *9*, 1959

Willer, A.: "Beiträge zur Kenntnis der Bandwurmseuche (Ligulosis) der Brachsen oder Bleie (*Abramis brama*)", Z. Fisch., *16*, 1912

Woker, H. and K. Wuhrmann: "Die Empfindlichkeit verschiedener Fischarten gegenüber Ammoniak, Blausäure und Phenol", Rev. Suisse de Zoologie, *57*, 1950

Wolf, K.: "Experimental propagation of lymphocystis disease of fishes", Virology 18(2), 1962

Wolf, K.: "Physiological salines for fresh-water teleosts", Prog. Fish-Cult. 25(3), 1963

Wolf, K.: "Lymphocystis disease of fish (revised)", Bur. Sport Fish. Wild. Fish. Leaf. No. 565, 1964

Wolf, K.: "Bacterial kidney disease of salmonid fishes", Bur. Sport Fish. Wild., Fish. Dis. Leaf No. 8, 1966

Wolf, K. and C. E. Dunbar: "Test of 34 therapeutic agents for control of kidney disease in trout", Trans. Amer. Fish. Soc. 88(2), 1959

Wolf, K., C. E. Dunbar and E. A. Pyle: "Infectious pancreatic necrosis of trout. II. Experimental infections with brook trout", Prog. Fish Cult. 23(2), 1961

Wolf, K., M. Gravell and R. G. Malsberger: "Lymphocystis virus: Isolation and propagation in Centrarcid fish cell lines", Science 151(3713), 1966

Wolf, K. and M. C. Quimby: "Established eurythermic line of fish cells in vitro", Science 135(3508), 1962

Wolf, K., M. C. Quimby and A. D. Bradford: "Egg associated transmission of IPN virus of trout", Virology 21, 1963

Wolf, K., S. F. Snieszko, C. E. Dunbar and E. A. Pyle: "Virus nature of infectious pancreatic necrosis in trout", Proc. Soc. Exp. Biol. Med. 104, 1960

Wood, E. M. and C. P. Larson: "Hepatic carcinoma in rainbow trout", Arch. Path. 71, 1961

Wood, E. M. and W. T. Yasutake: "Histopathology of Fish: V. Gill Disease", Prog. Fish-Cult. 19(1): 7–13

Wood, E. M. and W. T. Yasutake: "Histopathology of kidney disease in fish", Amer. J. Pathol., 32, 1956

Wood, E. M., W. T. Yasutake and W. L. Lehman: "A myxosis-like granuloma of fish", Jour. Infect. Dis. 97, 1955

Wood, J. W.: "A survey of tuberculosis in Pacific salmon and steelhead trout on Oregon streams in 1957", Bur. Sport Fish. Wild., Spec. Sci. Report No. 332, 1959

Wood, J. W. and E. J. Ordal: "Tuberculosis in Pacific salmon and steelhead trout", Contr. Fish Comm. State Oregon 25, 1958

Wood, J. W. and J. Wallis: "Kidney disease in adult Chinook salmon and its transmission by feeding to young Chinook salmon", Res. Briefs, Fish. Comm. Oregon, 6, 1955

Wuhrmann, K. and H. Woker: "Experimentelle Untersuchungen über die Ammoniak- und Blausäurevergiftung", Schweiz. Ztschr. Hydrobiol., 11, 1949

Wuhrmann, K. and H. Woker: "Die Giftigkeit von Phenol für verschniedene Fischarten", Schweiz. Ztschr. Hydrobiol., 12, 1950

Wunder, W.: "Über die Bekämpfung von Wasserschnecken in der Teichwirtschaft", Fisch.-Ztg., 29, 1926

Wunder, W.: "Die Dactylogyruskrankheit der Karpfenbrut, ihre Ursache und ihre Bekämpfung", Z. Fisch., 27, 1929

Wunder, W.: "Das jahreszeitliche Auftreten des Bandwurmes Caryophyllaeus laticeps Pall. im Darm des Karpfens (Cyprinus carpio L.)", Z. Paras., 10, 1939

Wunder, W. and H. Dombrowski: "Untersuchungen über die ansteckende Bauchwassersucht des Karpfens (Ascites)", Z. Fisch., 2, N. F., 1953

Wundsch, H. H.: "Eine besondere Art der 'Kiemenfäule' bei Hechten und Schleien", Z. Fisch., 27, 1929

Wundsch, H. H.: "Weitere Beobachtungen an Branchiomyces demigrans als Erreger der Kiemenfäule beim Hecht", Z. Fisch., 28, 1930

Wurmbach, H.: "Zur krankheitserregenden Wirkung der Acanthocephalen. Die Kratzerkrankung der Barben in der Mosel", Z. Fisch., 35, 1937

Wurmbach, H.: "Geschlechtsunkehr bei Weibchen von *Lebistes reticulatus* bei Befall mit *Ichthyophonus hoferi* Plehn-Mulsow", Arch. f. Entwicklungsmechanik, *145*, 1951

Zöbe, E.: "Histologische Untersuchungen über die Infektiöse Bauchwassersucht des Karpfens (*Cyprinus carpio* L.)", Diss. Tierärztl. Fak., Univ. München, 1952

Zwillenberg, L. O. and H. H. L. Zwillenberg: "Elektronenmikroskopische Untersuchungen an Regenbogenforellen mit infektiöser Nierenschwellung und Leberdegeneration", Arch. Ges. Virusforschung 14(3), 1964

Zwillenberg, L. O., M. H. Jensen and H. H. L. Zwillenberg: "Recherches de microscopie electronique et classification du virus de la septicemie hemorragique virale de la truite arc-en-ciel", 2. Symp. Comm. Perm. O.I.E. pour l'etude des maladies des poissons, Munich, 1965

INDEX

301

Date Due

NOV 1 8 2003			